Pathways to Peace

The Transformative Power of Children and Families

Strüngmann Forum Reports

Julia Lupp, series editor

The Ernst Strüngmann Forum is made possible through the generous support of the Ernst Strüngmann Foundation, inaugurated by Dr. Andreas and Dr. Thomas Strüngmann.

This Forum was supported by funds from the
Deutsche Forschungsgemeinschaft
(German Science Foundation)

Pathways to Peace

The Transformative Power of Children and Families

Edited by

James F. Leckman, Catherine Panter-Brick, and Rima Salah

Program Advisory Committee:

James R. Cochrane, James F. Leckman, Julia Lupp,
Catherine Panter-Brick, Rima Salah, Geraldine Smyth,
Diane Sunar, and Marinus H. van IJzendoorn

The MIT Press

Cambridge, Massachusetts
London, England

KH

Series Editor: J. Lupp
Assistant Editor: M. Turner
Photographs: U. Dettmar
Lektorat: BerlinScienceWorks

MIT Press books may be purchased at special quantity discounts
for business or sales promotional use. For information, please email
special_sales@mitpress.mit.edu.

The book was set in TimesNewRoman and Arial.
Printed and bound in the United States of America.

Library of Congress Cataloging-in-Publication Data is available.

ISBN: 978-0-262-02798-4

10 9 8 7 6 5 4 3 2 1

9/30/15

Contents

The Ernst Strüngmann Forum   vii

List of Contributors   ix

Foreword: The Culture of Peace   xiii
    Anwarul K. Chowdhury

Foundations for a New Approach

1   **Peace Is a Lifelong Process: The Importance of Partnerships**   3
    James F. Leckman, Catherine Panter-Brick, and Rima Salah

2   **Framing Our Analysis: A Dialectical Perspective**   19
    Robert A. Hinde and Joan Stevenson-Hinde

3   **Ecology of Peace**   27
    Pia R. Britto, Ilanit Gordon, William Hodges, Diane Sunar,
    Cigdem Kagitcibasi, and James F. Leckman

Human Biological Development

4   **Peptide Pathways to Peace**   43
    C. Sue Carter and Stephen W. Porges

5   **Epigenetics: Significance of the Gene-Environment Interface**   65
    for Brain Development
    Eric B. Keverne

6   **Group Identity as an Obstacle and Catalyst of Peace**   79
    Douglas P. Fry

7   **Human Biological Development and Peace: Genes, Brains,**   95
    Safety, and Justice
    Barak Morgan, Diane Sunar, C. Sue Carter, James F. Leckman,
    Douglas P. Fry, Eric B. Keverne, Iris-Tatjana Kolassa,
    Robert Kumsta, and David Olds

Early Childhood Events and Relationships

8   **Comparative and Evolutionary Perspectives**   131
    Dario Maestripieri

9   **The Problem of Institutionalization of Young Children and Its**   145
    Consequences for Efforts to Build Peaceful Societies
    Nathan A. Fox, Charles A. Nelson, and Charles H. Zeanah

10   **Prosocial Development and Situational Morality:**   161
    Neurobiological, Parental, and Contextual Factors
    Marinus H. van IJzendoorn and Marian J. Bakermans-Kranenburg

11   How Do Events and Relationships in Childhood Set the Stage   185
       for Peace at Personal and Social Levels?
       Howard Steele, Marinus H. van IJzendoorn,
       Marian J. Bakermans-Kranenburg, W. Thomas Boyce,
       Mary Dozier, Nathan A. Fox, Heidi Keller, Dario Maestripieri,
       Paul Odhiambo Oburu, and Hiltrud Otto

Challenges in Society

12   Mental Health and Development among Children Living in   213
       Violent Conditions: Underlying Processes for
       Promoting Peace
       Raija-Leena Punamäki

13   Structural Violence and Early Childhood Development   233
       Andrew Dawes and Amelia van der Merwe

14   Promoting the Capacity for Peace in Early Childhood: 251
       Perspectives from Research on Resilience in Children
       and Families
       Ann S. Masten

15   Healthy Human Development as a Path to Peace   273
       Daniel J. Christie, Catherine Panter-Brick, Jere R. Behrman,
       James R. Cochrane, Andrew Dawes, Kirstin Goth,
       Jacqueline Hayden, Ann S. Masten, Ilham Nasser,
       Raija-Leena Punamäki, and Mark Tomlinson

Program and Policy Implications

16   Interventions: What Has Worked and Why?   305
       Cigdem Kagitcibasi and Pia R. Britto

17   Linking Peacebuilding and Child Development: 323
       A Basic Framework
       Mohammed Abu-Nimer and Ilham Nasser

18   The Power of Media in Peacebuilding   339
       Lucy Nusseibeh

19   Creating Effective Programs and Policies to Reduce Violence   361
       and Promote Peace
       Pia R. Britto, Rima Salah, Mohammed Abu-Nimer,
       Jacqueline Bhabha, Anwarul K. Chowdhury, Gary R. Gunderson,
       Cigdem Kagitcibasi, Lucy Nusseibeh, Olayinka Omigbodun,
       Mikiko Otani, and Geraldine Smyth

Bibliography   385

Subject Index   445

The Ernst Strüngmann Forum

Founded on the tenets of scientific independence and the inquisitive nature of the human mind, the Ernst Strüngmann Forum is dedicated to the continual expansion of knowledge. Through its innovative communication process, the Ernst Strüngmann Forum provides a creative environment within which experts scrutinize high-priority issues from multiple vantage points.

This process begins with the identification of themes. By nature, a theme constitutes a problem area that transcends classic disciplinary boundaries. It is of high-priority interest, requiring concentrated, multidisciplinary input to address the issues. Proposals are received from leading scientists active in their field and selected by an independent Scientific Advisory Board. Once approved, we convene a steering committee to refine the scientific parameters of the proposal and select participants. Approximately one year later, we hold a central gathering, or Forum, to which circa forty experts are invited.

Preliminary discussion for this theme began in 2011, when Jim Leckman contacted me to explore the possibility of convening a Forum on the potential role of early childhood development in contributing to a more peaceful society. Impetus behind his request stemmed from discussions with the Mother Child Education Foundation (Anne Çocuk Eğitim Vakfı) in Istanbul, and their hypothesis that enhanced peace at the micro level of the family has the potential to facilitate peace at community and societal levels. After a period of development, a core concept for the Forum was delineated; the resulting proposal was approved to assess child development, in the context of familial and group relations, and its potential in peacebuilding. From September 30–October 2, 2012, the Program Advisory Committee met to transform the proposal into a framework that would support an extended discussion. The collective expertise and international experience of the committee members—James R. Cochrane, James F. Leckman, Catherine Panter-Brick, Rima Salah, Geraldine Smyth, Diane Sunar, Marinus H. van IJzendoorn—were instrumental in refining the issues for debate.

From October 13–18, 2013, the Forum was held in Frankfurt am Main. The activities and discourse that surround a Forum begin well beforehand and conclude with the publication of this volume. Throughout each stage, focused dialog is the means by which issues are examined anew. Often, this requires relinquishing long-established ideas and overcoming disciplinary idiosyncrasies which otherwise might bias or inhibit joint examination. When this is accomplished, a unique synergism results from which new insights emerge.

This volume conveys the synergy that grew out of a very diverse group of experts, each of whom assumed an active role, and it is comprised of two types of contributions. The first set provides background information on key aspects of the overall theme. Originally written in advance of the Forum, these chapters have been extensively reviewed and revised to provide current understanding on these topics. The second set (Chapters 7, 11, 15, and 19) summarizes the extensive group discussions. These chapters should not be viewed as consensus documents nor are they proceedings; their purpose is to transfer the essence of these multifaceted discussions, to expose the areas where opinions diverge and open questions remain, and to highlight topics in need of future enquiry.

An endeavor of this kind creates its own unique group dynamics and puts demands on everyone who participates. Each invitee contributed not only their time and congenial personality, but a willingness to probe beyond that which is evident, and I wish to extend my gratitude to all. A special word of thanks goes to the steering committee as well as the authors and reviewers of the background papers. The work of the moderators of the individual working groups (Sue Carter, Marinus H. van IJzendoorn, Catherine Panter-Brick, and Rima Salah) is gratefully acknowledged. In addition, I am especially grateful to the rapporteurs (Barak Morgan, Howard Steele, Daniel Christie, and Pia Britto): to draft a report during the Forum that takes into account the perspectives of all group members and bring it to a final form is no simple matter. Most importantly, I extend my sincere appreciation to Jim Leckman for bringing this theme to our attention. His commitment and that of his co-chairs, Catherine Panter-Brick and Rima Salah, ensured productive discourse.

A communication process of this nature relies on institutional stability and an environment that encourages free thought. The generous support of the Ernst Strüngmann Foundation, established by Dr. Andreas and Dr. Thomas Strüngmann in honor of their father, enables the Ernst Strüngmann Forum to conduct its work in the service of science. In addition, the following valuable partnerships are gratefully acknowledged: the Scientific Advisory Board, which ensures the scientific independence of the Forum; the German Science Foundation, for its supplemental financial support; the Frankfurt Institute for Advanced Studies, which shares its vibrant intellectual setting with the Forum; and the Mother Child Education Foundation of Istanbul (Anne Çocuk Eğitim Vakfı, or AÇEV), for its commitment to peace.

Long-held views are never easy to put aside. Yet, when this is achieved, when the edges of the unknown begin to appear and the resulting gaps of knowledge are able to be identified, the act of formulating strategies to fill them becomes a most invigorating activity. It is our hope that this volume will convey a sense of this lively exercise and inspire further scientific enquiry into the potential role of early childhood in contributing to a more peaceful world.

Julia Lupp, Program Director
Ernst Strüngmann Forum
Frankfurt Institute for Advanced Studies (FIAS)
Ruth-Moufang-Str. 1, 60438 Frankfurt am Main, Germany
http://esforum.de

List of Contributors

Abu-Nimer, Mohammed   International Peace and Conflict Resolution Program, School of International Services, American University, Washington D.C. 20016-8071, U.S.A.

Bakermans-Kranenburg, Marian J.   Center for Child and Family Studies, Leiden University, 2333 AK Leiden, The Netherlands

Behrman, Jere R.   Department of Economics, University of Pennsylvania, Philadelphia, PA 19104-6297, U.S.A.

Bhabha, Jacqueline   John F. Kennedy School of Government, Harvard University, Cambridge, MA 02138, U.S.A.

Boyce, W. Thomas   Faculty of Medicine, University of British Columbia, Vancouver, BC, V6T 1Z3, Canada

Britto, Pia R.   UNICEF, New York, NY 10017, U.S.A., and the Child Study Center, Yale University, New Haven, CT 06520, U.S.A.

Carter, C. Sue   Department of Psychiatry, University of North Carolina, Chapel Hill, NC 27599, U.S.A.

Chowdhury, Anwarul K.   Former Under-Secretary-General and High Representative of the United Nations, New York, NY 10010, U.S.A.

Christie, Daniel J.   Peace and Conflict Studies, Ohio State University, Delaware, Ohio 43015, U.S.A.

Cochrane, James R.   School of Public Health and Family Medicine, University of Cape Town, Rondebosch 7701, South Africa

Dawes, Andrew   School of Public Health and Family Medicine, University of Cape Town, Rondebosch 7701, South Africa

Dozier, Mary   Department of Psychology, University of Delaware, Newark, DE 19716-2577, U.S.A.

Fox, Nathan A.   Department of Human Development and Quantitative Methodology, University of Maryland, College Park, MD 20742, U.S.A.

Fry, Douglas P.   Department of Anthropology, University of Alabama at Birmingham, Birmingham, AL 35294, U.S.A., and the Department of Social Sciences, Peace, Mediation and Conflict Research, Åbo Akademi University in Vasa, 65101 Vasa, Finland

Gordon, Ilanit   Child Study Center, Yale University, New Haven, CT 06520, U.S.A.

Goth, Kirstin   Department of Child and Adolescent Psychiatry, University of Basel, CH-4056 Basel, Switzerland

Gunderson, Gary R.   Faith and Health, Wake Forest Baptist Medical Center, Medical Center Boulevard, Winston-Salem, NC 27137, U.S.A.

Hayden, Jacqueline   Institute of Early Childhood, Macquarie University, NSW 2109, Australia

Heinrichs, Markus   Department of Psychology, Albert-Ludwigs-University of Freiburg, 79104 Freiburg, Germany

Hinde, Robert A.   Sub-Department of Animal Behaviour, University of Cambridge, Madingley, Cambridge, CB3 8AA, U.K.

Hodges, William   Child Study Center, Yale University, New Haven, CT 06520, U.S.A.

Kagitcibasi, Cigdem   Department of Psychology, Koc University, Istanbul, Turkey

Keller, Heidi   Institute for Psychology, University of Osnabrück, 49076 Osnabrück, Germany

Keverne, Eric B.   Sub-Department of Animal Behaviour, University of Cambridge, Madingley, Cambridge, CB3 8AA, U.K.

Kolassa, Iris-Tatjana   Institute of Psychology and Education, University of Ulm, 89069 Ulm, Germany

Kumsta, Robert   Laboratory for Biological and Personality Psychology, University of Freiburg, 79104 Freiburg i. Br., Germany

Leckman, James F.   Child Study Center, Yale University, New Haven, CT 06520, U.S.A.

Maestripieri, Dario   Department of Comparative Human Development, The University of Chicago, Chicago, IL 60637, U.S.A.

Masten, Ann S.   Institute of Child Development, University of Minnesota, Twin Cities, Minneapolis, MN 55455, U.S.A.

Morgan, Barak   Department of Human Biology, Health Sciences Faculty, University of Cape Town, Fish Hoek, Western Cape 7974, South Africa

Nasser, Ilham   Early Childhood Education Program, College of Education and Human Development, George Mason University, Fairfax, VA, 22030, U.S.A.

Nelson, Charles A.   Boston Children's Hospital, Boston, MA, U.S.A.

Nusseibeh, Lucy   49 Nablus Road, P.O. Box 19322, East Jerusalem

Oburu, Paul Odhiambo   Department of Educational Psychology, Maseno University, Maseno, Kenya

Olds, David   Prevention Research Center for Family and Child Health, University of Colorado Denver, MS 8410, Aurora, CO 80045, U.S.A.

Omigbodun, Olayinka   College of Medicine, University of Ibadan, University College Hospital, Ibadan, Nigeria

Otani, Mikiko   Mita Branch, Foreigners and International Service Section, Tokyo Public Law Office, Minato-ku, Tokyo 108-0014, Japan

Otto, Hiltrud   The Martin Buber Society of Fellows, The Hebrew University of Jerusalem, Mount Scopus, Jerusalem 91905, Israel

Panter-Brick, Catherine   Department of Anthropology, Yale University, New Haven, CT 06511, U.S.A.

Porges, Stephen W.   Department of Psychiatry, University of North Carolina, Chapel Hill, NC 27599, U.S.A.

Punamäki, Raija-Leena   School of Social Sciences and Humanities, Department of Psychology, University of Tampere, FIM-33014 University of Tampere, Finland

Salah, Rima   Former Deputy Executive Director of UNICEF; Assistant Clinical Professor, Yale Child Study Center, New York, NY 10017, U.S.A.

Smyth, Geraldine   Irish School of Ecumenics, Trinity College Dublin, Milltown Park, Dublin 6, Ireland

Steele, Howard   Department of Psychology, New School for Social Research, New York, NY 10011, U.S.A.

Stevenson-Hinde, Joan   Sub-Department of Animal Behaviour, University of Cambridge, Madingley, Cambridge, CB3 8AA, U.K.

Sunar, Diane   Department of Psychology, Istanbul Bilgi University, Kazim Karabekir Cad. 34060 Eyüp Istanbul, Turkey

Tomlinson, Mark   Department of Psychology, Stellenbosch University, Matieland 7602, Stellenbosch, South Africa

van der Merwe, Amelia   Department of Psychology, Stellenbosch University, Matieland 7602, Stellenbosch, South Africa

van IJzendoorn, Marinus H.   Institute of Education and Child Studies, Leiden University, 2333 AK Leiden, The Netherlands; Center for Moral Socialization Studies, Erasmus University Rotterdam, Rotterdam, The Netherlands

Zeanah, Charles H.   Tulane University, New Orleans, LA 70118, U.S.A.

Foreword

The Culture of Peace

Anwarul K. Chowdhury

In 1945, after two world wars had exacted a devastating toll on humanity during the first half of the twentieth century, the combined will of 51 countries established an intergovernmental organization in an effort to spare future generations from the scourge of war. The United Nations was established "to reaffirm faith in fundamental human rights, in the dignity and worth of the human person, in the equal rights of men and women and of nations large and small; to establish conditions under which justice and respect for the obligations arising from treaties and other sources of international law can be maintained; and to promote social progress and better standards of life in larger freedom" (UN Charter, adopted June 26, 1945, preamble). To approach these goals, it was recognized that tolerance must be practiced and that living together in peace with one another as good neighbors was essential. This was not conceived to be the undertaking of a few nor was it to be a top-down process. To the contrary, it was envisioned that the combined strengths of humankind would be required to ensure long-term global peace and security.

In the nearly seven decades that have since transpired, it could be all too easy to think that not much has happened to progress toward these ends. One only needs to pick up the daily newspaper or to tune into a newscast to realize that many people live in settings that are far from secure and desirable. Universal peace is still a very distant goal.

Here, I wish to put forth a different perspective: The task of uniting the strengths and capabilities of billions of individuals, so as to ensure long-term peace and security in our world, is very much underway. Focusing on that which binds us together as human beings, a culture—a set of values, attitudes, traditions and modes of behavior and ways of life—is being created to support the eventual realization of these goals. For this to be successful, however, each individual must be empowered to act according to fundamental principles. These principles must be evident in our actions (both individual and societal), and they must form the very basis upon which policies are formulated at local, regional, national, and international levels. By immersing ourselves in a culture that supports and promotes peace, individual efforts will, over time, unite to enable sustainable peace and security to emerge.

The Process

Wars are fought to settle border disputes, control resources, and exert or retain dominance over others. Wars are also fought and conflict perpetuated to exact financial gain. In current political jargon, there is a preference to use the term "civil conflict" instead of "war." However there is nothing "civil" about genocide, rape, kidnapping, senseless killing, lynching, or the dismemberment of fellow human beings. The fact that such atrocities are often directed toward people who live in the same community or region as those who perpetrate such acts is most disturbing. All too often, hatred and intolerance drive such acts, skewing a person's ability to perceive others as equals.

As the Cold War was winding down, recognition emerged that the traditional ways of addressing conflict or war (i.e., mediation, humanitarian interventions, peacekeeping missions, diplomacy) were insufficient to create a lasting peace in the world. Conflicts erupt, problems get addressed, peace treaties are signed, but society never peels back the layers of a conflict to examine why it emerged in the first place. The United Nations' focus on promoting "international peace" (i.e., peace between nations) was understood to be the absence of war between states. However, to understand peace as the opposite of war is fallacious: the absence of war or conflict may bring about a cessation of hostilities, but it is not synonymous with peace.

> A peace based exclusively upon the political and economic arrangements of governments would not be a peace which could secure the unanimous, lasting, and sincere support of the peoples of the world…peace must therefore be founded, if it is not to fail, upon the intellectual and moral solidarity of mankind (UNESCO Constitution, adopted November 16, 1945, p. 1).

To abolish conflict or war as a viable option for action, a concept of peace needs to be embraced that is inclusive and sustainable. Theoretically, this should be possible, for the same species that invented war is surely capable of inventing peace (to paraphrase Margaret Mead).

To this end, my formal efforts began on July 31, 1997, when I approached the Secretary-General of the United Nations, Kofi Annan, in my capacity as the UN ambassador from Bangladesh, to request that the concept of a "culture of peace"[1] be included as an agenda topic for the plenary sessions of the UN General Assembly. As a result, in 1998 I was mandated by the President of the fifty-third regular session of the UN General Assembly, Mr. Didier Opertti of Argentina, to chair a committee, open to all member states, that would focus specifically on the concept of a culture of peace: its meanings and potential

---

[1]   The concept of the culture of peace was first proposed at the UNESCO International Congress on Peace in the Minds of Men in Yamoussoukro, Côte d'Ivoire, in 1989 (http://unesdoc.unes-co.org/images/0010/001058/105875e.pdf (accessed July 31, 2014). For further information, see http://www.culture-of-peace.info/index.html (accessed July 31, 2014).

implications for humanity. Given the mission of the United Nations—"to save future generations from the scourge of war"—it was felt that a fundamental conceptualization of peace—one that would be accepted by consensus—was crucially needed to address existing and emerging global realities.

As you might appreciate, achieving consensus among thinking individuals, let alone between delegates who represent diverse member states in an intergovernmental setting, can be a difficult and excruciatingly complex undertaking. Indeed, as the committee began its deliberations, initial difficulties became apparent as we tried to reach agreement on basic concepts and perspectives. In the background was the fear that the committee's efforts would divert focus and energies away from human rights issues or possibly be used to advance national interests.

In an international organization such as the United Nations, political reality can mean that the interests of any given government in power may take precedence over that country's fundamental principles. The voting cycle of elected governments and their term limits create additional challenges, as issues that require long time frames for realization are generally avoided.

The committee acknowledged these realities from the outset and endeavored to elevate the discussion on the culture of peace to a level that would transcend national boundaries and concepts of time. The challenge was to get member states to understand that a fresh conceptualization of peace was in the interest of every country, government, and administration: this issue is fundamental to all of humankind, present and future. Our goal was to advance a concept that would not reflect any particular intercountry conflict, that would redirect efforts toward peace as an attainable goal (and not merely the absence of violence or war), and that would surpass all national interests in the best interest of humanity as a whole.

After nine months of intense, concentrated efforts, the committee's results were presented to the fifty-third session of the UN General Assembly on September 13, 1999. The Assembly's adoption by consensus of the committee's negotiated text resulted in a landmark, norm-setting resolution: the "Declaration and Program of Action on a Culture of Peace" (UN Resolution A/RES/53/243, adopted Sept. 13, 1999).

The Declaration

The Declaration is a conceptual statement intended to guide governments, international organizations, civil society, and individuals. It lays forth fundamental principles of peace that derive from age-old values held in high esteem by all peoples and societies. It calls upon humankind to transform these principles into action, so as to promote a culture of peace in the new millennium.

It is important to note that *peace* is not understood to be merely the absence of conflict: It is a condition or state in which every person is empowered to develop to his or her full potential. It is a positive, dynamic participatory process wherein dialog is encouraged and conflicts are solved in a spirit of mutual understanding and cooperation.

The *culture of peace* is defined as "a set of values, attitudes, traditions, and modes of behavior and ways of life based on:

- Respect for life, ending of violence and promotion and practice of non-violence through education, dialog and cooperation.
- Full respect for the principles of sovereignty, territorial integrity and political independence of States and non-intervention in matters which are essentially within the domestic jurisdiction of any State, in accordance with the Charter of the United Nations and international law.
- Full respect for and promotion of all human rights and fundamental freedoms.
- Commitment to peaceful settlement of conflicts.
- Efforts to meet the developmental and environmental needs of present and future generations.
- Respect for and promotion of the right to development.
- Respect for and promotion of equal rights and opportunities for women and men.
- Respect for and promotion of the right of everyone to freedom of expression, opinion and information.
- Adherence to the principles of freedom, justice, democracy, tolerance, solidarity, cooperation, pluralism, cultural diversity, dialog and understanding at all levels of society and among nations; and fostered by an enabling national and international environment conducive to peace.

Clearly, for humanity to advance toward a culture of peace, corresponding values, attitudes, behavior, and ways of life are required. These must be realized and implemented by individuals, groups, and nations.

The development of a culture of peace is integrally linked to the peaceful settlement of conflicts, mutual respect, and international cooperation. To support this development, individuals need to have skills that promote dialog, consensus building, and peaceful resolution of differences. In addition, the following elements are crucial: Democracy is promoted as are human rights and fundamental freedoms. Participation in the development process must be accessible to all. Poverty, illiteracy, and inequalities must be eliminated; sustainable economic and social development must be promoted. Discrimination against women must cease, equal participation by women needs to be ensured on all decision-making levels, and the rights of children must be respected, promoted, and protected. Free flow of and access to information is imperative, as is the elimination of all forms of racism, racial discrimination, xenophobia, and related intolerances. In short, understanding, tolerance, and solidarity among all societies, peoples, and cultures must be cultivated and advanced.

The process of creating and sustaining a culture of peace is, by nature, participatory. Governments play an essential role in securing the institutional frameworks needed to promote and strengthen the culture of peace. However, civil society must be fully engaged. The media is well positioned to make integral contributions to inform and educate. Key roles must also be assumed by parents, caregivers, teachers, politicians, journalists, and religious leaders as well as by scientists, philosophers, artists, health workers, social workers, humanitarian agencies, and nongovernmental organizations.

The Declaration sets out the requisite norms, concepts, principles, and actors to the culture of peace, and the "Program of Action" delineates eight areas for prioritization at regional, national, and international levels:

1. Actions to foster a culture of peace through education.
2. Actions to promote sustainable economic and social development.
3. Actions to promote respect for all human rights.
4. Actions to ensure equality between women and men.
5. Actions to foster democratic participation.
6. Actions to advance understanding, tolerance and solidarity.
7. Actions to support participatory communication and the free flow of information and knowledge.
8. Actions to promote international peace and security.

Realizing the Culture of Peace

No one ever imagined that it would be simple to achieve a culture of peace. Humanity has a long history of resolving its differences through violence and has become used to a "culture of war." Transformation from this state to a culture of peace is not a matter of changing the mind-sets of groups of people or societies, but rather the mind-sets of individuals. By recognizing that peace begins with a single solitary person, we position ourselves better to accept the long-term scale that societal transformation may ultimately require. To transmute our individual thoughts, behavior, and actions, we must be able to address the challenges encountered in peaceful, nonaggressive ways. This requires each of us to be in a position of both opportunity and power to choose between options.

Violence and anger may be our first reaction to any hurdle; however, violence and anger do not always benefit us as individuals, especially when viewed on a long timescale. The attitudes and actions associated with violence and anger can actually work against us physically, mentally, and emotionally. Some of us may have grown up in environments where nonviolent solutions to conflicts with "others" were not taught. Indeed, the idea that unequal, intolerant treatment of certain people is a good strategy may actually be pursued in some settings. Thus, to acquire the necessary skills or transfer knowledge that can be used to revamp previous strategies or change old habits, education—in all of its forms—is essential. Education is needed to impart and instill fundamental principles. If our minds could be likened to a computer, then education provides the software with which to "reboot" our priorities and actions away from violence, toward a culture of peace.

Every individual is important to the transformation required to secure a culture of peace in our world. This means that each person must realize that nonviolent, cooperative action is possible. If a person succeeds in resolving a conflict in a nonviolent manner at any point in time, this individual has made a great contribution, for this singular act has succeeded in transferring the spirit of nonviolence and cooperation to another individual. When repeated, this spirit will grow exponentially—a practice that will become easier each time the choice is made to resolve a conflict nonviolently. Inculcating the culture of peace within yourself, as evidenced through your actions, gives a pleasure that is simple, possible, and completely independent from anyone else's actions. It is a good that belongs to you—one that you are able to transfer and share with others; that is with your fellow citizens.

Each one of us is undoubtedly a citizen of a particular community and country. However, we are also all global citizens in that we all live together on this planet and thus face the corresponding responsibilities that are bound up with our shared environment. As global citizens, we need to take a broad view of how our global community interacts. Globalization has created many levels of interdependence and interconnectedness—some which were unthinkable a few generations ago. This makes the pursuance of objectives marked solely by national, cultural, economic, religious or other limited interests counterproductive. What happens in one part of the world is linked to another; sooner or later unrest, violence, environmental degradation, and other calamities will affect us all.

As global citizens we need to look beyond the interests of our immediate surroundings and realize that we are intrinsically connected to each other. This does not mean that we are alike, in the sense of cultural identity. It simply means that the obstacles we face are encountered by others. Together we can meet such challenges.

Call to Action

To transform our societies to an enduring culture of peace requires concerted action on many levels. We must build on the awareness gained thus far and define clear-cut pathways to move forward. Well-informed, sensitive, and responsive programs are needed to assist all people at different levels.

On the global level, many groups and individuals are working to further the concept of the culture of peace. The Global Movement for the Culture of

Peace[2] is an example of an action-oriented coalition that has been successful in generating international attention to the issues, especially in terms of the roles that women and young people can assume. Pathways to Peace[3] and the Peace Education Resource Center[4] devote their efforts to making peace a practical reality at local and global levels. I believe that a global network should be created to connect organizations, groups, and individuals around the world, to offset geographical isolation as well as unite efforts around common goals.

At the national level, advocacy must remain an important goal. Given electoral cycles and changing representation among national leaders, the transcendent nature of the culture of peace must be continually communicated to decision makers. Equally important, nongovernmental networks and partnerships are crucial in broadening outreach to individuals. By integrating the fundamental principles of the culture of peace into coalitions and alliances, more might be able to be realized with the same amount of resources.

At the community level, local-level governance determines policies for those living within the community. It has the reach, authority, and capacity to enact change and can determine the tone and direction for its populace. In addition, it influences others who come into contact with the community, transferring the values and priorities associated with the community. Utilizing the culture of peace as a "compass for guidance and a lens to see and understand differently,"[5] the city of Ashland, Oregon (population: ca. 20,300), has recently undertaken a citywide attempt to integrate these principals into governance structures and educational organizations. Its goal is to shift mind-sets and behavior by "enabling deeper connections and wider collaboration in creating a peace culture through local efforts in business, education, government, and environment."[6] This is a collaborative project with Pathways to Peace, and it is hoped that the experiences gleaned from the Ashland attempt will serve to guide other municipalities.

At the level of the individual, early childhood provides a unique opportunity to address issues that would contribute to transform the culture of war to a culture of peace. Different types of programs or interventions are needed to support this, particularly those which would provide appropriate educational curricula. The events that a child experiences early in life, the education that this child receives, and the community activities and sociocultural mind-set in which a child is immersed all contribute to how values, attitudes, traditions, modes of behavior, and ways of life develop. Early childhood affords

---

[2] http://www.gmcop.org/ (accessed June 15, 2014).

[3] http://pathwaystopeace.org/ (accessed June 26, 2014).

[4] http://perc4peace.org/ (accessed June 26, 2014).

[5] http://media.wix.com/ugd/4ec65f_3c632514d1d6499dac23b9961ef9487d.pdf (accessed June 15, 2014).

[6] http://pathwaystopeace.org/collaborate/; see also http://www.cpi-ashland.org (accessed June 15, 2014).

a window of opportunity to instill the rudiments that each individual needs to become an agent of peace and nonviolence.

The task of uniting the strengths and capabilities of billions of individuals, so as to achieve long-term, sustainable peace and security in our world, is clearly underway. However at times, working toward this end can be frustrating and disappointing. It is easy to feel alone or to question if current affairs will ever change. Yet to alter the very foundation of an existing system requires time; transformation does not happen quickly. The key is not to be discouraged. Change will come through steadfast efforts.

As you read this volume, you will get a sense of the many different types of efforts that are underway to bring the experience of early childhood onto a path that will lead to a culture of peace. Many more efforts will undoubtedly be needed: Further evidence-based research will be imperative to inform the design of effective programs and interventions. The work of nongovernmental and international organizations will be crucial for such programs to be realized. Dedicated teachers and caregivers will be integral to implement these programs. Community leaders and policy makers are needed to ensure that the necessary frameworks are in place to support the transition toward the culture of peace. In support of all of these activities, the media could play an integral role.

In the end, however, this transformation is contingent upon each one of us. In everything we do, in everything we say, and in every thought that we have, there is an opportunity to create a culture of peace. Let us work each day to realize this. Let us choose strategies that require us to face each other with tolerance and mutual respect, viewing each other as fellow global citizens. Let us endeavor to build an inclusive world that respects and cherishes individual and group differences. And let us commit our efforts and resources to raise our children to be agents of the culture of peace.

Foundations for a
New Approach

1

Peace Is a Lifelong Process

The Importance of Partnerships

James F. Leckman, Catherine Panter-Brick, and Rima Salah

If we are to teach real peace in this world, and if we are to carry on a real war against war, we shall have to begin with the children....You must be the change you wish to see in the world.—Mahatma Ghandi (1869–1948)

In a real sense, all life is inter-related. All persons are caught in an inescapable network of mutuality, tied in a single garment of destiny. Whatever affects one directly affects all indirectly. I can never be what I ought to be until you are what you ought to be, and you can never be what you ought to be until I am what I ought to be. This is the interrelated structure of reality.—Martin Luther King, Jr. (1929–1968)

There can be no keener revelation of a society's soul than the way in which it treats its children. Education is the most powerful weapon which you can use to change the world.—Nelson Mandela (1918–2013)

The true measure of a community's standing is how well it attends to its children: their health and safety, their material security, their education, and sense of being loved, valued, and included in the families and communities into which they are born.—UNICEF (2007)

A Conceptual Journey

In 2013, the Ernst Strüngmann Forum convened a think tank to review a premise that has fascinating implications for research, practice, and policy: Do the ways we raise children hold promise for promoting peace in the world? The idea behind this Forum began to form in the spring of 2010, when James Leckman met with the Mother Child Education Foundation, known as AÇEV (Anne Çocuk Eğitim Vakfı), in Istanbul, Turkey. AÇEV wished to learn more about the biobehavioral systems involved in the formation of interpersonal bonds between parents and their offspring, and to receive a candid appraisal of their concept paper, "Building a Generation of Reconciliation: The Role of Early Childhood Development in Peace Building."

This paper reported on AÇEV's anecdotal experience with their father support program. This program, which began in 1996, brings together eight to ten fathers from poor areas of Istanbul as well as from rural regions of Turkey for 12–14 group sessions, to help them realize their importance in children's lives and to encourage them to take a more positive and active role in their children's development. In many of the groups, AÇEV observed that friendly relations were established between participating fathers despite their ethnic, religious, and ideological differences. Even more surprisingly, these friendships continued well after participation in the program ended. This led AÇEV to pose the question: Can early childhood interventions with families play a role in peacebuilding?

The need for an unbiased, scientific discourse was seen as integral. Thus, given James Leckman's earlier work with Julia Lupp, he approached her to see if the Ernst Strüngmann Forum would be able to help. After extensive review and development, support was granted and the Forum convened an interdisciplinary steering committee to refine the scientific scope of the proposal and select the participants, whose expertise ranged from those involved in the biobehavioral mechanisms of social bond development and early childhood, to the socioecological contexts that shape risk and resilience in the pursuit of social, physical, and mental well-being, to the international policy realm of interfaith dialog, peacebuilding, and conflict resolution. The goals established for this 15th Ernst Strüngmann Forum were to assess child development in the context of familial[1] and group relations and to examine its potential role in building pathways to peace. To approach these goals, four questions were posed, each of which was addressed by a specific working group (see Morgan et al., Steele et al, Christie et al., and Britto, Salah et al., this volume):

1. How does human biological development impact peacebuilding?
2. How do events and relationships in childhood set the stage for peace at personal and social levels?
3. Given multiple challenges in society, what kinds of early childhood interventions have potential for promoting peace?
4. How can we use new knowledge about child development and its contexts to create effective programs and policies that will reduce violence and promote peace?

In lieu of keynote speeches or presentations, papers were commissioned to provide entry points into the Forum. In light of the ensuing discussions and peer review, they have been extensively revised so as to communicate current thoughts on these topics. Most address specific aspects of the four focal questions. However, two chapters introduce overarching concepts: Hinde and

---

[1] Throughout this volume, the term "family" is used to describe a group of people bound together by bound together by kinship, roles in caring for each other, cultural traditions, or close affiliation.

Stevenson-Hinde (this volume) provide a framework for analysis and highlight the role of early childhood in creating individuals and societies with the values, motivation, and skills to foster peace for future generations. Britto, Gordon et al. (this volume) present an "ecology of peace" that builds on Urie Bronfenbrenner's ecological model of human development (Bronfenbrenner 1979) and expands the initial concept of AÇEV, regarding the potential of early child interventions to contribute to peace.

To our knowledge, this Forum represents the first systematic attempt to consider *whether the ways we raise children holds promise for promoting peace in the world*. In this chapter we wish to introduce you to the main topics of the Forum. We begin with a reflection on the concept of peace and examine what biology has to offer. Threats to human well-being are then examined and we review what has been learned from past early childhood interventions. Several ongoing initiatives are highlighted and the importance of partnerships emphasized. We argue that the current body of interdisciplinary evidence provides an ample call to action. To strengthen families and societies in ways that will reduce violence and promote peace across generations, new knowledge about child development must be transformed into effective pathways to peace. It is our sincere hope that this volume will stimulate further dialog and prompt concrete steps that will move humanity toward this ultimate goal.

What Is Peace?

Every language has a word to describe "peace" but defining it is hardly straightforward. In the English language, for example, the Oxford English Dictionary provides six primary definitions:

1. freedom from civil unrest or disorder; public order and security;
2. freedom from quarrels or dissension between individuals, especially in early use, between an individual and God; a state of friendliness; amity, concord;
3. freedom from anxiety, disturbance (emotional, mental, or spiritual), or inner conflict; calm, tranquility;
4. freedom from external disturbance, interference, or perturbation, especially as a condition of an individual;
5. absence of noise, movement, or activity; stillness, quiet; and
6. freedom from, absence of, or cessation of war or hostilities; the condition or state of a nation or community in which it is not at war with another.

Comparisons with other English-speaking dictionaries reveal additional definitions—a fact that becomes even more apparent when one broadens the review to include other languages. Throughout the Forum, we constantly confronted what it is that we mean when we use the word "peace": Is it the absence of "violence" or an entity itself? As we considered the closely related constructs of peacebuilding and peacemaking, the concept of peace proved even more elusive.

Given the multiple, yet related meanings, what do we mean by peace and its manifestations? We define peace through the following components (Figure 1.1):

- Peace is an *outcome* (e.g., it is assessed by the absence or cessation of violence).
- Peace is a *process* (e.g., peacebuilding is characterized by efforts to negotiate freedom from violence, through the creation of social bonds within and across groups of people).
- Peace is a *human disposition* (i.e., it is a personal and social orientation to secure freedom from distress and to foster a capacity to act, predicated on a fundamental recognition of freedom and dignity of all people).
- Peace is a *culture* (i.e., it is distinctive from a culture of violence, and fosters a sense of global citizenship).

Viewing the components of peace allows us to bridge approaches taken in the biological and neurological sciences (which strive to measure outcomes and processes in human development as they pertain to children and families) with approaches from the social and political sciences (which seek to understand shared goals and expectations that shape everyday human practices and the potential for change in policy, society, and everyday family life). This allows us to discuss the foundations of peace—in childhood, families, communities, and global policies—with the aim to initiate change across generations and engage children and families in pathways to peace.

When peace is viewed as a disposition (i.e., a state of mind that orients thoughts, behaviors, and principles of action), we recognize that it is also a

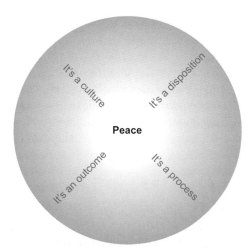

Figure 1.1   Multiple components of peace.

process conditioned by the historical, cultural, economic, and political contexts of people's lives as well as the microenvironments of their families and
communities. In an ideal world, peace is a source of freedom that allows individuals to pursue their lives in a meaningful way and to contribute to the
realization of universal human rights, justice, and oneness of humanity (Britto,
Salah et al., this volume). Yet beyond our own internal worlds, we must recognize that our lives are interdependent: every being influences and is influenced
by others, as the above quote from Martin Luther King reminds us. We are all
deeply interconnected with one another; our very survival depends on others. Aspects of this interconnectedness have their roots in the microsystems of
families; these roots extend to the very beginning of life *in utero* and are deeply
influenced by how we are raised as children (see Keverne; Maestripieri; Fox et
al.; and van IJzendoorn and Bakermans-Kranenburg, all this volume).

The word "peace" and its adjective form "peaceful" could be interpreted as
reflecting a degree of passivity or docility in response to injustice and discrimination (Christie et al., this volume). However, such a view distorts our argument. The pursuit of peace leads to giving voice and taking action to make our
world a better place (see Punamäki; Dawes and van der Merwe; Masten; and
Christie et al., this volume). Well-recognized exemplars of global citizenship
can be found in the lives of Mahatma Gandhi, Nelson Mandela, and Martin
Luther King, who espoused nonviolence as a means to achieve social justice.
Equally, however, others can be found in the actions of those who continually
grapple with issues of violence and social justice, who through their actions
bring agency in voice and action to considerations of peace and its linkages
with society, families, and children.

We view *peaceful children* as individuals who are committed to relational
harmony and social justice, resting on a steadfast attentiveness to human dignity, with the power to promote this human disposition across generations.
Healthy children form secure attachments, have well-developed social skills,
and exercise the capacity to reason and communicate. *Peaceful* children, however, have additional capabilities: the capacity for empathy, respect for others,
commitment to fairness, and trust in relationships with other people (Christie
et al., this volume). Having these peacebuilding capabilities goes beyond the
creation and maintenance of harmonious relationships: they lead to the expression of a *peaceful* disposition, which enables individuals to think and act in
ways that will promote equity, safety, and well-being for all people.

What Can Biology Teach Us?

The biobehavioral systems that underlie the development of selective social
bonds between sexual partners and parent-child dyads are ancient and deeply
rooted in mammalian evolution. Our threat-detection and stress-response systems have been evolutionarily conserved and are closely interconnected with

the biobehavioral systems associated with the formation and maintenance of social bonds. The neuropeptides oxytocin and vasopressin and their receptors are key elements within this system. They appear to influence, and be influenced by, many of the mental states and behaviors that directly pertain to peace, including trust, cooperation, and empathy (see Carter and Porges; Fox et al.; van IJzendoorn and Bakermans-Kranenburg, all this volume). Despite ever-expanding coverage in the scientific literature, unresolved questions remain concerning the interplay of the central and peripheral components of this complex biobehavioral system that dynamically engages the brain as children and caregivers interact over the course of human development.

In terms of brain structure and function, there can be no doubt that severe, early socioemotional deprivation can have a profoundly negative impact on an individual. There is also increasing evidence that there are "sensitive periods" of development that have a foundational effect on a broad range of skills and competencies (Fox et al., this volume). While the negative effects of institutionalization can be permanent, data from the Bucharest Early Intervention Project, the English Romanian Adoptees Study, and other studies of children adopted from institutional settings all indicate that some degree of remediation following adoption is possible, particularly when the adoption occurs before the age of two years and when the child has been with their adoptive family six years or more. These findings, along with data from other studies of children who were malnourished, neglected, and/or abused in their early years, provide compelling evidence that early experience matters and is an important determinant of brain structure and function as well as the children's cognitive and social behaviors (see Morgan et al. and Christie et al., this volume). Multiple childhood adversities, from socioeconomic disadvantage to war-related violence, leave their mark on well-being that lasts well into adulthood (Kessler et al. 2010; Mitchell et al. 2014). These data give way to *a call for action*: What can we do to intervene on behalf of these children? More importantly, what can we do to prevent early adversity?

Epigenetics—the study of changes in the regulation of gene activity and expression that are not dependent on gene DNA sequence (Keverne, this volume)—is another area of biological science that is potentially relevant to peace. Animal studies have demonstrated that future parental behaviors can be shaped by epigenetic modifications and can have a lasting influence on patterns of gene expression in the developing brain, starting at fetal development. For example, investigators have documented that high versus low levels of licking and grooming behaviors by Norwegian mother rats during the first few days of postnatal life are associated with epigenetic modifications of the regulatory regions of a number of genes that can produce enduring effects on gene expression, leading to individual differences in stress response and future maternal behavior by the pups (Meaney 2010). These studies also indicate that *individual differences in maternal behavior matter and can be transmitted across generations*. If this finding is confirmed in humans, this will provide a solid foundation for the assertion that interventions to strengthen families and to improve the cognitive and socioemotional well-being of children have *transgenerational consequences*. This possibility is a source of genuine excitement among well-informed policy makers: it points to the huge, potential long-term benefits that would result from efforts to refine and implement, in a sustainable fashion, early childhood education and family support programs of proven value.

Despite an ever-growing body of research, much remains to be done before we fully understand the role of the epigenome in shaping human behavior across generations. At present, we know that early-life adversity in primates and humans is associated with distinct patterns of methylation across the entire genome. For example, a recent study examined whether, in rhesus macaques randomly divided into two groups at birth, differential methylation in early adulthood was associated with different early-life social and rearing experiences (Provençal et al. 2012). "Mother-reared" monkeys were raised by their biological mother in a social group, whereas "surrogate peer-reared" monkeys were reared with an inanimate surrogate as well as daily socialization periods with age-matched peers. Provençal et al. (2012) found that differential rearing led to differential DNA methylation in both the prefrontal cortex and peripherally circulating immune cells. These differentially methylated promoters tend to cluster by both chromosomal region and gene function. Studies in humans also support the hypothesis that, in response to early-life adversity, there are system- and genome-wide changes in methylation patterns in peripheral cells that directly impact our stress-response and immune systems (Bick et al. 2012; Naumova et al. 2012; Labonté et al. 2013).

In humans, the timing, nature, and plasticity of these epigenetic modifications may be especially important and complex. The recently completed ENCODE project (ENCyclopedia Of DNA Elements) provides evidence that variation in the regulation of gene expression during development, rather than variation in protein sequence, is almost certainly the dominant factor in human brain evolution (Pennisi 2012). These changes in the sequence of the "regulatory" portions of the human genome appear to have led to the creation of new combinatorial expression patterns during development, which in turn may be responsible for uniquely human aspects of brain circuitry and connectome[2] (Kang et al. 2011; Seung 2012). One plausible hypothesis that is currently being explored maintains that these epigenetic modifications may reflect evolutionarily conserved and broadly represented physiological processes that translate specific environmental information at different stages of development to "program" gene co-expression networks to adapt to specific external environments (Karatsoreos and McEwen 2013; Szyf and Bick 2013). Emerging evidence also indicates that there may be parental environmental legacies through the male/female germ lines (sperm and ova) (Barouki et al. 2012; Soubry et al. 2014).

---

[2] A connectome is a comprehensive map of prominent neural connections within a nervous system.

Although challenging, future studies will need to examine these issues, particularly concerning the timing and plasticity of epigenetic modifications when the nature of the external environment is enriched. What is fixed and what can be reprogrammed? The use of animal model systems and the employment of random assignment to different rearing conditions, which change over the course of development, will likely be necessary (see Carter and Porges; Keverne; and Maestripieri, this volume). However, the ENCODE findings clearly indicate that the epigenetic modifications seen in our primate relatives may only hint at the complexity that is likely to exist in humans. In addition, while epigenetic modifications can often be developmentally sensitive and regionally specific, genomic imprinting is another set of epigenetic modifications that results in less variability in gene expression (e.g., the inactivation of large portions of the X chromosome in females) (see Keverne, this volume).

The underlying biology of groups constitutes another largely unexplored area relevant to "peace" (see Fry; Morgan et al.; and Steele et al., this volume). The influence of groups greatly impacts how individuals function in the world: we are born into groups; groups often provide the means by which we take care of each other, work and play, create and destroy; from groups we learn about our own identity and our beliefs about others. Social dominance hierarchies are nearly ubiquitous within groups and can directly influence the extent to which a society is despotic or egalitarian. Although groups at times can foster "us vs. them" social identities, there are many examples of neighboring societies where the identity of the in-group ("us") expands to include external individuals ("them"; see Fry, this volume). Efforts to understand the underlying neurobiology of groups are just beginning (Jordan et al. 2013; Gordon et al. 2014) and should be prioritized in the future.

Threats to Well-Being in Societies Today

Many, if not a majority, of the world's children live in environments that provide grossly inadequate foundations for good health, nutrition, and cognitive, language, and socioemotional development (Christie et al., this volume; UNESCO 2010; UNICEF 2012). Although poverty reduction is a central feature of the international development agenda, vast asymmetries exist in terms of income, access to food, water, health, education, housing, and employment. These inequalities produce and reproduce multiple deprivations and violations to basic human rights. Indeed, global health[3] action has firmly shifted attention away from the narrow goal of poverty elimination to the broader goal of equity promotion (D'Ambruoso 2013).

---

[3]   Global health addresses the persistence of harmful and unfair health outcomes, and views equity (or fairness) in social, economic, and political structures as an essential pathway to achieve health and well-being for all.

What are the main threats to well-being in relation to peace? On the occasion of the Nobel Peace prize in 1966, Mohammed Yunnus stated succinctly in his acceptance speech: "Poverty is a threat to peace." In this volume, we extend this viewpoint to include violence, insecurity, and inequity as significant and additional threats to peace. Violence and discrimination create injurious harm to communities, families, and children, while disparities within and across communities have been demonstrably linked to poor health (Galtung 1996; Farmer et al. 2006; Wilkinson and Pickett 2009). In conflict-affected countries, widening income and ethnic inequalities are now understood to be significant drivers of violence and barriers to sustainable peace (Langer et al. 2012). Thus peace is not only linked to poverty, it is also inextricably linked to equity (i.e., fairness).

Peace and violence are often viewed as two sides of the same proverbial coin. Dawes and van der Merwe (this volume) discuss two primary forms of violence and injurious discrimination—direct violence and structural violence—and debate how these might be transformed by efforts to secure equity and justice. Without doubt, the most visible form of direct violence that inflicts harm on families and children is war-related violence (Punamäki, this volume). It is estimated that over one million children today live in countries affected by wars, armed conflicts, and military violence (Attanayake et al. 2009). It is important to understand that war-related violence cascades across generations, impacting households to subvert and overwhelm everyday family life in ways that threaten the health and well-being of both caregivers and children (Panter-Brick et al. 2014b). In Afghanistan, for example, children and families must negotiate several layers of interrelated violence; the stress of widening inequalities and shattered infrastructure, related to war-related violence, results in "everyday violence," as manifested in persistent domestic quarrels and fierce disputes between neighbors. In the context of pervasive violence and weak governance, families prove to be children's first line of defense.

Structural violence—an insidious, often invisible form of political, legal, social, and economic discrimination—produces persistent, unfair, and harmful health outcomes due to disparities in access or quality of resources by ethnic, socioeconomic, religious, or other backgrounds (see Dawes and van der Merwe, this volume; Galtung 1996). Similar to direct forms of violence, exposure to structural violence can initiate a series of unfortunate developmental consequences, which compromises full developmental potential. For example, children are less likely to develop the capacities and motivation required to be empathetic to the needs of others, to become productive members of society, and to work toward the goals of peace and equity. They may be more likely to engage in violent conduct (Walker et al. 2007). Later, should they become parents, these individuals raise not only children but also the expectations (social, political, economic, and legal) of their children, thereby inculcating thoughts and behaviors that shape the capacities to act.

Increasing evidence suggests that under conditions of severe life adversity, understanding pathways to resilience matters just as much as understanding pathways to risk in human development. Why and how children and families overcome violence and discrimination is just as important to understand as why and how "developmental cascades" may trap children into vulnerability (Masten, this volume). The concept of resilience as a holistic process—one that allows not only coping but transformation as well—provides a new paradigm to focus attention on the developmentally and culturally relevant leverage points necessary to foster healthy human development (Panter-Brick and Leckman 2013). In a similar vein, understanding "pathways to peace" and their connections to the everyday lives of children and families offers a perspective that extends understanding beyond what it means to minimize violence.

Given the existing global inequalities in children's environments and opportunities, as well as the potential power that is inherent in early child development, what interventions, at the family and community levels, show promise for promoting peace in the world?

Lessons Learned

Early childhood is known to be the optimal period in which human capital is developed and formed; consequently, investments in early childhood enrichment programs provide the greatest potential for economic and human returns (Heckman and Krueger 2003; Heckman and Kautz 2013). Emerging evidence also indicates that investments in early childhood can substantially boost adult physical health (Campbell et al. 2014). By investing in early childhood intervention and family support programs, communities contribute to an enhancement of their social capital and gender equity (Coleman 1988). In addition, there is the potential for family-based intervention programs to permeate not just individual homes but entire communities. These interventions provide a bottom-up approach at the family level which can create cumulative change in communities and societies (Britto, Gordon et al., this volume). A particularly important feature of these programs is that they facilitate the formation of diverse in-groups. By focusing on commonalities among families, these programs provide an opportunity for productive relationships to be formed across ethnic, cultural, and religious divides (see Kagitcibasi and Britto, this volume).

Early childhood interventions aim to enhance the development and well-being of children during the early years of life and to improve family environments. These interventions encompass a range of programs across multiple dimensions (Britto et al. 2013):

- age of the child (e.g., infancy, toddlers, preschool ages),

- foci of intervention (e.g., health, nutrition, protection, education, the social capital of the parents),
- generation(s) being served (e.g., children or caregivers, or both),
- mode of implementation (e.g., home-based, center-based, one-on-one training vs. group-based interventions), and
- sponsorship of the program (e.g., government, nongovernmental organizations, private for profit).

A number of programs show promise, and a few have demonstrated long-term benefits. Notable examples of studies from the United States that have shown positive long-term outcomes into adulthood include the High/Scope Perry Preschool Project, the Chicago Longitudinal Study, and the Abecedarian Project (reviewed in Kagitcibasi and Britto, this volume). The Turkish Early Enrichment Project (Kagitcibasi et al. 2001) and Jamaica Study (Grantham-McGregor et al. 1991b)—two of the few longitudinal studies conducted outside of the United States—have assessed the impact of overall development and cognitive/achievement outcomes that early childhood intervention programs have had on the participants in adulthood. These two projects share a number of common elements: both work with at-risk children, involve direct parent and child engagement, and use an experimental design. Most importantly, these two studies, like the U.S. studies, demonstrated measurable gains for the child into adulthood as a result of their participation in the program.

The Turkish Early Enrichment Project involved both center-based preschool environmental enrichment and home-based training for mothers in a quasi-experimental design. Mothers were trained to support their preschool-age children's overall development, including preparation for school. At the end of the first stage of study, benefits were noted in virtually all areas: the child's cognitive abilities, school adjustment and performance, social acceptance by peers, level of autonomy, and decreased use of aggressive behavior (Kagitcibasi et al. 2001; see also Kagitcibasi and Britto, this volume). As the participating children moved into adolescence, sustained benefits were noted with regard to cognitive development, school achievement, educational attainment, socioemotional development, and social integration. Secondary benefits were also observed: mothers and families benefited from better family relations and the intrafamily status of women increased. At the second stage of the study, carried out in young adulthood, the following long-term benefits were noted in young adults who had participated and/or whose mothers had participated: increased educational attainment (including university education), better cognitive performance, higher occupational status, and greater social participation (Kagitcibasi et al. 2009). Two other promising elements of this intervention should be noted: (a) interaction between parents promotes the creation of social bonds across ethnic, cultural, and religious boundaries; (b) program sustainability is reliant on the involvement of government officials at both local and national levels, which should be cultivated from the onset. Both elements highlight the importance of *partnerships* to achieve jointly held goals.

One of the biggest limitations to ongoing work is the lack of any direct assessment of relevant peace promotion variables. Although we were able at the Forum to create conceptual links between outcomes of better executive function, increased empathy, better social communication skills, reduced violence, and peacebuilding, these have not been rigorously tested in diverse contexts. To do this, we must decide how to *measure* peace, in terms of outcomes, processes, disposition, or cultural values. Ideally, metrics should be developed for use in national surveys and early intervention programs. Some of the possibilities that have yet to be explored include measuring dyadic and triadic parent-child interactions in the home, using video recordings, before and after early intervention programs. If peace is regarded as a state of mind, then monitoring the dyadic interactions between parent and child in real time could offer a good approach. Other possibilities include the use of biomarkers, such as salivary oxytocin and hair cortisol (Feldman et al. 2013), immune competence (Panter-Brick et al. 2008), or telomere length (Mitchell et al. 2014) as well as indicators of future risk for cardiovascular and metabolic diseases (Campbell et al. 2014). A range of social science methods is also essential to gain a fuller appreciation of the effectiveness, relevance, and long-term impact of these programs on children and their families. Given the potential for transgenerational effects of interventions, it is crucial for participants of early childhood intervention programs to be evaluated when they become parents, so that the nature of parenting can be evaluated when it is their turn to raise children. In addition, the design of evaluations needs to be more robust before we can know for certain what impacts specific programs have on child development or family dynamics.

Global Citizenship

Throughout the Forum, the concept of global citizenship and the culture of peace (see the Foreword, this volume) directed discussion on efforts to strengthen families and improve the lives of children. As set forth by the United Nations, "a culture of peace is a set of values, attitudes, traditions and modes of behavior and ways of life" that "reject violence and endeavor to prevent conflicts by tackling their root causes to solve problems through dialogue and negotiation" among individuals, groups and nations (UN 1999). The UN declaration resonates with Hinde's perspective set out in his recent book, *Changing How We Live: Society from the Bottom Up* (Hinde 2011; see also Hinde and Stevenson-Hinde, this volume): What changes are necessary so that each of us takes responsibility for looking after each other and our planet? As an evolutionary biologist and peace activist, Hinde (2011) highlights two basic propensities of human nature: *selfish assertiveness*, which leads to behaviors that primarily benefit the actor, and *prosociality*, which leads to behaviors that benefit others as well as one's own self.

What better place to start than childhood? What needs to be done to develop and empower the next generation of Mahatma Ghandis, Martin Luther Kings, and Nelson Mandelas? To this end, Abu-Nimer and Nasser (this volume) offer a framework that links peacebuilding with child development, and Nusseibeh (this volume) reviews the potential role that the media could play in peacebuilding. Potential exemplars, such as the Panwapa initiative, exist that empower children across the globe to interact with one another and become global citizens (Lee and Cole 2009).

Next Steps

Assessing whether the ways we raise children holds promise for promoting a more peaceful world is an ongoing process (e.g., Panter-Brick and Leckman 2013; Sunar et al. 2013; Panter-Brick et al. 2014a) predicated on relevant knowledge, careful evaluations, strong partnerships, and fundamental interdisciplinary collaborations to bridge and assimilate expertise from academic, practitioner, and policy worlds. Our journey has now led to the specific hypothesis that early childhood development *is* relevant to peacebuilding (Sunar et al. 2013; Panter-Brick et al. 2014a). Based on the current body of interdisciplinary evidence, a clear call for action is warranted and initial steps have been taken.

The Early Childhood Peace Consortium was established "to advocate for investment in young children as a way to promote peace in homes and communities and, ultimately, as a strategy for peacebuilding."[4] At its launch in September 2013, over 140 partners from multiple sectors (e.g., civil society, the social and mass media, government officials, multi- and bi-lateral agencies, practitioners, academic researchers) took part in activities focused on "creating a legacy of sustained peace drawing on the transformative power of early child development." Currently, the consortium is striving (a) to achieve the key goals related to the global peacebuilding agenda,[5] by recognizing the transformative power of early development to promote prosociality, diminish selfish assertiveness, and reduce and prevent violence; (b) to create a platform to advocate for change, using bottom-up approaches and to inform future research, policy agendas, and programs; and (c) to strengthen established and emerging networks around children and peace.

In addition to the Early Childhood Peace Consortium, work is underway with UNICEF, AÇEV, the UN Alliance of Civilizations, the Fetzer Institute, and Sesame Workshop to build global strategies that will promote pathways to peace—pathways that will involve children and their families at the community

---

[4] http://www.unicef.org/earlychildhood/index_70959.html (accessed June 15, 2014).

[5] http://www.un.org/en/peacebuilding/pbso/pbun.shtml (accessed June 15, 2014).

level. This work will involve policy makers, government officials, academic partners, and, importantly, the media (see Nusseibeh, this volume).

We also wish to direct attention to an ongoing program in South Africa: Ilifa Labantwana. This program, described in detail by Dawes and van der Merwe (this volume), operates on a large scale, is multifaceted and funded completely by donors. It is based on the recognition of the structural inequities that face the majority of South African children and those who care for them. Its main goal is to provide the evidence necessary to inform changes in government policy and provisioning for early childhood development, thus enabling scale up of essential services to ensure that children thrive, grow, and are ready to learn when they reach school.

Common to each of these examples is the clear focus on early child development. By working, first and foremost, with families (and then, by extension, with the communities and governing bodies in which they reside), important steps can be taken to promote both *healthy* and *peaceful* child development. In turn, *healthy* and *peaceful children* will provide the necessary, if not wholly sufficient, foundations for peace.

We do not advocate a one-size-fits-all view of community engagement, family structure, or child development; roles and configurations of what it means to be a family or a parent vary substantially within and across cultures. Regardless of their configuration, families are an important locus for the biological and social care of children. Consequently, families provide significant entry points to promote healthy and peaceful child development through interventions that reduce violence, vulnerabilities, or harm as well as interventions that build peace, resilience, and equity in health.

Engaging with families is not the sole option. Resilience, equity, or peace can also be promoted within schools and/or at the community level. Families, however, represent a sensible and effective place to start. Furthermore, engaging with families is not equivalent to engaging mothers alone, since other caregivers have a demonstrable impact on family dynamics and healthy child development (Cowan et al. 2009; Panter-Brick et al. 2014a).

If we are to move consciously toward peace, our ways of being must incorporate a culture and a disposition toward peace that will shape processes and outcomes for future generations. In this volume, various "pathways to peace" are explored, based on the biological and social underpinnings of child development, to promote harmonious and equitable relations in families and across generations. There are, no doubt, many others. Thus, in the spirit of the Ernst Strüngmann Forum, we wish to enlist your involvement in this discussion, in future programs, and in new research endeavors. If concrete progress is to be made, intersectorial partnerships between stakeholders (e.g., government agencies, policy makers, funders, service providers, researchers, community leaders, families, children) must be created and sustainably maintained, for the task requires the efforts of all.

Acknowledgments

Many partnerships contributed to this project: We wish to thank Sue Carter and Julia Lupp for their help and input in drafting the original proposal. We express our gratitude to the Ernst Strüngmann Forum for its support and partnership over the last two years. We are grateful to James Cochrane, Geraldine Smyth, Diane Sunar, and Marinus van IJzendoorn for their work on the steering committee.

To prepare for the multifaceted discussions that constituted this Forum, the efforts of the authors of individual chapters deserve special mention. These people laid the groundwork for the Forum and revised their contributions extensively thereafter to ensure that the arguments could be effectively passed on to you, the reader. The moderators of the discussion groups—Sue Carter, Marinus van IJzendoorn, Catherine Panter-Brick, and Rima Salah—as well as the rapporteurs—Barak Morgan, Howard Steele, Daniel J. Christie, and Pia Britto—worked together to ensure lively and productive discussions during the focal meeting and concise summary reports thereafter (see Chapters 7, 11, 15, and 19). Most importantly, we thank each participant for their time and invaluable expertise.

Supplemental funding was received from the German Science Foundation and in-kind support was provided by the Frankfurt Institute for Advanced Studies. In closing, we are enormously grateful to the Ernst Strüngmann staff for their tireless efforts associated with this think tank, as well as with the editing and production of this book.

2

Framing Our Analysis

A Dialectical Perspective

Robert A. Hinde and Joan Stevenson-Hinde

Abstract

This chapter presents a framework (Figure 2.1) to examine dialectical relations between successive levels of analysis. It represents dynamic processes, with bidirectional influences and continuous change over time, and is particularly relevant to child rearing, where parental adaptation to change is essential. Attachment theory and research indicate how early parent-child interactions lead to the development of an attachment bond, and how the quality of this attachment lays a foundation for the child's socioemotional development. Finally, viewing behavior within the context of our common evolutionary past leads to the assumption of two basic propensities: selfish assertiveness, which primarily benefits the actor, and prosociality, which benefits others. These propensities remain with us today and suggest the need to provide contexts that promote more prosociality and less selfish assertiveness, both within our own groups as well as toward other groups.

Introduction

This chapter provides a dialectical framework for integrating various levels of analysis in this book. Although a particular chapter may focus on only one or two levels, each level may be understood within the broader context of the framework as a whole.

As an example, at the level of early relationships, the development and implications of a secure attachment bond will be outlined. Consistent with the thrust of this volume, the emphasis within attachment theory and research is on a "bottom-up" approach. However, as Figure 2.1 illustrates, "top-down" influences will also be operating, including those of context. It is not difficult to see how unsettled contexts, occurring across too much of our world today, may bear down on any path to peace.

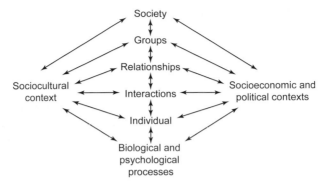

Figure 2.1 Framework indicating some of the dialectical relations between successive levels of analysis.

A Dialectical Perspective

Early childhood can be viewed as the beginning of a developmental pathway that may produce individuals and societies with the values, motivation, and skills to foster harmonious relationships and negotiation rather than aggression. Such a pathway involves successive, interacting levels of social complexity. Figure 2.1 outlines dialectical relations between various levels, ranging from interacting internal biological and psychological processes to individual behavior, interactions, relationships, groups, and society (Hinde 1987).

Each of these levels influences and is influenced by context, including the *socioeconomic context*. This involves the availability of resources such as food, healthcare, education, work, and social mobility. The *sociocultural context* subsumes an aspect particularly relevant to early childhood, namely the concept of a *developmental niche* (Super and Harkness 1986). This consists of three interacting components:

1. The *physical and social settings* in which the child lives: with whom the child interacts, sleeping practices, the balance between work, play or rest, and schooling arrangements, if any.
2. Culturally regulated *customs* of child care and child rearing, seen within a culture as the "natural" thing to do: from daily routines, such as back carrying, to practices such as circumcision rituals.
3. The psychological "ethnotheories" of caretakers referring to the rich cross-cultural variety of parents' *shared beliefs* about children's social and emotional development.

Primary developmental themes across the Asian continent are emotional interdependence between a mother and her children, as well as empathy and harmony within the social group. In Latin America, themes involve obedience, responsibility, and good manners, whereas in the United States the focus is on cognitive qualities and independence (Super et al. 2011; see also Chen and Rubin 2011).

Within the framework of Figure 2.1, each level has emergent properties that are not relevant to the level below. For example, although built upon antecedent behavioral interactions, relationships are more than a simple sum of interactions, involving perceptions, fears, and expectations. Unlike interactions, relationships continue over time, even during separations. Additionally, "the nature of a personal relationship is affected not only by its constituent interactions, but also by the group in which it is embedded......Furthermore, each of the levels of complexity affects, and is affected by, the sociocultural structure of the ideology, beliefs, values, norms, institutions and so on more or less shared by the individuals in the group or society....Each level must thus be treated not as an entity but as involving processes of continuous creation, change or degradation through the dialectical influences within and between levels" (Hinde 1999:19–20).

As an example, consider attitudes toward divorce. Before World War II in most Western countries, divorce was barely respectable: both moral attitudes and legal obstacles had to be overcome, and divorced individuals were regarded with reservation. In the United Kingdom, prejudice was so strong that it caused a King to abdicate. However, during World War II many couples were separated from each other, many men and women joined the Forces or went out to work, and in both cases were introduced to new ways of living. For these and other reasons, many husbands and wives drifted apart after the war, and divorce became more frequent. As divorce became more prevalent it became less disreputable, and as it became less disreputable it became even more frequent. The ramifications of the resulting changes in societal values were immense.

Thus Figure 2.1 represents dynamic processes, with bidirectional influences and continuous change over time. The basic concept is not unlike that of family systems theory, which focuses on continuous cycles of interactions within a flexible family system (e.g., Minuchin 1985). Transactional models and dynamic systems theory, involving a continuous process of change with innovative outcomes, are particularly relevant to child rearing. As stated by Kuczynski (2003:7) in his review of bidirectional frameworks: "The task of parenting is to rear a rapidly changing organism; therefore, adaptation to change rather than stability is an essential element of successful parenting" (for a thorough discussion of dialectical models of socialization, see Kuczynski and De Mol 2015).

Such a framework, with a hierarchy of levels ranging from the individual to the cultural and physical contexts, may serve at least two purposes within the present volume: (a) to locate which level(s) any particular chapter is addressing, and (b) to make one aware of levels *not* considered, with potential intralevel and interlevel dynamics overlooked. Sameroff (2009) pointed out that individuals are constrained by underlying biological processes and are embedded in networks of relationships. Groups and social institutions provide roles that children come to fill, and cultures provide meaning systems for their practices. Indeed, the same behavior may have different meanings, or different behaviors the same meaning, in different cultures. Furthermore, individuals are limited by the availability of economically related resources, which determine whether or not they can realize their potential.

Attachment

At the heart of Figure 2.1 is *relationships*, a misleadingly brief term for an ever-expanding network of different types and different levels of commitment. Attachment theory is particularly relevant here, since it focuses on an aspect of our earliest relationships and indicates how these may lay a foundation for subsequent socioemotional development. By choosing this exemplar, we are not suggesting that attachment is the only aspect of a close relationship, or the only developmental path to peace.

John Bowlby postulated that experiences within early close relationships lead to an "internal working model" of the self in relation to others that acts as a guide for future interactions. With a secure working model comes the expectation of *gaining* support when it is needed and, in turn, *feeling worthy* of such support. A secure attachment relationship is associated with an ability to communicate emotions in an easy, open manner and to appreciate the feelings of others. If continued into adulthood, this sense of "felt security" should enable an individual to communicate effectively and form trusting relationships with others. To the extent that such characteristics lead to harmonious rather than conflicted interactions and relationships, attachment security may be seen as an initial step on the path to peace.

The basics of attachment theory can be outlined as follows. First, at the level of *interactions*, consider *attachment behavior* toward a caregiver, defined as any form of behavior that attains or maintains proximity to a caregiver in times of need or stress. Attachment behavior begins at birth and appears to be universal, with the evolutionary function of protection from harm (Bowlby 1969, 1982). "During the course of time, the biologically given strategy of attachment in the young has evolved in parallel with the complementary parental strategy of responsive caregiving, the one presumes the other" (Bowlby 1991:293; for an overview of attachment, see Cassidy 2008). It was in a non-Western culture that Bowlby's colleague, Mary Ainsworth, first fully appreciated and documented infants' attachment behavior toward the mother and the use of her as a "secure base" from which to explore (Uganda: Ainsworth 1967; Ainsworth 1977; see also Posada et al. 2013).

Second, Ainsworth went on to develop a method for assessing the quality of the child's *attachment relationship* with the mother. This involved a standard laboratory procedure (the Strange Situation) in which attachment behavior was elicited by two brief separations from the mother. The *organization* of attachment behavior and emotions expressed (or not) toward the mother upon reunion provided the basis for assessing aspects of the attachment relationship, such as the degree of security (rated from 1–9, low to high) and "pattern of attachment." Ainsworth's seminal Baltimore study showed that infant-caregiver interactions observed in homes over the first year of life lead to the development of an attachment relationship, with its own emergent properties (Ainsworth et al. 1978).

Third, the above quality of the child's attachment relationship depends crucially upon antecedent maternal interactions. In Bowlby's words, "what is happening during these early years is that the pattern of communication that a child adopts toward his mother comes to match the pattern of communication that she has been adopting toward him" (Bowlby 1991:295–296). Thanks to Ainsworth, maternal "sensitive responsiveness," defined as reading signals accurately and responding appropriately, has been related to security of attachment in cultures ranging from Baltimore (Ainsworth et al. 1978) to Indonesia (Zevalkink 1997; see also van IJzendoorn and Sagi-Schwartz 2008). A meta-analysis over many studies, including non-Western cultures with various caregiving arrangements, has shown significant associations between maternal sensitivity and infant security of attachment (De Wolff and van IJzendoorn 1997), and intervention studies indicate the causal link between the two (Bakermans-Kranenburg et al. 2003). A recent special issue of the journal *Attachment & Human Development* focused on the centrality of Ainsworth's concept of maternal sensitivity to the development of security (Grossmann et al. 2013). It also reviewed findings that sensitivity is not independent of internal factors such as maternal state (e.g., anxiety or depression), other interactions and relationships (e.g., within the family), or external contexts (e.g., traumatic experiences).

Thus the main tenets of attachment theory appear to be universal, with an interplay between the levels of *interactions* and *relationships,* namely: (a) the phenomenon of infants showing attachment behavior toward caregivers from birth, leading to (b) the formation of an attachment bond with one or more specific caregivers, with (c) the security of that bond dependent upon the "sensitive responsiveness" of the caregiver to infant's signals.

Of special interest to a discussion on peace, *security* is associated with a variety of (theoretically predictable) positive outcomes, such as a sense of self-worth, resilience, empathy, and social competence (reviewed in Weinfield et al. 2008; Thompson 2008; Groh et al. 2014).

Finally, it must be emphasized that our early attachment relationships, formed during a sensitive period of development and regarded as a foundation for later relationships, are not indelibly fixed over time. Bowlby postulated an "internal *working* model" of close relationships that tends to be self-fulfilling but open to change. All of this suggests that close relationships, and the security that may derive from them, are susceptible to change, from the bottom up or top down, and need to be nourished across the life span (e.g., Parkes et al. 1991).

Evolutionary Considerations

Human behavior must be seen in the context of our common evolutionary past. For heuristic reasons, let us assume the evolution of two basic propensities: selfish assertiveness leading toward behavior that primarily benefits the actor, and prosociality leading toward behavior that primarily benefits others (Hinde 2011). It has long been a mystery how natural selection could have produced prosociality, which benefits not the actor but others who may be potential competitors. It now seems, however, that several processes were involved, one of which depended on competition between groups. Competition does not necessarily imply violent conflict, but can imply effectiveness in acquiring scarce resources. Since early humans were faced with shortages of resources, competition must have been ubiquitous, occurring between individuals within a group as well as between groups. Selection would have favored groups in which the individuals behaved predominantly prosocially and cooperatively toward each other. For example, if netting small animals was involved in gaining food resources, hunting would have been more efficient if individuals spread their nets in a continuous line and then shared the catch, than if the nets were placed here and there with gaps between them.

Thus, as depicted in Figure 2.2, cooperation (as an aspect of prosociality) toward members within any one group (i.e., the in-group) would have been selected, but not toward members of different groups (i.e., the out-group). Within a group, a balance between selfish assertiveness and prosociality must have been maintained. A group in which the individuals had no propensity to look after their own interests would not be viable, as it would be exploited by free-riders. A group of individuals who were wholly selfish would explode.

We suggest that rules of morality were developed within groups as a means of supporting a viable balance between prosociality and selfish assertiveness. Furthermore, the culture developed within groups also tended to favor discrimination against out-groups. Figure 2.2 points to the lack of natural or cultural selection for a pathway promoting prosociality toward a perceived out-group.

Such tendencies remain with us today. Although morality may hold the balance between prosociality and selfish assertiveness *within* groups, when it comes to interactions *between* groups, rules are rarely effective, either in preventing conflict (*jus ad bellum*) or in regulating conflict once it has begun (*jus in bello*). Negotiations between groups are more likely to be successful if they start with individual representatives discussing shared concerns and goals. An appreciation of how much is held in common may serve to blur the distinction

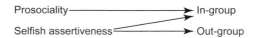

Figure 2.2 Differential influences of natural and cultural selection on the direction of prosocial and selfish propensities toward the "in-group" versus an "out-group."

between in-groups and out-groups, thereby enabling prosocial behavior toward the latter.

Conclusion

To change society, and we believe that this must be our aim, we need to give our world outlook a nudge toward more prosociality and less selfish assertiveness in our interactions and relationships, within our own groups as well as toward other groups. Experience shows that this requires us to work both from the bottom up and the top down (Hinde 2011). Changes in divorce conventions, mentioned earlier, resulted primarily from practice (i.e., bottom up) and were at first resisted by the law. More usually, however, change is imposed from above. For instance, the compulsory wearing of helmets implemented by legislation[1] (i.e., top down) was initially strongly resented by motorcyclists in the United Kingdom. However, since it made such obvious sense, acceptance quickly spread through the motor-cycling community. This may have been facilitated by the fact that the helmet became accepted as a badge of belonging to a select and daring group (i.e., one that could straddle and control a powerful machine). Smoking provides a similar case. The discouragement and regulation of smoking was first seen as an attack on personal freedom, but attitudes changed after the public became aware of overwhelming scientific evidence of health risks (perhaps aided by well-publicized lurid illustrations). Historical examples, such as the end of the use of British ships to transport slaves, the cessation of dueling, and the end of foot-binding for Chinese women, have been carefully documented (Appiah 2010).

There can be little doubt that individual violence and war must be tackled at the level of individuals as well as at the governmental level. In the United Kingdom, and in the particular case of eliminating war, both levels are being pursued. British Pugwash is a leading branch of the Pugwash Conferences on Science and World Affairs,[2] an international network of scientists and others concerned about the social impact of science, with particular emphasis on abolishing weapons of mass destruction and war. It works through politicians, providing them with data and acting as go-betweens in crisis situations (e.g., preparation for U.S.-Palestine relations meetings in Ramallah before President Obama's visit in March 2013). The Campaign for Nuclear Disarmament,[3] which advocates unilateral nuclear disarmament, as well as the Movement for the Abolition of War,[4] which endeavors to spread the belief that the abolition

---

[1]   Motor Cycles (Wearing of Helmets) Regulations (S.I., 1973, No. 180), February 7, 1973.

[2]   http://www.pugwash.org (accessed June 15, 2014).

[3]   http://www.cnduk.org/ (accessed June 15, 2014).

[4]   http://www.abolishwar.org.uk (accessed June 15, 2014).

of war is both desirable and possible, are examples of groups in the United Kingdom that operate at the grassroots level.

In a similar way, we can act from the bottom up as well as from the top down toward the goal of long-term altruism rather than short-term greed. Such a goal is essential to promote the well-being of all of us, including the youngest and most vulnerable, with whom our future lies.

3

Ecology of Peace

Pia R. Britto, Ilanit Gordon, William Hodges,
Diane Sunar, Cigdem Kagitcibasi, and James F. Leckman

Abstract

Peace is a state of being that encompasses harmonious international as well as intra- and interpersonal relationships, directly impacting an individual's safety and prosperity. For an individual, peace is a positive "state of mind" conditioned by our histories and context. The concept "ecology of peace" is introduced to capture these vast interconnected ecosystems that extend from our internal biology to our subjective sense of self (i.e., our thoughts, emotions, and behaviors) to the environments in which we live. It is our thesis that positive, stimulating, and harmonious early childhoods can contribute to peace and human security, and that early-life interventions have transformative power which may help lay the foundations for conflict resolution and peace in future generations. As such, we posit that these interventions can contribute to "peacebuilding" (actions that promote sustainable peace by supporting the prosocial skills needed for peace) as well as "peacemaking" through the enhancement of positive reciprocal communication within families, communities, and nations. This chapter reviews (a) neurobiological foundations of peace, including genetic, epigenetic, hormonal, developmental, and social factors that shape young brains; (b) the importance of parenting and early learning for peacebuilding; and (c) the place that early childhood can play in bridging the gap between peacebuilding and peacemaking. Evidence from available developmental neurobiology as well as social and economic studies suggests that change in favor of peace can be initiated not only from the top down, through official policies and agencies, but also from the bottom up, by supporting the physical, emotional, and social development of children and the well-being of their families and communities.

Introduction

Scientific evidence in the field of early childhood development has demonstrated that the early years of life are crucial for all aspects of adult functioning, including competencies, attitudes, and skills (Britto et al. 2013; Steele et al., this volume). For example, Duncan et al. (1998) concluded that the effect of poverty on cognitive skills and educational attainment is greatest in early childhood. In contrast, child abuse, neglect, and psychosocial deprivation have been shown to have profound negative impacts on all aspects of socioemotional and cognitive development (Nelson et al. 2007; Fox et al., this volume). Thus, the nature and quality of early childhood are among the strongest predictors of later human development. Given the profound importance of early childhood and the devastating consequences that violence has on individuals, communities, and societies, it would be surprising if the events that an individual experiences in early years did not have fundamental implications for the propensity to peace or violence later on in life (Punamäki, this volume). Globally, efforts to build peace in communities and among nations tend to involve top-down approaches, beginning with the setting of policies and national security agendas. Largely unexplored are alternate approaches that begin with the individual and the family unit at a crucial stage of human development; namely, from conception through early childhood.

The concept "ecology of peace" is introduced to signify that humans are part of vast interconnected ecosystems that extend from our internal biology to our subjective sense of self (i.e., our thoughts, emotions, and behaviors) to the environments (families, communities, societies) in which we live, and that actions and interactions at each level are both affected by and help to determine whether or not the condition of peace is present. It is our thesis that positive, stimulating, and harmonious early childhoods can contribute to peace and human security and that early-life interventions have transformative power which could help lay the foundations for conflict resolution and peace in future generations (see Leckman et al., this volume). In this chapter we discuss the significance of potential associations between early childhood development and both peacebuilding (i.e., actions that promote sustainable peace by supporting the prosocial skills needed for peace) and peacemaking through the enhancement of positive reciprocal communication within families, communities, and nations. We explore the question of whether these interventions can contribute to peacebuilding as well as peacemaking, drawing on ongoing work of the Mother Child Education Foundation, known as AÇEV (Anne Çocuk Eğitim Vakfı).[1]

Definition of Constructs

Early Childhood Development

Early childhood development[2] refers to the dynamic interplay between the child and the proximal environment that influences development. At the level of the child, it spans the prenatal period to the transition to school, which is generally completed by age eight or nine years (Convention on the Rights of the Child

---

[1] http://www.acev.org/en/anasayfa (accessed June 15, 2014).

[2] In this chapter, early childhood development includes the care and education to which the individual is exposed during this stage of development.

1989:3; McCartney and Phillips 2006; Britto et al. 2013). Development during these stages occurs across several interrelated domains: physical health and motor development; cognitive skills; social and emotional functioning; competencies in language and literacy; ethical and spiritual development; sense of group membership; and identity within families, communities, and cultures (Britto and Kagan 2010). At the family and community levels, context is an important determinant of the achievement of developmental potential. Within the first few years of life, as they interact with their environment, typically developing children make rapid strides in all aspects of development (Shonkoff and Phillips 2000; Richter 2004; Irwin et al. 2010; Richter et al. 2010). When we consider the theoretical models and practice-oriented frameworks of early childhood development from an ecological perspective, it is clear that a host of contextual factors are involved, including proximal (e.g., family) and distal contexts (e.g., international policies) (McCartney and Phillips 2006; Hodgkin and Newell 2007; Britto and Ulkuer 2012; Britto et al. 2013). Early childhood development is foundational to later human development as well as to the stability of character skills expressed in adulthood (Heckman and Kautz 2013). From the age of three years, if not earlier, children normally develop a "sense of self" that is conducive to the development of "creative freedom" (a "world to explore") and the moral order (a "justice order") that accompanies it (Snyder et al. 1980). Children as young as three years of age have a preference for specific cultural symbols; they affiliate and identify with particular communities and, in the context of a divided society, show a tendency to make sectarian statements (Connolly et al. 2002). Thus it follows that attitudes relevant to "peaceableness" versus conflict and actions of peacebuilding versus violence are formed during early childhood development.

Peace and Violence

Peace as a psychological concept has typically been described in the context of human behavior and is often characterized as the absence of negative experiences. Consistent with other perspectives in this volume (e.g., Leckman et al. this volume), we define peace as a positive state of mind that can influence and be influenced by relationships within families, communities, and nations to affect ultimately the future of our globe.

Violence is categorized as direct or structural; direct violence refers to conflict that harms individuals, whereas structural violence results from social, political, and economic structures and processes, ranging from poverty to overcrowding to discriminatory laws and social practices that lead to oppression within a society (see Dawes and van der Merwe, this volume). The root causes of structural violence include systematic deprivation, unfair political systems, and powerful, inequitable social hierarchies. Structural violence can beget direct violence through various paths, from neurobiological effects during development to rebellion against injustice. Both have deleterious effects on human health and well-being. Similarly, efforts to achieve peace can be categorized as two different processes: peacebuilding and peacemaking (Christie et al. 2001; Christie et al., this volume). Peacebuilding addresses the root causes of violence by reducing structural violence and establishing a rule of law; it has a proactive focus with an emphasis on the development of an effective infrastructure to sustain social justice, health care, and economic development. Peacebuilding is multidimensional and interactive, with legal, cultural, political, medical, and socioeconomic components (Galtung 1969). According to AÇEV, peacemaking is the process of resolving conflict and reducing or preventing direct violence, whereas peacebuilding is the process of establishing a basis for sustainable peace by maximizing justice, equality, and harmony. Both aim to reduce and prevent violence. In this conception, peacemaking involves the reduction of direct violence through conflict resolution and other nonviolent means; it is temporally and spatially constrained by the situation—a reaction in response to the threat or the anticipation of violence (MacNair 2003).

The Ecology of Peace: How Early Childhood Development Is Related to Peace

The ecology of peace is a conceptual framework for exploring the multiple relationships between early childhood development and peacebuilding. Both early childhood development and peacebuilding are complex constructs that are expressed at multiple, interrelated levels: individual, family, and community. The associations among these levels are dynamic, varied, and elaborate. To understand the relationships between early childhood development and peacebuilding fully, each level needs to be closely examined. Such an examination suggests the following hypotheses.

1. Early experience, as determined by the interaction between the developing child's brain and the immediate environment (specifically caretakers and other household members), lays the foundation for violent or peaceful relations and behaviors in later life.
2. Interventions that target either the family or the developing child can impact the child's propensity for violent or peaceful relationships and behaviors in later life.
3. Support for the development of human capital (i.e., realization of a child's potential) can contribute to peace in the community and beyond; in other words, measures that contribute to peacebuilding can also contribute to peacemaking.

In the following discussion, three components—the neurobiology of peace, the promise of parenting and early childhood intervention programs, and the path from peacebuilding to peacemaking—are identified that are crucial elements underlying each of these three hypotheses. By separately addressing these components, we are able to examine, explore, and analyze, to some degree, specific relationships without diffusing or conflating other relationships in the framework. This also leaves open the issue of "emergent properties" produced by nonlinear interactions between the different levels of the framework (Lewin 1943; Kim 2006). For example, biology can be viewed as an emergent property of the laws of chemistry which, in turn, can be viewed as an emergent property of particle physics. Similarly, psychology could be understood as an emergent property of neurobiological dynamics. At a macro level, intergroup relations may be an emergent feature of familial and intragroup dynamics. We also acknowledge the importance of "top-down" effects within these interactive domains. At the end of each section, gaps in knowledge are identified and key questions posed that need to be answered by future research.

Component 1: The Neurobiology of Peace

The first component delineates the pathway between biology and behavior at the level of the child; specifically, early neuronal development may be an important ingredient in peacebuilding. A primary point of interest in neuroscience research is how early-life experiences (especially the initial bonds formed between infants and their caregivers) can set the stage for future interactions. Here we point to two domains: (a) the role of environment-dependent epigenetic modifications that can have a lasting influence on gene expression in the developing brain and somatic tissues, and (b) the biobehavioral system associated with the neuropeptide oxytocin.

Epigenetics

Individual differences in maternal behavior can be transmitted across generations via *epigenetic* mechanisms (see Keverne, this volume). Based on the results of the recently completed ENCODE (Encyclopedia of DNA Elements) project, it is clear that variation in regulation of gene expression during development, rather than variation in protein sequence, is almost certainly the dominant factor in human brain evolution (Pennisi 2012). Epigenetics refers to the study of changes in the regulation of gene activity and expression that are not dependent on the gene DNA sequence. Epigenetic variation includes chemical modification of the DNA by methylation and hydroxymethylation, as well as structural modifications of histones (the proteins that are the building blocks of chromatin) which, in turn, affect DNA packaging within the nucleosome (Razin and Riggs 1980; Razin 1998). The potential relevance of epigenetics to the neurobiology of peace first became apparent through the work of Michael Meaney and his team at McGill University; they documented that high versus low levels of licking and grooming behaviors in mother rats were associated with epigenetic modifications of the promoter region of a gene that is critically involved in the stress-response pathway. Specifically, they found that differential patterns of methylation at this site in the genome had enduring effects on gene expression, leading to differences in stress response and future maternal behavior by the pups (Weaver et al. 2004). Epigenetic modifications have now been documented throughout the human genome. Some are directly related to environmental stressors, including child abuse (Labonté et al. 2012).

Oxytocin Pathways

Parent-child dyadic interactions and pair bonding in later life are regulated, in part, by oxytocin and the closely related neuropeptide, vasopressin. They form core elements in an integrated and dynamic biobehavioral system within the developing brain that is crucially involved in early-life bonding (Carter 2014 and this volume; Garrison et al. 2012). Recent discoveries point to the extensive involvement of the oxytocin system in behaviors that pertain to peace, including trust and cooperation, empathy among in-group members, and the ability to read the mental states and empathize with the feelings and experiences of others (Domes et al. 2007; Guastella et al. 2009; Bartz et al. 2010b; De Dreu et al. 2011; van IJzendoorn and Bakermans-Kranenburg 2012b). The oxytocin system is thus a prime candidate to pursue in peacebuilding research, because of the complex neural and somatic systems that it influences during the emergence of intimate dyadic relationships throughout development. In addition, preliminary data point to the importance of epigenetic modifications of the oxytocin receptor gene (Kumsta et al. 2013). When studying the neurobiology associated with peacebuilding, it is crucial to examine components that are directly involved in the behavioral building blocks of peace (e.g., early-life bonding) as well as to focus on how these systems interact with other biobehavioral systems. For example, the oxytocin system is not only involved in processes of bonding, sexual and maternal behavior, salience, and reward pathways, it also interacts with stress response, anxiety, reward, feeding behavior and energy homeostasis, pain cognition, and the immune system (Maccio et al. 2010; Gordon et al. 2011; Ho and Blevins 2013). Indeed, recent data indicates that oxytocin plays a pivotal and multidirectional role in the microbiome-gut-brain-immune system network (Poutahidis et al. 2013). All of this points to the importance of the central role that the oxytocin system plays at the dynamic interface of physical and mental health, as well as to the need for further research, both generally and with a specific focus on peacebuilding.

The existing literature has many gaps, and many important questions remain to be answered by future research on epigenetic modifications of the human genome and the oxytocin biobehavioral system and their impact on bonding in early life. The following areas for investigation are worth noting:

- How does stress in early life (via family and/or environment) lead to epigenetic modifications? How widespread, tissue-specific, and alterable are these modifications?

- What is the developmental trajectory and function of the oxytocin system throughout embryonic, fetal, and infant development? How is this complex biobehavioral system influenced by epigenetic modifications?
- Which behavioral, neurophysiological, genetic, and epigenetic mechanisms inform parent-infant oxytocin synchrony?

Affiliative Bonding in Early Life

Here the focus is on the pathway between biology (at the level of the child) and parenting behavior (as part of the family context)—specifically, early bonding as a precursor to behaviors associated with peacebuilding. Numerous studies that assess the involvement of the oxytocin system in human bonding have examined the expression of microlevel social behavior in each partner, during dyadic or triadic interactions, through the dimensions of gaze, proximity, arousal, touch, affect, exploratory behavior, and vocalizations (Carter and Porges, this volume; van IJzendoorn and Bakermans-Kranenburg, this volume; Gordon et al. 2011). The expression of these behaviors in various social contexts (e.g., face-to-face interactions, exploratory play, interactions between children or adolescents and their best friends or a peer group, and exchanges between romantic partners) has been assessed in relation to peripheral measures of oxytocin. Such microlevel behaviors are integrated into meaningful behavioral constellations with distinct temporal patterns and can advance understanding of the intricate relationships between the oxytocin biobehavioral system and attachment processes in humans. Neuroimaging studies of new mothers also point to the involvement of oxytocin-related circuitry in sensitive caregiving (Strathearn et al. 2009; Kim et al. 2011; van IJzendoorn and Bakermans-Kranenburg, this volume). With respect to early childhood development and peacebuilding, the role of oxytocin needs further clarification (Carter and Porges 2013). For example, further work is needed to explain the degree to which the oxytocin biobehavioral system plays a role in the emergence and maintenance of relationships that extend beyond dyadic relationships to in-groups to the wider community and intergroup relations. Likewise, efforts to understand the interrelationship between epigenetic modifications and the functioning of the oxytocin biobehavioral system are just beginning (Labonté et al. 2012; Provençal et al. 2012; Peña et al. 2013). However, these recent findings, which link parental behaviors with relatively stable peripheral levels of oxytocin, raise a number of questions that must be resolved:

- How are stable oxytocin concentrations maintained in the periphery?
- How is this related to events in the brain?
- Is somatodendritic release and diffusion sufficient, or is maintenance of peripheral oxytocin due to a release from axon collaterals extending into the forebrain from magnocellular hypothalamic neurons?

- How does the distribution and sensitivity of oxytocin receptors change over the course of development, and what role do epigenetic modifications play in mediating (reflecting) patterns of parent-infant bonding?
- How valuable are peripheral measures of oxytocin as well as blind ratings of parent-child dyadic interactions as "biomarkers" for evaluating early childhood interventions?
- How can genome-wide studies of an individual's methylome be valuable and relevant within early childhood studies?
- How stable is a child's genome-wide methylome, and can it be modified as a consequence of an early childhood intervention?

Component 2: The Promise of Parenting and Early Childhood Intervention Programs

The pathway between family context and behavior at the level of the child—specifically, understanding the impact of parenting programs and child-focused interventions on parent and child peacebuilding behaviors—is the focus of the second component.

Parenting and Peacebuilding

The way that caregivers meet a child's physical, cognitive, socioemotional, and moral needs provides the foundation for a child's development. Responsiveness and care in addressing these needs are critical to healthy growth and development (Bornstein and Putnick 2012), and optimal parenting is every child's need and right. Parenting can be defined as the interactions, behaviors, knowledge, beliefs, attitudes, and practices associated with child health, development, learning, protection, and well-being that are passed on to a child by primary caregivers (Britto et al. 2013). As such, primary caregivers (e.g., parents, grandparents, community elders, older siblings) determine the environment in which children grow, develop, and learn. Based on existing literature (Bradley and Corwyn 2005), there are five distinct and identifiable elements of parenting: caregiving, stimulation, support and responsiveness, structure, and socialization. Each element manifests in the behaviors, knowledge, and/or attitudes of primary caregivers. Research consistently demonstrates that violence against children is highly prevalent and has severe developmental and physical consequences (Mikton and Butchart 2009). A child's protection should be primarily secured by the family, but studies of violence in the home (measured across 24 low- and middle-income countries) indicate that nearly two-thirds of children under the age of four years experience mild physical and psychological aggression by their parents (Lansford and Deater-Deckard 2012). Tolerance of violent behavior is learned in early childhood, often by witnessing violence in the home. Through such early exposure, violence can become established as the accepted or normal method for resolving conflict in later life.

Early childhood intervention programs designed for parents aim to improve any or all aspects of parenting (Moran et al. 2004; Kaminski et al. 2008; Shulruf et al. 2009). These programs can be offered through a variety of modalities, including home-based individual services and group-based sessions, and can vary greatly in focus and scope. The vast majority of these programs have been implemented in high-income countries, and there is a clear need to adapt, implement, and refine similar programs in low- and middle-income countries. Emerging results from parenting interventions in the early years of a child's life have demonstrated positive results, reducing harsh discipline and partner violence, and improving family cohesion and harmony (Al-Hassan and Lansford 2010; Feinberg et al. 2010; Love et al. 2005). These findings point to the following questions:

- From a developmental perspective, is there a critical window in which an early childhood intervention should begin to maximize the positive impact of the program? How can the influence of the timing of different interventions be measured to compare, for example, those that begin at conception[3] (see also Slade et al. 2005) with those that begin during the preschool years (Kagıtcıbasi et al. 2001; Koçak and Bekman 2009)?
- How crucial will it be to involve fathers? (Pruett et al. 2009; Sunar et al. 2013; Panter-Brick et al. 2014a)?
- How strong are intergenerational patterns of parenting? To what degree are they influenced by epigenetic modifications?
- How do negative experiences such as early trauma, abuse, and bullying influence brain development in children? How does psychological conflict in the family setting affect the mental health outcome of children?
- How does resilience (i.e., the process of harnessing biological, psychosocial, structural, and cultural resources to sustain well-being) fit within the peacebuilding framework (Panter-Brick and Leckman 2013)?
- What new research is required to produce empirically valid data to fill the current gaps in knowledge regarding the association between intrafamily relationships and peacebuilding in early childhood?

Early Learning and Peacebuilding

Here the focus is on the relationship between early childhood programs and behavior at the level of the child; that is, the association between early learning programs and peacebuilding (Kagitcibasi and Britto, this volume). Early childhood programs (e.g., preschools, kindergartens, childcare centers) represent

---

[3] See the Nurse-Family Partnership at http://www.nursefamilypartnership.org/about/program-history (accessed June 15, 2014).

the first microcosm of society for many young children in high-income countries. Consequently, in these contexts, children start to develop their own social identity, attitudes toward others, and dominance hierarchies in relationships (Astuto and Ruck 2010; Boyce et al. 2012a; Carretero 2011). These contexts, therefore, can strongly influence the development of stereotypes and attitudes as well as reinforce existing interpersonal relations among groups (Davies 2008). Data clearly indicate that the investments in early childhood programs have the greatest return in terms of a society's economic benefits (Heckman 2009; Heckman and Krueger 2003; Heckman and Masterov 2007). Six dimensions of early learning programs have been identified in the literature (Bowman et al. 2001) and can be used to delineate the theoretical foundation for examining the relationship between early childhood development and peacebuilding: holistic child outcomes; responsive interpersonal relationships between key caregivers or teachers and children; training and capacity of service providers; curriculum; school and home relationship and interactions; and presence of provisions for children in higher risk situations.

Application of these dimensions to peacebuilding initiatives has yet to be tested. Although several theoretical frameworks have been proposed, and a series of case studies have been conducted in conflict zones on early childhood interventions, none have been rigorously evaluated (Connolly and Hayden 2007). A variety of questions must be answered with regard to the association between early learning programs and peacebuilding:

- Where does peace fit into the accepted domains of development (e.g., motor, physical, linguistic, cognitive, social, and emotional)? Does peace consist of traits that are part of these given domains, or should peace be considered a separate domain of development?
- How can we support the development of morally responsible sensibilities and prosocial behavior in young children that would enhance pathways to peace throughout their lives?
- On a societal or interfamilial level, how is peace understood? How does this correspond to the relevance that peace holds in the domains of development (see above)?
- How much do contextual factors such as poverty, poor nutrition, ongoing violence, and conflict in the larger community influence the efforts of early childhood and family interventions?
- Can a set of standards be generated to evaluate the effectiveness of early childhood development programs for peacebuilding?

Component 3: The Path from Peacebuilding to Peacemaking

This component connects the level of the child to the outermost societal contexts; that is, the association between individual-level outcomes and community- and societal-level functioning. Most parenting and early learning programs target the individual and the family. In some contexts of peace nomenclature, this translates to the peacebuilding level. However, the ecology of peace framework goes further by exploring how families can influence communities and how peacebuilding can be translated into peacemaking. Therefore, this component encompasses the macro level (i.e., the social, cultural, political, and economic contexts).

The first way to explain how peacebuilding transitions to peacemaking involves the development of human capital. Since early childhood is known to be the optimal phase during which human capital is formed, investments in early childhood programs provide the greatest return on investment (Heckman and Krueger 2003). By investing in early childhood programs, communities enhance social capital and gender equity (Coleman 1988). A second mechanism involves the outcomes of family-based intervention programs that permeate entire communities, not just individual homes (Britto, Salah et al., this volume). This path, which suggests a bottom-up approach, promotes the idea that grassroots changes at the family level create cumulative change in communities and societies. A particularly important feature of such programs is that they facilitate the formation of diverse in-groups. By focusing on the commonalities among families, these group programs promote the development of friendships across ethnic, cultural, and religious divides. Other such mechanisms need to be evaluated and tested to demonstrate whether the path from peacebuilding to peacemaking can be achieved through early childhood programs. Many questions remain to be answered:

- Can peace within the family contribute to peace within the community? Most models of family and community interactions examine whether community-level factors influence family functioning. Here we argue the opposite: How does individual family functioning influence the larger community?
- From a socioecological and political perspective, can person-to-person approaches alter the biology of the brain and transform combatants/competitors into good neighbors? Or, are culturally informed narratives and self-interest too strong? For example, in regions of chronic conflict, can person-to-person initiatives which focus on enhancing child development reduce hostility between warring groups?
- Is there a set of principles that can guide the translation of science into useful material for diverse audiences (e.g., educators, community leaders, mass media, international development agencies, national-level policy makers) who need this information for program and policy development? How does a country hold together the micro and the macro levels of policy making with a focus on peace and human rights in early childhood?

Human Biological Development

4

Peptide Pathways to Peace

C. Sue Carter and Stephen W. Porges

Abstract

Humans are capable of premeditated aggression and warfare. In a war-torn world, it is tempting to forget that we are highly affiliative primates, whose survival as a species may have been based on the capacity to live and reproduce in groups (Hrdy 2009). War and peace are dependent on human behaviors, which rely on interactive and over-lapping physiological substrates. Despite experiences of aggression, abuse, or neglect, most humans have sufficient mental resources to exhibit positive social behaviors, social cognitions, and motivation for social attachment. Our physical survival and mental health requires "others." This apparent paradox, as well as the search for social safety, arises because the nervous system and behavior of contemporary humans are products of evolution. The purpose of this essay is to examine specific neuroendocrine pathways that may influence the positive social behaviors necessary for peace, when peace is defined as social safety within a society. This definition emphasizes the enabling power of social safety in promoting positive "states" associated with individuals interacting, socially connecting, and being mutually responsible for each other. Peptide pathways, including those reliant on oxytocin and vasopressin and their receptors, function as an integrated system mediating states of social safety. These endocrine and genetic pathways are at the center of a network that permitted the evolution of the human nervous system and allowed the expression of contemporary human sociality. Affiliation, pair bonds, and other forms of prosocial behaviors are not simply the absence of aggression. As reviewed here, we now understand that the prerequisites for peace, including prosocial behaviors and social safety, are built on active peptide systems. Knowledge of neurobiological mechanisms that form the foundations of social bonds and restorative behaviors offers a rational perspective for understanding, preventing, or intervening in the aftermath of adversity, and for enabling the emergence of peace in human societies.

Introduction

Since the end of the Second World War, 248 armed conflicts have been active in 153 locations worldwide (Themner and Wallensteen 2012). The current civil conflict in Syria provides a snapshot of the effects of an unsafe environment, which may be particularly disastrous for children. For example, on August 23, 2013, the number of children registered as refugees from Syria hit the one million mark. Child psychologist Dante Cicchetti (2013:403–404) summarizes the lasting implications of maltreatment for early child development as follows:

> Child maltreatment constitutes a severe, if not the most severe, environmental hazard to children's adaptive and healthy development…Specifically, maltreated children are likely to manifest atypicalities in neurobiological processes, physiological responsiveness, emotion recognition and emotion regulation, attachment relationships, self system development, representational processes, social information processing, peer relationships, school functioning, and romantic relationships…These difficulties pose significant risk for the development of substance abuse and psychopathology across the life course…Furthermore, there exists an increased risk for abused and neglected children to perpetuate maltreatment with their own offspring.

Nonetheless, contemporary humans are adaptive and reproductively successful in ways that few other large mammals can match. The interplay between social and aggressive traits of humans permitted the survival of *Homo sapiens* under historically difficult conditions. It has been proposed that our Neandertal cousins became extinct because they were less able than humans to create viable social groups (Pearce et al. 2013).

In 2011, the human population of the world surpassed 7 billion and by 2024 it is expected to exceed 8 billion. The development of agriculture and the industrial revolution have allowed the human population to explode. Humans are fundamentally social. However, war, rapidly expanding populations, and other adversities can challenge the capacity of humans to be social and cooperative.

The Biological Origins of War and Peace

Behaviors that are described as threatening or aggressive can be cognitive and comparatively non-emotional, such as the decision to use chemical warfare or deliver bombs in unmanned missiles. Alternatively, they may be highly emotional and defensive, sometimes leading to direct physical aggression and homicide. However, even emotionally motivated aggression does not necessarily lead to war (Fry and Soderberg 2013; Fry, this volume). The feelings and states that lie at the heart of defensive or reactive aggression probably have somewhat different biological and genetic substrates than planned "strategic" forms of aggression. Although the neurobiology of human aggression is beyond the scope of this chapter, defensive behaviors are central components of human sociality. Thus, it is difficult to separate the biological substrates of peace from those of war and aggression. Multidisciplinary perspectives from evolution, phylogeny, neuroendocrinology, genetics, and the development of the mammalian nervous system are critical to understanding both positive and negative patterns of behavior. Studies linking positive behaviors to the anatomy and physiology of the nervous system have increased dramatically, especially over the last two decades. A new and more positive perspective on human behavior is emerging from these studies. This perspective is built upon the hypothesis that prosocial behaviors, including social bonds and loving relationships, have distinct biological substrates (Carter 1998; Porges 1998; Carter and Porges 2013).

Peace as a psychological concept has generally been considered in the context of human behavior and is often described as the absence of negative experiences. However, as with aggression and other negative experiences, the positive behaviors and psychological states that are associated with peace are also based on ancient biological systems. We will argue here that hormonal and neural processes allow the emergence of states, experienced as peaceful, which are shared among social mammals. Consistent with other chapters in this volume, we will focus on the individual, defining peace as a positive state of mind derivative of social safety and emotional experiences associated with feeling calm and tranquil. The emotional states and experiences of the individual translate into relationships and have consequences for families, communities, and nations, ultimately affecting the future of our globe. To provide context, a few foundational assumptions that guide this perspective are offered below.

Working Hypotheses and Assumptions

Evolution and Development

In response to conditions of extreme adversity and maltreatment, individual variation is common, and some individuals are resistant to the lasting effects of trauma, even in early life (Ellis et al. 2011; Cicchetti 2013). Adaptation and resilience in the face of adversity have biological causes and consequences, including effects on growth and development. In addition, adaptation and resilience are often described in terms of differential activity in the hypothalamic-pituitary-adrenal (HPA) axis, as well as differential responsivity to adversity (sometimes termed diathesis stress) (Hostinar et al. 2013). Research from a variety of sources suggests that some individuals seem to respond primarily to and are shaped by positive experiences, rather than by adversity. The sources of these individual differences are not well identified, but are at least partly biological, with genetic/epigenetic underpinnings.

Understanding the evolutionary and developmental origins of the mammalian nervous system provides critical insights into the variations in social and emotional behaviors that characterize contemporary humans. Across evolutionary time, these systems responded to the adaptive demands of individual survival and reproduction (genetic survival). In the current human population, broad variation exists in behavioral phenotypes, including the responses to positive or negative environmental conditions. These are presumed to reflect individual differences in "differential susceptibility," based, at least in part, on individual differences in the "neurobiological sensitivity to context" (Ellis et al. 2011). Such variations may be adaptive depending on environmental context and demands. As described below, mechanisms for these differences may be found in an understanding of two ancient peptides: oxytocin and vasopressin. We propose that knowledge of these processes could lead to a new science of child development—a perspective that is shared by others (reviewed by Feldman 2012; Hostinar et al. 2013).

Genetics, Epigenetics, and Behavior

Human behavior is, in part, a product of inherited genetic codes, which in turn guide the assembly of biochemical molecules into tissues including the nervous system. At least some processes, presumably adaptive at some point in our evolutionary past, are retained in our anatomy and physiology. Among the products of our genes are hormones, neurotransmitters, neuromodulators, and receptors which regulate the functions of those tissues.

The mammalian nervous system and genome can be physically and functionally altered by behavioral experiences, especially in early life. However, studies that directly connect *specific* behavioral experiences to *specific* neuroanatomical or neuroendocrine changes remain scarce. Much of what we know about development and behavior is based on correlations that do not prove "causation."

Short- and Long-Term Perspectives on Neuroplasticity and Adaptation

The human body, and especially the nervous system, adapt in response to a changing and challenging environment. Included in the genome are genetic programs that influence the capacity of the nervous system to modify itself. Rather than being "hard-wired," mammals, and especially humans, have inherited a nervous system with "plastic" components that appear designed to be changed, both through "learning" and comparatively long-lasting, epigenetic processes which allow us to incorporate new information into the genome.

Both positive and negative social behaviors rely on neural substrates that were inherited, in part, from our premammalian ancestors. In the face of extreme stressors, older systems, based on our phylogenetic past, may take precedence. For example, the "shutdown" adaptations that emerge in the face of trauma rely on ancient neural systems that are not easily addressed by our modern cognition (Porges 1998, 2011). Evolutionarily older components of the nervous system, especially in the brainstem, may be less capable of adaptation than more modern neocortical systems. However, even ancient systems can be profoundly affected by both positive and negative experiences.

The developing nervous system is physically and biochemically sculpted by social interactions. Experiences, especially in early life, can epigenetically regulate gene expression (Champagne 2012; Zhang et al. 2013; Kumsta et al. 2013). Social experiences during sensitive periods, including prenatal, perinatal, and adolescent development, may be of special significance to social and emotional behavioral traits in later life. In addition, acute versus chronic responses to challenge differ physiologically. Reactions to stressful or negative experiences may in the short term appear advantageous. However, chronically negative and stressful experiences are costly on a longer timescale, creating vulnerability to emotional and physical diseases (Cicchetti 2013; Tol et al. 2013).

Research in monkeys or humans reared without a mother or consistent caretaker (Fox et al., this volume) confirms the hypothesis that appropriate parenting is important for primate social and emotional development. Social interactions are beneficial throughout life, and the absence of social support or a perceived sense of loneliness increases vulnerability to many forms of mental and physical disorders.

Stressful early experiences can produce a variety of changes, such as a smaller body size or atypical sociality in later life. Such changes might be deleterious in some environments, but adaptive in others, depending on individual differences, experience, resources, and context (Ellis et al. 2011). Understanding evolutionary and contemporary context is critical to evaluating the impact and mechanisms for a given experience (Bartz et al. 2011).

Neuroendocrine Perspectives on Mammalian Social Behavior

The Social Nervous System

Positive social behaviors are not simply the absence of aggression or other forms of pathology (Carter 1998). Rather, neural structures and mechanisms form the basis for active behavioral responses that lead to affiliation, selective social attachment, empathy, and other prosocial behaviors. These behaviors include the willingness to approach and trust others, and to use other people to manage emotions, such as fear or trauma in the presence of maltreatment or stressful experiences (Feldman et al. 2014).

Embedded in the human brain is a circuitry that has been described as the "social nervous system" (Adolphs 2009). Mammals also have an evolved "social engagement system," with the biological and behavioral capacity for both positive social behaviors and physical and behavioral reactions to threat (Porges 2011). The social engagement system includes nerves that calm our hearts and regulate facial expression, ingestion, vocalizations, and listening. This system, which is essential for social expression and communication, has the capacity to inhibit autonomic states that promote fight or flight behaviors. The social engagement system is an integrated system with common brainstem areas regulating visceral state (through vagal pathways) and the striated muscles of the face and head (through special visceral efferent pathways embedded in several cranial nerves). Innervation of this system relies on at least some of the same hormonal processes that are also implicated in the central and autonomic regulation of social behavior. Accessibility of this system is dependent on cues in the environment that trigger (a) a sense of safety to promote social connectedness, (b) a sense of danger to promote fight/flight behaviors, or (c) life threat responses associated with fainting, defecating, and dissociation.

The Autonomic Nervous System and Physiological Adaptations Linking Sociality and Health

The same neural systems that regulate emotional behaviors and social communication also regulate the physical body. Understanding basic physiological processes allows us to reconceptualize social behavior and the social nervous system as core features of the body's integrated system of health and restoration. Of special importance to both survival and social and emotional behaviors is the autonomic nervous system (Porges 2011). Older brainstem and autonomic systems, including the vagus, are necessary for vegetative and growth processes. These autonomic systems supply oxygen and energy to the brain via cardiovascular, respiratory, and metabolic pathways, and also regulate the immune and reproductive systems.

The mammalian nervous system is constructed upon a hierarchical template with evolutionarily older systems having impact on more recently evolved systems. The demands of ancient vegetative systems, including those that support life and reproduction, may override those of the more cognitive or rational neocortex. These phylogenetically ancient systems also serve the survival and reproduction of the species and help account for behavioral states and traits.

In a safe environment, the healthy human nervous system generally exhibits positive social behavior. In an unsafe or threatening environment, defensive or aggressive behaviors are more likely to appear. Mammalian sociality is based on evolved anatomical and neurochemical substrates that serve social communication and cognition. These systems are regulated by both the central and autonomic nervous system, integrating voluntary and involuntary expressions of social cues and emotions (Porges 2011). Humans are especially responsive to facial cues and acoustic signals. Because these can express social safety or threat, they may be particularly powerful channels of communication.

Mammalian Reproduction and Motherhood Shape the Nervous System

Placental mammals provide nurturance for their offspring throughout gestation and during lactation. In some species, prolonged maternal care exists, including defense of the offspring during the postpartum period. The unique physiological adaptations of placental mammals are associated with high levels of social behavior and may support the development of a comparatively larger neocortex. The placenta is regulated by the paternal and maternal genome, allowing the parents to further influence the growth and size of their offspring (Keverne, this volume).

The intense maternal investment that is provided by mammals, especially by human mothers, has the consequence of supporting the development of the young during periods of vulnerability. In humans, lactational hormones can be contraceptive, allowing birth spacing and thus increasing the access of offspring to their biological mother and her resources. Even among primates, humans have an exceptionally long period of maturation. Developmental processes, including growth of the neocortex, can continue past reproductive maturity (Carter 2014). Under optimal conditions this allows a protected period during which the neocortex can develop. During this period, various forms of learning, including social cognition and the formation of social networks, may be facilitated (Hrdy 2009). Social synchrony between caretakers and children can also be emotional learning experiences for the offspring, enhancing both prosocial behavior and the capacity for emotion regulation in later life (Feldman 2012). Furthermore, family or group living facilitates successful reproduction and fitness.

Maternal Behavior as a Prototype for Social Behavior

It can be argued that maternal behavior is a biological and behavioral prototype for other forms of sociality (Carter 1998). At the endocrine center of social behavior are oxytocin and vasopressin. The same hormones that facilitate birth and lactation also promote maternal behavior and maternal defense of the young. Small mammals, such as mice, are capable of birth and maternal behavior even in the absence of oxytocin. However, milk ejection and nursing are not possible in mice mutant for the gene for oxytocin or its receptor, suggesting that lactation is a fairly recently evolved trait and is dependent on oxytocin.

Lactation is unique in mammals and may depend on physiological functions of oxytocin that arose during the evolution of mammals (Carter 1998). In addition, milk contains a variety of hormones, including oxytocin and probably vasopressin, which may be involved in tuning the nervous system of the offspring to adapt to environmental changes. In milk, for example, high levels of oxytocin might be associated with periods of resource abundance, whereas high levels of vasopressin might reflect periods of stress or limitations of resources such as water or food. Lactation—especially frequent and nocturnal nursing—has the capacity to regulate maternal physiology and suppress the return to ovarian cyclicity after birth. Because lactational suppression of ovulation can be contraceptive, it contributes to spacing births, with indirect consequences for resource allocation. Mothers who are gestating or rearing fewer babies can contribute more to the physical, emotional, and cognitive development of a given offspring.

Hormones in human milk may serve as a form of social and endocrine communication between mother and baby. The lactating mother also has reduced reactivity to stressors (Carter 1998). These adaptations increase the behavioral flexibility of the parent in the face of the demands of child rearing and can modify the behavior and physiology of the infant, with consequences that vary according to environmental demands and with the history of the mother.

The neurobiological substrates for a long gestation, forceful birth, and postnatal nutrition in the form of lactation allowed the emergence in mammals of an increased brain size. The mammalian birth process accommodates the enlarged primate nervous system, whereas increased parental investment is necessary to nourish and protect the immature offspring and to support the elaboration of the primate nervous system (Keverne, this volume). Delivering a large baby, which involves prenatal maternal investment, cervical stimulation, and the release of oxytocin as well as stress and pain in birth, may increase the attachment between the mother and child. Furthermore, it is likely that these same processes were critical in permitting the evolution of modern human social cognition and language (Carter 2014).

Oxytocin and Vasopressin Pathways

Properties of Oxytocin

Oxytocin is a nine amino acid peptide hormone composed of a six amino acid ring and a three amino acid tail. At least some of the functions of oxytocin and vasopressin may be explained by the dynamic biological properties of the sulfur bonds that create the ring in oxytocin. These bonds allow the oxytocin molecule to form temporary and long-lasting unions with other chemical entities, with dynamic functions that remain to be described (Martin and Carter 2013).

Receptors for oxytocin are localized in areas of the nervous system that regulate social and adaptive behaviors, including the HPA axis and the autonomic nervous system. Only one oxytocin receptor (OXTR) has been described, which is present in neural tissue and other parts of the body, including the uterus.

Variations in the gene for the oxytocin receptor (*OXTR*) have been associated with variation in social behaviors, including the atypical behaviors that characterize autism spectrum disorders (Jacob et al. 2007), but also in healthy individuals (van IJzendoorn and Bakermans-Kranenburg, this volume). In addition, hypermethylation of the OXTR, which may silence that gene, has been detected in autism spectrum disorders (Gregory et al. 2009). The capacity of the OXTR to be genetically and epigenetically regulated (possibly by early-life experiences) brings up important questions about the origins of individual differences in social behavior and in the sensitivity to social context and adversity. For example, certain single nucleotide polymorphisms (SNPs) in *OXTR* have been associated with heightened sensitivity to social cues or their absence (Riem et al. 2013b; Hostinar et al. 2014; Dadds et al. 2014; Feldman et al. 2014) and more empathetic emotional and physical responses to the pain of others (Smith et al. 2014).

Oxytocin is found in high concentrations in the paraventricular (PVN) and the supraoptic nuclei (SON) of the hypothalamus. Following synthesis in the PVN and SON, oxytocin is transported to the posterior pituitary, where it is released into the blood stream. Oxytocin is also released within the brain, reaching targets throughout the nervous system with direct behavioral consequences (Neumann and Landgraf 2012). Outside of reproduction, the exact nature of the stimuli that release oxytocin is poorly understood. However, it is known that oxytocin can be released in response to a variety of social experiences and under circumstances that are both positive and negative (Ebstein et al. 2012; Feldman 2012; Neumann and Landgraf 2012).

Oxytocin is normally produced tonically, and individual blood levels tend to be consistent across time (Dai et al. 2012; Feldman 2012). Oxytocin release can also be pulsatile; unique plasticity in oxytocin-synthesizing cells allows physical transformation in response to social and hormonal stimulation. Stimulation of the oxytocin system can "feed forward" to release more oxytocin. Oxytocin can be released in a coordinated fashion, within the brain and at the posterior pituitary, into the general circulation (Neumann and Landgraf 2012). It is likely that the ability of oxytocin to have broad and synchronized behavioral and physiological consequences, increasing connectivity among brain areas, is related to this capacity for movement throughout the brain and body.

Oxytocin is exceptionally abundant in blood and brain. The messenger RNA for oxytocin has been reported in rats to be the most abundant transcript in the hypothalamus (Gautvik et al. 1996), presumably translating into very high concentrations of the oxytocin peptide in the brain and blood. Measurement of oxytocin by mass spectrometry indicates that this peptide is sequestered on plasma proteins, possibly available for local release as needed (Martin and Carter 2013). Levels of oxytocin in blood and brain vary across species, and individual differences in oxytocin are common. These have been related to individual traits, including social behavior and some of the novel patterns of behaviors associated with autism spectrum disorders, schizophrenia, or unique behavioral phenotypes, such as the hypersociality seen in Williams Syndrome (Dai et al. 2012).

Functions of Oxytocin

Oxytocin plays a major role in positive social behaviors and sensitivity to social cues. In general, oxytocin has been associated with social interactions that involve positive sociality and contact, such as female sexual (Carter 1998; Porges 2011) and maternal behaviors (Feldman 2012). Oxytocin receptors are abundant in pathways that serve ancient visceral components of mammalian reproduction. However, oxytocin may directly or indirectly influence more modern neural systems necessary for social engagement, allowing the high levels of social sensitivity and attunement necessary for human sociality and for rearing a human child. The behavioral patterns associated with oxytocin specifically include "immobility without fear," which is critical to several forms of positive social and reproductive behaviors in mammals (Porges 1998). Concurrently, oxytocin may reduce anxiety, reactivity to social stressors, and aggression. Under optimal conditions, oxytocin may reduce fear, serving as a biochemical metaphor for safety (Carter 2014).

Ties That Bind

Selective social behaviors and social bonds or attachments are components of emotionally loving relationships and healthy families in human societies. Social bonds often develop between family members or sexual partners. Whether human social bonds can be formed in the absence of oxytocin is not known. However, animal research, originally conducted in sheep (Keverne, this volume) and in the socially monogamous prairie vole (Carter 1998), suggests that oxytocin is necessary but perhaps not sufficient for social bond formation.

Oxytocin can, in general, encourage emotional states which allow the use of others as emotional support during periods of stress and restoration (Hostinar et al. 2013, 2014; Feldman et al. 2014). Oxytocin may help to protect both mother and infant from the memory of pain associated with childbirth, thus further promoting attachment. Maternal oxytocin may protect her from postpartum depression (Stuebe et al. 2013), which has serious negative consequences for child development and family relationships.

Oxytocin Facilitates Growth and Healing

Oxytocin has therapeutic consequences that are only now being discovered, including protective and healing effects on injured tissue. Among the restorative processes that oxytocin can affect are neurogenesis, cellular growth, differentiation, death or motility, and inflammation. The most complete work in this area has been done in the heart (Gutkowska and Jankowski 2012). In rodents, apoptosis (programmed cell death) in heart tissue can be inhibited by oxytocin, especially by the precursor or "fetal" form of oxytocin. Oxytocin holds the potential to literally heal a broken heart.

The effects of oxytocin may help to explain the well-documented association between social support and prevention or recovery from many disorders of brain and body, including trauma (Carter 1998; Olff et al. 2013). Among the mechanisms for both social support and the beneficial effects of oxytocin are actions of this peptide on the autonomic nervous system, which in turn has consequences for sensory, visceral, metabolic, and smooth motor systems. In addition, through actions on the autonomic nervous system, oxytocin may play a role in the maintenance of the blood supply to the cortex, thus allowing consciousness (Porges 2011).

Oxytocin is synthesized in the hypothalamus in an area known as the PVN. Because the PVN is a major site of convergence and integration for the HPA axis and autonomic function, oxytocin is positioned for a role in stress and emotion. Oxytocin is also co-localized with corticotropin-releasing factor (CRF), which regulates the HPA axis. CRF has been implicated in some of the detrimental effects of chronic stress. Thus, the co-release of oxytocin and CRF may be adaptive, allowing both mobilization in the presence of a challenge, followed by coping responses, including possibly increases in social motivation.

Across the life span, oxytocin probably increases social sensitivity and modulates reactivity to stressors. Oxytocin dynamically moderates the autonomic and immune systems, with antioxidant and anti-inflammatory effects. These actions of oxytocin may help to explain the adaptive consequences of social behavior for emotional and physical health. Both directly and indirectly, oxytocin might facilitate the use of both prosocial and rational, versus emotional or aggressive, strategies in the face of challenge.

Properties of Vasopressin

Vasopressin is also a nine amino acid peptide with a six amino acid ring and a three amino acid tail. Vasopressin is structurally similar to oxytocin, with only two amino acids distinguishing the two molecules. Both arose from a common ancestral molecule. Like oxytocin, vasopressin is synthesized in the PVN and SON, although oxytocin and vasopressin are usually not present in the same cells. Vasopressin is found in several other brain regions, including the medial amygdala, bed nucleus of the stria terminalis, and lateral septum. In this axis, the effects of vasopressin are androgen dependent and thus usually male biased (Carter 2007). In addition, vasopressin is found in the suprachiasmatic nucleus.

Three receptor subtypes have been identified for vasopressin. Of these, the V1a receptor, which is found in the brain, has been associated with social behavior, engagement, and pair bond formation, especially in males. Both individual and species differences in V1a receptor distributions have been identified. Among the sources of these differences are species-typical variations in the promoter region of the gene for the V1a receptor (Hammock and Young 2005).

Functions of Vasopressin

Vasopressin is associated with active forms of coping and defense at several levels. The primitive functions of vasopressin were probably water retention and other forms of adaptive defense of cells from environmental challenges, such as dehydration. In mammals this behavioral motif may have eventually been co-opted at the level of the organism to include defensive behaviors and some forms of aggression (Ferris 2008; Neumann and Landgraf 2012). As the functions of vasopressin evolved in more complex organisms they included defense of self, mate, offspring, and resources. Vasopressin may be especially critical for forms of sociality that require mobilization and defensive arousal (Carter 1998). Vasopressin in the suprachiasmatic nucleus plays a central role in biological rhythms, helping to coordinate activity with rest and restoration.

Vasopressin (and oxytocin) may permit social approach in the presence of a novel conspecific, possibly by increasing social "bravery." Vasopressin is also important to autonomically mobilized forms of male parental behavior (Kenkel et al. 2012a, 2013). Oxytocin and vasopressin systems seem to function in concert to allow selective social behaviors and male parental behavior, which involve social approach, nurturance, and in some cases autonomic arousal, potentially in defense of a sexual partner or offspring or when new relationships are initially forming (Carter 1998; Porges 1998).

Vasopressin may synergize with CRF to activate the HPA axis, potentially permitting stress reactivity, anxiety, and territoriality. Increased central vasopressin and reductions in oxytocin have been associated with defensive aggression and, in human males, with emotional dysregulation (Lee et al. 2009). Vasopressin, CRF, and other central hormones might help to create emotional states that reduce the capacity to use cognitive or "top-down" strategies to manage stressful experiences. Overactivity in the vasopressin system would in theory lower the threshold to impulsive forms of aggression, although studies administering either oxytocin or vasopressin suggest that males and females respond differently to these peptides. Vasopressin elevates blood pressure and cardiovascular activity and may be implicated in the arousal associated with posttraumatic stress disorder (PTSD).

Interactions between Oxytocin and Vasopressin

Vasopressin and oxytocin have the capacity to bind to each other's receptors, and under normal conditions they are probably dynamically interacting. Under conditions of stress, both peptides may be released together or in tight synchrony. These interactions may facilitate rapid changes in behavioral and emotional states (Neumann and Landgraf 2012). Under some conditions (and especially with regard to behavior, emotional arousal, mobilization, and autonomic functions), the behavioral effects of oxytocin and vasopressin can be opposing (Carter 1998). However, in other circumstances the effects of both peptides seem to be functionally similar (Kenkel et al. 2013). For example, exogenous oxytocin and vasopressin can both facilitate initial social approach and pair bonding in prairie voles. Whether the endogenous peptides have similar effects is less clear, especially since central vasopressin is androgen dependent and associated with defensive behaviors in males, but less so in females (Carter 2007).

In adult males, including humans (Feldman 2012) and prairie voles (Kenkel et al. 2012a), oxytocin and vasopressin may be released by infants and can facilitate parental behavior. The release of oxytocin in males by stimuli from the infant could facilitate coping in response to the complex needs of the infant.

However, when reproductively naive males are exposed to an infant, they transition to a physiological state characterized by activation of both the sympathetic and parasympathetic branches of the autonomic nervous system. This somewhat novel physiological state, which probably depends on interactions between oxytocin and vasopressin, allows the simultaneous appearance of nurturing and active protective forms of social behavior (Kenkel et al. 2013).

The Effects of Oxytocin Are Not Always Prosocial

The arousal-enhancing effects of oxytocin, and presumably the release of oxytocin, differ widely among individuals and are likely influenced by genetics, context, and social history. In the absence of a supportive rearing experience or the presence of a history of adversity, the effects of exogenous oxytocin may no longer appear prosocial or positive (Bartz et al. 2011). For example, neutral stimuli may be perceived as threatening. In the presence of a challenge, the release of endogenous oxytocin might initially support arousal, including activation of the sympathetic nervous system and other components of the HPA system. For example, there are indications that perceived loneliness or isolation in early life could alter the physiological consequences of exogenous oxytocin (Norman et al. 2011). Early maltreatment has also been associated with an increase in endogenous oxytocin (Seltzer et al. 2014). However, some individuals are much more sensitive than others to the consequences of maltreatment (Hostinar et al. 2014) or trauma (Feldman et al. 2014), and presumably to oxytocin as well (van IJzendoorn and Bakersman-Kranenburg, this volume).

Another example of the apparently paradoxical effects of high levels of oxytocin is seen in Williams Syndrome, a genetic condition characterized by hypersociality but also anxiety. In this syndome, high levels of oxytocin are associated with maladaptive social behaviors (Dai et al. 2012). Whether this atypical behavioral phenotype can be directly attributed to oxytocin, vasopressin, or interactions between these and other neurochemicals remains to be determined.

Without knowledge of the status or sensitivity of the oxytocin or vasopressin receptor, or other physiological variables, we can only speculate about the possible mechanisms or effects of high levels of endogenous or exogenous oxytocin. For example, oxytocin appears to facilitate fear conditioning in humans (Acheson et al. 2013), and local effects of oxytocin in the septum of mice facilitate fear conditioning (Guzman et al. 2013). Large amounts of oxytocin may activate vasopressin receptors, further supporting mobilization and potentially defensive responses. This might help to explain the tendency toward parochial behavior and "out-group" rejection described in some studies after intranasal oxytocin (De Dreu 2012).

As with early-life experiences in general (Ellis et al. 2011), the response to peptides, of either exogenous or endogenous origins, are likely to be context dependent and individualistic (Bartz et al. 2011; Feldman et al. 2014). Context, in turn, may influence other physiological process, such as those regulated by sex steroids, opioids, catecholamines, and inflammatory cytokines. Patterns of autonomic response would also be expected to differ among individuals and by context (Porges 2011). Emotional context is influenced by autonomic sensations (Norman et al. 2011), and autonomic systems are targets for the actions of oxytocin (Carter et al. 2009; Carter and Porges 2013; Kenkel et al. 2013).

Developmental Consequences of Oxytocin and Vasopressin

Of particular importance to child development are the effects of oxytocin and vasopressin during early development. Oxytocin present during the perinatal period can tune the central nervous system, potentially supporting adaptive patterns of physiology and behavior in later life. Oxytocin helps to protect the brain and heart from hypoxia, especially during birth. Circulating oxytocin acts as a signaling mechanism between the mother and fetus and may help to protect and mature cortical cells during development (Khazipov et al. 2008; Tyzio et al. 2006, 2014; Kenkel et al., submitted). Through lactation and prolonged periods of postnatal nurture, oxytocin shapes the physical development of the brain, with a role in the genetic regulation of the growth of the neocortex, which is permissive for human cognition (Carter 2014).

In a series of experiments in prairie voles, we examined the effects of manipulations of oxytocin during the first days of life (Carter et al. 2009). In general, exposures to low doses of oxytocin were associated with later increases in social behavior, whereas higher doses of oxytocin or treatments that blocked oxytocin were likely to interfere with normal patterns of social behavior, including the capacity for pair bonding. Alterations in social behavior were seen when mothers and infants were exposed to differential amounts of handling. Either repeated manipulations or reductions in stimulation could interfere with the later appearance of typical social behavior. In general, male voles appeared to be more sensitive than females to the long-term consequences of early experiences, possibly through alterations in the vasopressin systems. Alternatively, females may be resistant to some of the detrimental effects of early experiences, possibly due to protective epigenetic consequences of oxytocin (Carter et al. 2009).

When exposed to exogenous vasopressin during the first week of life, prairie voles of both sexes showed increased aggression in adulthood. This effect was stronger in males than females (Stribley and Carter 1999).

Synthetic forms of vasopressin, which reduce urine production, are sometimes used to treat bed-wetting in children, with unexamined behavioral effects. Mechanisms for the developmental effects of peptides need further exploration, especially in light of the widespread clinical applications of synthetic oxytocin to induce or augment labor (Kenkel et al., submitted).

Sex Differences and Psychiatric Implications
of Oxytocin and Vasopressin

Sex differences in the vasopressin system may have particular consequences for behaviors that are sexually dimophic, including male-biased disorders such as autism spectrum disorders (Carter 2007). Early onset schizophrenia is also more likely in males. In women diagnosed with schizophrenia (and receiving medication), there was an association between higher levels of oxytocin and fewer psychotic symptoms. In a separate study in unmedicated women experiencing a psychotic episode, vasopressin levels were elevated (Rubin et al. 2013). The effects of medications and gender on both oxytocin and vasopressin deserve further study.

Posttraumatic Stress Disorder

Of special relevance to understanding the consequences of early-life trauma, adversity, and war-related experiences across the life cycle is the clinical syndrome known as PTSD. Understanding the behavioral and emotional consequences of trauma requires awareness of the evolution of the mammalian nervous system (Porges 2011). Withdrawal of the myelinated vagus may leave an individual vulnerable to sympathetic overarousal and mobilization. The responses that taken together comprise PTSD may reflect activity in older parts of the nervous system, including unmyelinated vagal pathways, which involves a passive "shutdown" strategy and immobilization. While adaptive in some contexts, the reactions which follow are traumatic or highly stressful and can be disruptive to social engagement and other prosocial behaviors, when manifest as either overactivation or "immobilization with fear" (Porges 1998). Thus, individuals who experience PTSD may exhibit limitations in their abilities to regulate subsequently their emotional state in response to environmental challenges.

PTSD can occur in both sexes. However, the phenotype of PTSD may be sexually dimorphic. Males may show a more aroused or mobilized form of response to trauma, whereas women can be differentially vulnerable to immobilizing or "shutting down" in response to trauma. Preliminary studies suggest that blood levels of endogenous oxytocin may be altered in PTSD, with profound individual differences that may manifest as individual differences in the peptide or receptor (Seng et al. 2013; Olff et al. 2013). The mechanisms for individual vulnerability in disorders such as PTSD often include an early history of adversity and might be associated with differential sensitivity in the oxytocin receptor (Feldman et al. 2014). It is also possible that the absence of adequate maternal stimulation in early life can produce overactivity in the synthesis of vasopressin (Zhang et al. 2012) or altered sensitivity in the vasopressin receptor.

Although in early stages, research on the functions of oxytocin and vaso-pressin in emotional responses and coping holds promise for understanding individual and sex differences in a more general sense. It is unlikely that males and females use oxytocin pathways in identical ways (Carter 2007), and one of these mechanisms for individual variations may be based on sex differences in the epigenetic consequences of early experiences.

Methodological Limitations

Interactions between oxytocin and vasopressin are an essential component of the capacity of these peptides to support dynamic behavioral change (Carter 1998; Neumann and Landgraf 2012). However, at present, studies attempt-ing to address real-time interactions between biochemical changes and social behavior have to be taken in the context of methodological limitations. For example, among the most directly translational approaches to studying human behavior are psychophysiological methods, such as continuous recordings of autonomic functions that appear to be comparable across species (Porges 2011; Carter et al. 2009). However, interpreting physiology in terms of complex be-havioral experiences and emotions offers additional challenges.

Variable adaptive strategies allow some individuals to flourish most fully in good times, whereas others may survive and even prosper under adversity (Ellis et al. 2011). It is possible that the physiological basis of these response patterns will be shown to be based, at least in part, on sensitivity or respon-sivity to oxytocin- and vasopressin-based systems. Research testing this hy-pothesis in humans is now emerging. At present these are based primarily on individual variations in genes that regulate responses to oxytocin (Hostinar et al. 2014; Feldman et al. 2014). However, a more in depth understanding of the role of peptides in human behavior requires knowledge of not only receptor genetics, but also epigenetic modifications and the dynamics of the release and actions of the oxytocin and vasopressin peptides.

Animal research was the original source of most of our understanding of the peptide pathways described here. Historically, attempts to describe the role of peptides in behavior have been based on pharmacological manipulations using drugs that stimulate or block specific receptors' genetic manipulations. For example, in knockout mice, a gene for a hormone or receptor is permanently or temporarily inactivated. In a few cases endocrine measurements are made by dialysis of tissue-specific hormonal changes. However, because a comparative-ly large sample volume is needed to assay these hormones, the sampling rate is rarely frequent enough to match the pace of behavioral changes (Neumann and Landgraf 2012). In some cases elegant, tissue-based methods (usually done in rats) have been used to describe tissue-specific endocrine changes (Stoop 2012). Although all of these methods have limitations, taken together they sup-port the assumption that the functions of oxytocin and vasopressin are both intertwined and in general rapidly changing, possibly approximating the time course of behavioral events, such as approach or avoidance.

The therapeutic importance of oxytocin is supported by reports of treatments for mental disorders including autism spectrum disorders, schizophrenia, PTSD, and addiction. Those findings are not described here but are detailed in other reviews (e.g., Ebstein et al. 2012; MacDonald and Feifel 2013; Acheson et al. 2013; Buisman-Pijlman et al. 2013).

Of course, pharmacological approaches have many limitations and are not ideal for producing social change. Thus, the important goal for future research is to understand the naturally occurring mechanisms that regulate biological mechanisms and to use this knowledge to create a science of peace and safety.

Questions and Challenges for Future Research

As we seek the biological foundations of peace or war, we face a variety of challenges. Understanding the contrasting physiology and health consequences between experiences of social safety and aggression is a major task for the behavioral and neural sciences in the twenty-first century. Many questions are still mired in our incomplete understanding of the fundamentals of mammalian biology. Others are based on methodological and theoretical limitations. Of particular importance to the concept of "peace" is the capacity to extract physiological patterns and predictors relevant to human social and emotional experiences, especially within groups. A few examples of these are described here.

Methodological Challenges

Many practical and ethical considerations restrict the methodologies that are available for the analysis of behavioral physiology. The most common unit of analysis for behavioral research is the individual. However, social behavior inherently involves one or more individuals—or a mental representation of another. Social behavior is dynamic and ideally reciprocal, thus creating daunting levels of complexity. Against this background, measurements of endocrine processes typically depend on samples taken at single or infrequent time points. The act of collecting endocrine samples can disrupt both physiology and behavior. Noninvasive and more frequent methods for collecting data will be critical to understanding the biological basis of social behaviors. The time courses possible for collecting endocrine or other physiological measurements may not necessarily correspond to the time course of behavioral changes in question. Physiological events may precede behavior by time periods which are variable.

What is the developmental time course of endocrine processes, including peptides and their receptors relevant to a sense of peace? How do the developmental changes in peptides interact with the changing and usually expanding access to others? Are endocrine processes relatively stable across time, equating to "traits," or perhaps more variable in the face of environmental demands, possibly more equivalent to "states"?

Measurement of Peptides Has Proven Challenging

Questions have been raised regarding the reliability and validity of current assays for peptide hormones, including oxytocin and vasopressin. The most common assays rely on polyclonal antibodies and preparation of samples which can be variable across methods. Within the limitations of these methods, competently conducted radioimmunoassays or enzyme immunoassays typically provide replicable data within and across subjects, and in some cases across studies. Dozens of studies using these methods support the hypothesis that measurements of peptides in bodily fluid can be related to behavioral outcomes (Ebstein et al. 2012; Weisman and Feldman 2013; Weisman et al. 2013).

For example, we have recently compared plasma levels of oxytocin and vasopressin as measured by enzyme immunoassays in individuals suffering from psychosis and their first-degree relatives. This study revealed that sources of variance ("heritability" or "familiality") related to family membership strongly predicted individual differences in plasma peptides (Rubin et al. 2014). Antibody-based assays provide an index of hormone levels, but do not precisely describe the molecular concentrations of a given peptide. In addition, the degree to which peptides are biologically available may vary considerably, especially if samples are first "extracted" using other chemical or physical procedures. New evidence from a more exact quantitative method, mass spectrometry, indicates that the levels of oxytocin and vasopressin in blood are much higher than previously assumed, probably because peptides are sequestered on common proteins such as albumin (Martin and Carter 2013), and thus removed and discarded by extraction. Other binding proteins, including the neurophysins, which are synthesized in conjunction with oxytocin and vasopressin, may also have a role in determining the functional effects of these peptides. Even within blood samples studied *ex vivo,* the functional dynamics of peptides remain incompletely described (Martin and Carter 2013).

Functional Sources and Targets for Hormones Are Difficult to Specify

Many fundamental questions have not been successfully addressed. For example, what are the sources of functional and behaviorally active peptides? Outside the brain, oxytocin-synthesizing cells have been identified in a variety of tissues, including the heart, skeletal muscle, enteric nervous system, pancreas, the adrenal medulla, thymus, gonads, and placenta. Are the oxytocin and vasopressin levels measured in bodily fluids, including plasma and saliva, derived primarily from the hypothalamus via the posterior pituitary, or do these somatic sources also contribute significantly, with consequences for behavior? If peripheral sources of peptides do contribute to behavior, what regulatory mechanisms guide this process, and do they differ depending on gender, age, or social context? What role do sensory afferents and the autonomic nervous system play as we seek to understand the brain-body interface and the functions of these neuropeptides in the development of affiliative or defensive behaviors?

Individual and Sex Differences and Context

Every individual has a different set of genes and a different life history. Even in identical twins, experience and epigenetic variation can alter gene expression, and eventually physiology and behavior. Genetics and epigenetics contribute to these. In the context of the physiology of both positive social behaviors and aggression there is increasing evidence for sex differences. Theorizing about sex differences has been focused historically on the actions of sex steroids. However, sex differences exist in oxytocin and vasopressin pathways, the origins of which are not fully understood. Male-female differences are particularly apparent in response to early-life experiences as well as in the face of severe challenge or trauma in later life (Carter 2007; Carter et al. 2009). The consequences of a given peptide hormone also may be context dependent (Bartz et al. 2011; van IJzendoorn and Bakersman-Kranenberg, this volume). In turn, context and experience interact with genetics and gender. Comparisons of males and females, in the context of individual differences in life history, will be necessary to permit a sophisticated analysis of the biological and developmental foundations of both peace and war.

The Value of Animal Models

Physiological responses in modern humans are the consequence of evolution acting upon biological and neural substrates, some of which are shared across species. Thus, cross-species comparisons can inform our understanding of physiological mechanisms underlying positive or negative experiences. However, social and physiological systems differ among species. Some animal models may be more relevant than others because they share with humans evolved social systems or behavioral traits, such as the capacity to form lasting social relationships and dependence on others (Carter et al. 1995; Carter 2014). As one example, socially monogamous prairie voles share with humans a reliance on social interactions, as well as the capacity to form life-long social bonds; they exhibit biparental and alloparental care of the young, produce high levels of oxytocin, and maintain high levels of parasympathetic activity (Carter et al. 2009). Studies which focus on the capacity for social relationships and on neural systems, such as the autonomic nervous system (Porges 2011) and oxytocin and vasopressin, that are shared among mammals are offering powerful insights into the neurobiology of social behavior (Hostinar et al. 2013).

Neurotransmitter-Peptide Interactions

Among other critical elements in the emerging biochemistry of socioemotional states are peptide interactions with systems involving dopamine, serotonin (van IJzendoorn and Bakersman-Kranenburg, this volume), and inhibitory neurotransmitters such as GABA. As one recent example from animal models, GABA plays a critical role in behavioral regulation, and the development of the GABA system has been shown to be sexually dimorphic. The maturation of the GABA system is influenced by the presence or absence of oxytocin at the time of birth, with consequences for social and emotional behaviors in later life (Tyzio et al. 2006, 2014). In addition, GABA is involved in the communication among brainstem nuclei involved in autonomic regulation, especially through vagal pathways (Wang et al. 2002). Although beyond the scope of this review, studies of these interactions will be important to the future understanding of the capacity for peace.

Peptide Interactions Are Expected

Oxytocin and vasopressin systems have dynamic functional interactions with each other (Carter 1998; Neumann and Landgraf 2012). What is the nature of these interactions? Is it valid to study only one of these processes at a time? Does the relationship between oxytocin and vasopressin vary during sensitive periods of psychosocial development, in the face of environmental challenges, context, or between the sexes? The features of these interactions are poorly understood, especially in humans. It is possible that interactions between these two peptides can help to explain the capacity of oxytocin to have "paradoxical" behavioral consequences, including both positive and negative behavioral outcomes (Bethlehem et al. 2014; Weisman and Feldman 2013).

Sensitive Periods May Be Epigenetic and Interact with Sex

There is increasing evidence that experiences, especially in early life, can have lasting behavioral and epigenetic consequences (Champagne 2012; Zhang et al. 2013). Developmental periods, including gestation, infancy, and childhood, contain sensitive periods for tuning emotional and social behaviors. The very act of being born, which may take on many forms, is epigenetic. However, manipulations of endogenous and exogenous oxytocin are routine during birth, with largely unknown consequences for later physiology and behavior (Carter et al. 2009). The nature of the molecular processes associated with experience-associated changes in behavior is only now becoming apparent, and many questions remain.

Modeling Human Experiences

Recently, the Mother Child Education Foundation (Anne Çocuk Eğitim Vakfı, AÇEV), based in Turkey, suggested that family- and community-based programs designed to enhance early child development can alter patterns of decision making within the families and communities, so that there is greater "peace" and less conflict within families as well as within the larger community. The identification of physiological substrates, such as peptide pathways, associated with different patterns of social organization may generate data relevant to the physiological basis of these differences in sociality. However, the extrapolation from biological studies to constructs derived from human cognition is difficult. For example, do the behavioral states or experiences described as "social behavior" in animals correspond to broad human constructs such as "peace" or "love" (Carter and Porges 2013)?

There is increasing evidence that oxytocin acts on neural substrates necessary for a sense of safety (Porges 2011). In the search for the biological basis of peace, it may be helpful to focus on less anthropomorphic constructs, perhaps using terms such as emotional or physical "safety." Oxytocin may have a context-dependent capacity to serve as a kind of physiological metaphor for "safety" (Carter 2014).

Humans are capable of experiencing a sense of purpose, in some cases showing acts of bravery or self-sacrifice. In the context of individual survival, such behaviors appear "irrational." Perhaps the novel behavioral effects of peptide hormones may help to explain not only our capacity for reproduction and life, but also our capacity to face death with valor. Could the surges of oxytocin which allow women to survive the trauma of birth, also permit humans to die with a sense of peace and safety? Do changes or individual differences in peptide pathways help to explain the individual phenomenology and time course of responses to trauma (Olff et al. 2013; Seng et al. 2013; Feldman et al. 2014)?

The Promise of Formative Childhoods

Specific pathways, involving oxytocin and other biochemical systems, can influence the expression of behavioral states that would support social structures associated with peace. Peptide pathways are active across the life span. However, the developmental effects of peptides are of particular importance to individual and sex differences in temperament and to the capacity for peace. Early nurturing can alter human behavior through formative and epigenetic effects on peptide pathways. Uncovering the deeper biology of these pathways can offer a fresh perspective on the role of formative childhoods in human behavior. Although we are in the early days of the search for a science of peace, we propose here that the evidence is strong that the most efficient and enduring routes to peace are through formative childhoods.

Acknowledgments

Meetings supported by the Fetzer Institute (Kalamazoo, MI) on the role of formative childhoods in peacebuilding created a context from which this review emerged. Studies from the authors' laboratories were primarily sponsored by the National Institutes of Health. Many colleagues and students, whose ideas and data inform the perspective offered here, are gratefully acknowledged. We are especially grateful for feedback from Dr. Sarah Hrdy, and for the detailed review provided by James Leckman of an earlier version of this essay. Our attempts to respond to Dr. Leckman's probing questions molded this chapter, but also leave little doubt that we have at present far more questions than answers.

5

Epigenetics

Significance of the Gene-Environment Interface for Brain Development

Eric B. Keverne

Abstract

Brain development in humans extends over a very lengthy time period, initially *in utero* and subsequently embracing attachment interactions with the mother, social interactions with peers, and the emotional turmoil of puberty. Puberty is a period of development when those cortical regions concerned with forward planning and emotional control undergo synaptic pruning and reorganization of connection strengths. Each of these life phases is developmentally important in shaping and being shaped by the maternal and social environments. Although genetics forms the scaffold for brain development, the detail of connectivities is determined by the kind of environment in which the brain functions. The brain, more than any other organ, is a product of gene-environment interaction.

The *in utero* environment is the most protected of environments and has evolved strong maternal-fetal coadaptations. The fetal placenta hormonally interfaces with and regulates the mother's brain (hypothalamus) at a time when these same parts of the fetal brain (hypothalamus) are themselves developing. This transgenerational coordinated development is under the control of epigenetically regulated imprinted genes. Since the maternal hypothalamus controls all aspects of care and provisioning, offspring in receipt of such quality care will themselves be both genetically and epigenetically predisposed to good mothering of the next generation. However, impairments at the placental level caused by stress, toxins, or poor nutrition may impact adversely on the developing hypothalamus, and hence mothering of the next generation. A peaceful, secure environment is thus of paramount importance to a mother for securing a successful pregnancy and for the security of well-being in raising her offspring. Further, we need to take into account how events experienced *in utero* also shape the outcome of future generations, since epigenetic reprogramming of future oocytes (matrilineal contribution to grandchild) occurs at the earliest (epiblast) stages of *in utero* ovarian development.

The postnatal formative years of the brain are strongly influenced by mother-infant interactions. The brain's mechanisms for reward that subserve mother-infant-mother affiliation subsequently extend to the reward process of social interaction later in life. Throughout the first two decades of development, functional contacts are made across the brain's billions of neurons, involving trillions of synapses such that no two brains are the same, not even those of genetically identical twins. Since consolidation of neural connectivities is activity dependent, the environments that generate this activity determine the functional details of these structural connections. Our brains are very much a product of the pre- and postnatal niche in which they develop and survive.

Introduction

The impact of our environment may have effects across generations, effects that are difficult to explain through Mendelian inheritance. Recent work has focused on epigenetics as a possible mechanism for gene-environment interactions (Szyf 2013b). Epigenetics is underpinned by the noncoding regions of DNA that regulate the timing and tissue-specific regulation of gene expression. In this way, a single cell (fertilized egg) can develop into many different cell types which possess identical genomes. Epigenetics provides the code for gene expression, which not only differs in different cell types but also across different individuals and, in the brain, it even provides for differences between monozygotic twins (Haque et al. 2009). It is becoming clear that epigenetics can, in some contexts, confer stable heritable genomic modifications (genomic imprinting); in other contexts, epigenetic modifications are dynamic, adaptable changes that are transgenerationally erased (Morgan et al. 2005).

The essence of all biological systems is that they are encoded as molecular descriptions on their genes. Some ten years ago, the human genome was sequenced and approximately 20,000 genes were identified that encoded for the protein-building blocks of every cell. This represented a mere 1.5% of total DNA and the rest was labeled as "junk DNA," nucleotides that were remnants of our past evolutionary history. We now know that embedded in these noncoding sequences is the DNA that determines where, when, and how this protein-coding DNA is itself regulated. Such gene regulation is determined by the spatiotemporal, highly specific transcriptome; that is, transcription factors which bind to DNA (protein-coding regions) in a combinatorial fashion to specify the on and off state of genes. These transcription factors bind in distinct combinations and may even bind differentially to the two parental alleles.

Not all genes are active at any one moment in time, and although transcription factors are necessary to bring about this activation, genes may also be actively silenced and not available for transcription as a consequence of DNA methylation. This primarily occurs at promoters rich in cytosine-guanine di-nucleotides (CpGs). The human genome contains approximately 29 million CpGs, the methylation of which influences transcription factor/DNA interactions, gene expression, chromatin structure, and stability (Deaton and Bird 2011). Thus DNA methylation contributes to the epigenetic regulation of many important developmental processes. Methylation and silencing of DNA can be brought about by methyltransferase proteins (DNMT3B). DNA is itself associated with the nucleosome, a bead-like structure of enriched histone proteins that are involved with the tight chromatin packaging of DNA that is transcriptionally inactive, whereas diffuse chromatin is associated with DNA that is actively transcribed. The different histones are themselves subject to methylation (silent chromatin) and acetylation (active chromatin) thereby effecting transcriptional regulation. The signature chromatin histone mark H3K4Me3 interferes with DNA methylation. Indeed, three histone modifications are associated with repressed genes (H3K27Me3, H3K9Me3, H4K20Me3) whereas two histone modifications are associated with active transcription (H3K4Me3, H3K36Me3).

Histone modifications underpin a code of their own: the histone code of gene transcription. However, transcription is not this simple; during development some gene promotors may have both activating and repressive marks available simultaneously. How these different tiers of gene regulation are deployed represents the field of epigenetics, which is crucial to understanding development and how this may be influenced by the environment. These multiple levels for gene expression point to far-reaching influences on development and disorders beyond the well-established mutations and small nucleotide polymorphisms that are recognized as part of heritable dysfunctions. The multitude of epigenetic regulatory modifications to the genome, which occur in the lifetime of individuals, is mainly advantageous to that individual. However, some environments, particularly those created by humankind, are not advantageous and can create relatively long-term pathological changes to DNA function (e.g., warfare, child abuse, social neglect) (Szyf 2011). Fortunately, many of these changes are not transgenerationally heritable due to germline reprogramming of the epigenetic marks to achieve the totipotency required for development of the following generation (Morgan et al. 2005). Specifically, in the haploid reproductive cells of males (sperm) and females (ova) the preexisting gene expression patterns have to be erased (DNA demethylation) and subsequently established differently. Many regulatory elements can evade zygotic demethylation, such as retrotransposed elements, which are potentially hazardous (Smallwood and Kelsey 2012). It has recently been demonstrated that some maternal regulatory elements may also escape systematic DNA demethylation in the maternal germline, providing a potential mechanistic basis for transgenerational epigenetic inheritance. This has been shown to be the case for one of the genes (SRRM2) involved with Parkinson disease (Hackett et al. 2013). Not only is there a bias for epigenetic inheritance through the matriline but from the very earliest stages of germ cell production, germ cell reprogramming, decidualization, transfer of mitochondrial DNA, DNA repair mechanisms and postfertilization placentation, such are the selection pressures introduced by viviparity that have endowed the matriline with a biased contribution to reproductive success and fetal survival. Thus, *in utero* development has not only provided a safe environment for fetal development, but also one in which the matriline plays a dominant role. Importantly, the coexistence of three generations of matrilineal genomes in a mother has provided a special evolutionary dynamic for enabling forward planning and adaptation at the epigenetic level (Keverne 2014). However, this transgenerational coadaptive process provides a potential for maladaptive methylation changes to take place created by traumatic environmental events, such as warfare.

Severely adverse environments may disrupt developmental planning, producing maladaptive consequences. Maternal malnutrition, food shortage, or smoking results in low birth weight babies, predisposing these infants to diabetes (type 2), obesity, and heart disease (Maccani and Knopik 2012). Longitudinal studies have found transgenerational correlations that go beyond the first generation, linking food supply during the early life of grandparents with cardiovascular disorders and diabetic deaths of grandchildren. The mechanisms responsible for this are not known, but the coexistence of three genomes in one individual (mother, child, and developing female germline for the third generation) may hold some of the clues. Epigenetic studies based on people born around the time of the Dutch famine (1944–1945) have shown that exposure to famine during World War II at any stage of gestation was associated with diabetes later in life. Exposure to famine in early gestation was associated with coronary heart disease, increased stress responsiveness, and obesity (Roseboom et al. 2006). It has also been shown that some six decades after the famine, the imprinted gene, Igf2, was less methylated than in control subjects, thus providing evidence for epigenetic influences of early-life environment conditions (Heijmans et al. 2008). However, lower levels of Igf2 methylation may actually suggest an adaptive response for those individuals exposed to famine (i.e., increasing Igf2 expression to increase subsequent growth). Measurements made some six decades after exposure to famine could introduce an aging variable impossible to control. Although the cause of methylation differences later in life are not clear, this remains an interesting epigenetic finding. How we raise our children undoubtedly impacts on behavioral outcomes but the environment to which we expose them in the mother's womb, and even in the grandmother's womb, can change their metabolic profile, brain development profile, and a propensity for psychiatric dysfunctions.

Genomic Imprinting

Genomic imprinting is a gene-dosage regulatory mechanism that provides for transgenerational epigenetic inheritance for a subset of genes that are monoallelically expressed according to parent of origin. In other words, these genes are haploid dominant with the same maternal or paternal allele being expressed in all tissues. The genes themselves (i.e., their coding sequence) are remarkably stable, under purifying selection, and with few evolutionary changes across mammalian species (O'Connell et al. 2010). They are epigenetically regulated by differentially methylated regions (DMRs). These DMRs (also called imprint control regions, ICRs) are heritable and reprogrammable; they undergo demethylation in the maternal germline and are re-methylated on the maternal allele postfertilization at the earliest stages of fetal development. The matriline is thus primarily responsible for controlling gene dosage, thereby avoiding errors which might otherwise jeopardize reproductive success and potentially the mother's own survival.

Many of the imprinted genes are themselves regulators of other genes producing complex expression networks, representing differences between maternal and paternal specific networks. Some 4,798 transcription factor targets are predominantly maternally or paternally regulated targets (Gerstein et al. 2012). As the degree of combinatorial regulation increases, so too does the number of target genes, and these genes appear to be under negative selection. In other words, they represent gene networks that have monoallelic expression with greater stability. Most of the imprinted genes are not unique to humans; as mammals evolved, the reorganization of nonimprinted genes around the methylated ICRs also resulted in their monoallelic expression. Thus many of the genes and indeed, the DMRs, that are imprinted in humans are not imprinted in the phylogenetically older mammals. The longer *in utero* development lasted and the more complex placentation became, so more genes were recruited to this tight imprinted regulatory mechanism of gene dosage. The downside to this epigenetic regulation is that failure of ICR methylation brings about complex pathological syndromes, involving many genes which are themselves structurally normal (e.g., Prader-Willi Syndrome, Angelman Syndrome, Silver-Russell Syndrome) (Berdasco and Esteller 2013). The well-established postnatal nurturing issues (see Fox et al. as well as van IJzendoorn and Bakermans-Kranenburg, this volume) have consequences for the next (second) generation primarily through development of the brain, but also through nutritional inadequacies that effect growth and metabolism. Low-dose ionizing radiation, which can influence DNA methylation, is particularly relevant to genomic reprogramming in the matriline, which occurs at earliest stages of epiblast oocyte development. The consequences of this exposure appear in the following (third) generation.

In Utero Influence on Transgenerational Brain Development

In utero placental development introduces a new dimension to understanding how the environment influences brain development of the next generation through regulatory influences on maternal behavior of the current generation. The primary motivated behaviors of sex and feeding, which are regulated by the maternal hypothalamus, become reorganized by the influence of hormones from the fetal placenta, together with the regulation of postpartum delivery of milk, warmth, and maternal behavior (Keverne 2007). Progesterone, in

particular, suppresses fertility and increases maternal food intake in anticipation of subsequent fetal demands in the later stages of pregnancy. The same
feto-placental hormone promotes synthesis of maternal hypothalamic oxytocin
in anticipation of its requirements for parturition, maternal behavior, and milk
ejection (Keverne 2006).

Placental progesterone is also a precursor for the production of the remarkably high concentration of allopregnenalone in the mother's brain as well as
in the fetal brain, and shows a rapid decline with placental loss at birth (Hirst
et al. 2008). Progesterone and allopregnenalone have neuroprotective properties against ischemia and lack of oxygen in the brain by acting at the GABA
receptor (Knight et al. 2012). These placental steroids are also alleviators of
maternal stress. Allopregnenalone restrains the responses of the hypothalamic-
pituitary-adrenal axis to stress activation of neural opioids which also prevents
any premature secretion of oxytocin (Brunton and Russell 2011). In contrast,
glucocorticoids, which are produced by chronic prenatal stress of the mother,
are associated with the programming of disease in the fetus (metabolic, cardiovascular, and psychiatric) (Harris and Seckl 2011). In short, the fetal genome
determines its own destiny via the placenta, hormonally regulating the maternal hypothalamus to serve the interests of the fetus which, at the same time, is
developing its own hypothalamus.

Two questions arise: How does the developing fetal genome "know" the
optimal way of regulating the adult maternal hypothalamus, and how does the
adult mature hypothalamus know how to respond to future demands of the next
generation? These transgenerational coadaptive events also require coadaptations across the maternal and fetal genomes, the success of which is epigenetically carried forward to the next generation through genomic imprinting. The
same imprinted genes which develop both the fetal hypothalamus and fetal
placenta do so at a time when the placenta is instructing the maternal hypothalamus for provisioning the fetus. In this way, the developing hypothalamus
and placenta serve as a template upon which positive selection pressures for
good mothering operate, driven by the effectiveness and success of placental
interactions with the adult maternal hypothalamus. Thus, offspring that receive
optimal nourishment and improved maternal care will themselves develop a
hypothalamus that is both genetically and epigenetically predisposed to good
mothering. Unfortunately, these adaptive transgenerational effects carry the
risk for transgenerational maladaptive consequences in the context of warfare.

Mechanistically, imprinted genes have played an important role in the
mother-infant coadaptive process. Many of these genes are coexpressed at critical times in the developing placenta and developing hypothalamus. Mutations
to these genes in the placenta produce remarkably similar functional deficits
when the same gene is selectively mutated in the developing hypothalamus.
Indeed, the convergent phenotypic outcomes strongly support the coadaptation of hypothalamus and placenta. Because the placenta and hypothalamus
are developmentally synchronized, the placenta is in a pivotal position for

providing resources for fetal hypothalamic development at the same time as commandeering the adult maternal hypothalamus to provide these resources. Challenging this developmental linkage of hypothalamus and placenta with 24-hour food deprivation in animal studies results in disruption to coexpression of imprinted genes, primarily by affecting placental gene expression (Broad and Keverne 2011). Conversely, placental-specific deficiency of the imprinted gene Igf2 changes the developmental adaptations to under-nutrition (Sferruzzi-Perri et al. 2011). One imprinted gene in particular (*Peg3*) decreases in the placenta with food deprivation as do many of the downstream genes regulated by *Peg3* expression. Such genomic dysregulation does not, however, occur at the late stages of pregnancy in the developing hypothalamus. On the contrary, *Peg3* expression increases with food deprivation late in pregnancy. These changes in gene expression are consistent with the fetal genome maintaining hypothalamic development at a cost to the placenta. This biased change to gene dysregulation in the placenta is linked to autophagy and ribosomal turnover which sustains, in the short term, nutrient supply for the hypothalamus (Broad and Keverne 2011). Thus the fetus controls its own destiny at this late stage in pregnancy by short-term sacrifice of the placenta to conserve brain development.

Yet another linkage between the placenta and hypothalamus is the finding that placental stem cells from human term placenta can be induced to differentiate into neurons (Portmann-Lanz et al. 2010). Other studies have shown the placenta itself to be a source of the neurotransmitter serotonin (Bonnin et al. 2011). Whether or not serotonin can affect fetal brain development is not known; however, serotonin has been shown to increase placental aromatase activity. Placental aromatase is a key enzyme controlling placental steroids, which have important actions on the hypothalamus during pregnancy.

Neocortical Development and Environmental Influences

The brain is a very specialized organ endowed with the unique ability to respond to the environment, reshaping its connections according to what it has experienced. How the brain develops is influenced not only by the relatively stable *in utero* environment but, more importantly, by its extended postnatal growth and development, lasting some twenty years in humans during a time of instability in an ever-changing social environment. Since the making and consolidation of neural connections is activity dependent, the kind of environment that creates this activity has an impact on the connections and their consolidation of strengths through epigenetic regulation of gene transcription. The vast majority of epigenetic marks are reprogrammed in the germline, thereby providing each new generation with a DNA "open reading frame." Transgenerational inheritance, especially in humans, is primarily achieved through the way in which the postnatal social environment shapes the epigenetic regulation of the developing brain of this next generation. This is particularly true of the neo-cortex, which develops into the largest component of the human brain. Much of this developmental time is spent under the protective environment of the family, the mother becoming a particularly important attachment figure who provides a secure base from which other relationships develop and social horizons broaden.

This dependence on adaptive epigenetic changes for normal brain development may also produce dysfunction if the environment is chronically stressful (Harris and Seckl 2011). Most of these experiences are transient and readily overcome. Others are more durable, especially those which are a consequence of warfare at the time of brain development, and which are subject to epigenetic modification (Mehta et al. 2013). Animal studies have shown a causal relationship between early-life adversity and changes in methylation to those genes expressed in the brain. Methylation silencing of gene expression in rhesus monkeys is influenced in the prefrontal cortex by surrogate mother rearing (Provençal et al. 2012). Other studies have shown distinct histone methylation signatures in the frontal cortex of schizophrenic brains and DNA methylation differences assessed from the blood in identical twins discordant for schizophrenia (Kordi-Tamandani et al. 2013). Interpreting these methylation findings from blood samples may not reflect what occurs in the brain; however, since human brain samples are problematic to obtain, they may provide an indicator for further consideration.

Supporting evidence from animal studies have shown that offspring born from stressed mothers (cf. controls) show increased levels of DNA methyltransferase preferentially expressed in GABAergic neurons of the frontal cortex, accompanied by decreases in reelin and gad67. In line with this finding, postmortem studies of psychotic patients have also found a down-regulation of GABAergic genes (GAD and Reelin) associated with DNA methyltransferase overexpression in GABAergic neurons. Human studies have further found direct causal effects of point mutations in the methyl transferase (MeCP2) gene in autism of subjects with Rett Syndrome (Miyake et al. 2013). Transfection experiments in mice show that MeCP2 can repress gene transcription by an interaction with the histone deacetylase complex. These findings suggest that MeCP2, which represses transcription, is targeted to specific neocortical genes via DNA methylation. Moreover, these transfected mutant animals have their symptoms reversed by transfection with the MeCP2 genes regulated by a neuron specific promoter.

In addition to epigenetic methylation of DNA and histones in gene expression regulation, mRNAs may also be methylated and silenced. mRNAs carry the code from the transcribed DNA in the nucleus to the cytoplasmic ribosomes for protein synthesis. Reversible mRNA methylation, analogous to DNA and histone modifications, affects gene expression and cell fate during development. The fat mass obesity association protein (FTO) is a m6A RNA demethylase that shows a strong association with obesity and is expressed in the brain. Genetic variations in this gene result in reduced regional brain volume in the elderly. Recent studies have examined polymorphisms in the FTO gene and causally determined phenotypes associated with Alzheimer disease (Reitz et al. 2012).

In addition to the cortex, FTO is expressed in adipose tissue, and insulin has been identified as a key factor in its expression. Carriers of the FTO risk allele have some 20 differentially methylated genome sites associated with obesity that influence adipocyte development as well as the hypothalamic production of the feeding appetite hormone, NPY (Tung et al. 2010). Tracing the network of genes and the pervasive nature of m6A demethylase, the tissue variants of this network, and how they are influenced by the environment, requires further work. M6A demethylase is known to be influenced by insulin, which is also affected by diet and stress, so there is clear potential for linking the environment into these various phenotypes.

Some of the better evidence for epigenetic modification to the adult brain is found in studies of addiction that is associated with histone modifications and DNA methylation (Nestler 2013). Chronic morphine decreases the expression of a specific histone methyl transferase (H3K9me2) in the nucleus accumbens, an important region of the brain that processes reward. These epigenetic changes have long-lasting effects that are difficult to reverse. Another adult disorder, posttraumatic stress disorder (PTSD), affects only a small percentage of individuals exposed to trauma and is a good example of dysfunction caused be gene-environment interaction (Domschke 2012). Thus polymorphisms in the risk allele of the stress response gene (FKBP5) does not in itself predict PTSD, but it does interact with childhood stress to predict an increased risk of adult PTSD due to demethylation of this gene in children exposed to trauma. FKBP5 suppresses glucocorticoid receptor activity promoting resistance to the glucocorticoid stress hormones. Thus an early-life stressful experience is associated with long-term effects on behavior through epigenetic reprogramming of the glucocorticoid receptor located in a part of the brain, the hippocampus, which is involved in learning and memory (Suderman et al. 2012). The methylation profiles surrounding the glucocorticoid receptor reveal hundreds of DNA methylation differences associated with early-life experiences. In particular, childhood maltreatment is associated with decreased expression of the hippocampal glucocorticoid receptor and increased predisposition to stress in adulthood (Zhang et al. 2013). There is also evidence for an association of childhood physical aggression with differential DNA methylation in cytokines that influence the immune system (Guillemin et al. 2014; Provençal et al. 2013)

Evidence is thus rapidly accumulating that demonstrates how adverse environments can bring about epigenetic changes in the brain and other tissues. The human brain is especially vulnerable due to its long postnatal development, involving widespread frontal and temporal neocortical reorganization at puberty (Sowell et al. 2001). Indeed, human puberty is itself changing in the modern era due to changes in diet and lack of physical exercise. Although we tend to think of adverse nutritional environments as those which provide lean resources, it is also the case that an excessive availability of rich high-caloric food can also be problematic in advancing the onset of puberty. At the start of the twentieth century, puberty occurred at 16–17 years of age, but it has become progressively earlier (12–13 years of age) in modern-day Western populations. Malnutrition is associated with delayed menarche: obese girls experience menarche earlier than lean girls. This is in part due to the increase of the hormone "leptin," which originates in fatty adipose tissue and signals the basal parts of the brain (hypothalamus) to undertake maturation of the reproductive system. Physiologically, if the human body has sufficient energy reserves to reproduce successfully, then puberty will occur early. However, the cortical regions of the brain have not matured, and these are important to establish and manage peer relationships, to regulate emotions through knowledge of self, and to develop high self-esteem. Foreshortening this long brain developmental period through readily available and inexpensive diets rich in fat and sugar may provide an environment just as maladaptive for brain development as malnutrition is for body and brain development. Puberty is a vulnerable period for the development of numerous behavioral problems, including eating disorders, onset of depression, obsessive-compulsive behavior, addictive behavior, depression, and schizophrenia. Epigenetic mechanisms undoubtedly contribute to these disorders and presumably depend on adverse environments, which are effective at critical periods in development.

Conclusions

It is now 25 years since David Barker put forward the hypothesis that the risk for diseases in human adults is related to the environmental conditions that were experienced during gestation and early childhood. Over the past decade, epigenetic mechanisms have become a focus for explaining this phenomenon. Epigenetic modifications, unlike genetic mutations, are potentially reversible; however, serious pharmacological barriers exist for specificity of target tissues and, indeed, specificity of targeting specific DNA loci to change methylation status. Research in the field of epigenetics is moving at a very fast pace and is the focus for new drugs which can influence chromatin methylation. Targeting specific chromatin regions is problematic, and although lithium and valproate (histone deacetylases) have been used in the past for treating schizophrenia, they target broad areas of chromatin. Future targeting of specific histones may prove possible for making DNA accessible to other drugs to bring about gene transcription. These may take decades to develop and will be expensive. However, education and the realization of the all-pervading influence of warfare on the well-being and health of generations to come is an area of knowledge that should serve as preventative medicine.

Knowledge of our biological heritage is essential to an understanding of the predispositions and constraints that have operated on the development of the brain and the influence this has had on behavior. *In utero* development, which provides a stable environment in terms of oxygen, nutrient supply, and constant temperature, also embraces the coexistence of two genomes, maternal and fetal, together with a third that undergoes reprogramming in the developing germlines of the fetus. These three sets of DNA in the same individual functionally interact in the pregnant female, providing the potential for coadaptation. The regions of the brain that regulate primary motivated behavior and autonomic responses are the major beneficiaries of this *in utero* coadaptation. Thus the fetal genome determines its own destiny via the placenta, hormonally regulating the maternal hypothalamus to serve the interests of the fetus which, at the same time, is developing its own hypothalamus.

Such transgenerational coordinated development enables forward planning by instructing increased maternal food intake in advance of fetal demands, thereby ensuring adequate reserves for growth in the last trimester of pregnancy. The success of this transgenerational coadaptation is epigenetically carried forward to the next generation through genomic imprinting. The same imprinted genes that are engaged in the development of both the fetal hypothalamus and fetal placenta are coactive at a time when the placenta is instructing the maternal hypothalamus for provisioning of the fetus. In this way, the developing hypothalamus and placenta serve as a template upon which selection pressures operate, driven by the effectiveness and success which these same genes have on placental interactions with the adult maternal hypothalamus. In this way, offspring that have received optimal nourishment and improved maternal care will themselves develop a hypothalamus that is both genetically and epigenetically predisposed to good mothering. Unfortunately, these adaptive transgenerational effects carry the risk for maladaptive consequences, such as in the context of warfare. Women, children, and grandchildren who do not participate in war are nevertheless susceptible to the consequences of modern warfare through trauma, stress, malnutrition, and lack of support (monetary and social). A peaceful environment is thus of paramount importance to the mother for a successful pregnancy, for the security of well-being in raising her children, and for the security of her daughter's future children that result from developmental genome reprogramming, which occurs during the early stages of *in utero* oocyte development. How we raise our children, even in the times of peace, is important for successful brain development, but the environment of warfare is uncontrollable and leaves its epigenetic mark for generations to come.

The very early phase of *in utero* life normally provides a stable environment that enables a more deterministic genetic control of development. This is a period when tight control over gene dosage is required and achieved by genomic imprinting and monoallelic gene expression. Most of the epigenetic marks that regulate imprinted monoallelic gene expression have become heritable and are reprogrammed in the germline, such is their importance. With imprinting, it is always the same allele that is expressed further, tightening up gene dosage by avoiding allelic polymorphisms. Pathologies can and do occur when this kind of gene regulatory control is impaired, producing low birth weight and preterm death and, in the case of brain development, the production of complex developmental disorders (Prader-Willi Syndrome, Angelman Syndrome, autism spectrum disorders, Silver-Russell Syndrome).

The neocortex is the largest part of the human brain and those regions (frontal and temporal cortex) which are uniquely enlarged in human species are the last to develop and refine their interconnections in the postpubertal period until 22 years of age. Thus, the early maternal environment progressively becomes one small part of an ever-expanding social world as age progresses. The complexity of the interconnections made by the neocortex (i.e., the millions of neurons and billions of synapses) make developmental errors inevitable. However, those neurons which fail to make the proper connections at the right time undergo programmed cell death. Of course, there is no hard-wired genetic program that ordains when and where cell death occurs; this is an epigenetic process. Moreover, all cortical neurons make contact with other neurons that undertake the same process. Since consolidation of neural connectivities is activity dependent, the environment that generates this activity is important. Thus no two brains are exactly the same, and although genetic programs play an integral part in brain development, the epigenetic regulation of gene expression also ensures that severe or chronic adverse conditions are "imprinted" into DNA transcription.

Since the kind of environment which is generating neural activity determines the trajectory for its functional development, infants reared in extremely deprived environments, such as that of the Romanian orphans, fail to develop language or locomotor control. With interventions and persistent attention, these children did develop locomotor control, although they were considerably delayed compared with the normal toddler age. Abnormal brain connectivities were also found in the children experiencing severe socioemotional deprivation (Eluvathingal et al. 2006). Neurophysiological assessment of these orphans verified cognitive impairments and impulsivity, with structural changes in the cortical connections (uncinate fasciculus) between temporal and frontal cortices. Other studies have found abnormalities in language and limbic connection pathways of the brain at ten years of age in children with histories of early social deprivation (Kumar et al. 2014). Most of life's adverse experiences are transient and forgotten. However, experiences that are traumatic and never forgotten epigenetically predispose the brain's circuitry to general emotional arousal, even in contexts that are mildly reminiscent. Some of these contexts may even be generated by the imaginary recollections of the brain itself.

Since the early theories of attachment and bonding, developmental science has provided insights as to how these lifetime interactions have shaped neurobiological outcomes. Following the sequencing of the human genome, an intense interest developed as to how genetics may have contributed to this understanding of development. Small nuclear polymorphisms and point mutations became a focus for attention, but revealed very little other than the kind of complexities that might arise. This is not surprising when an evolutionary comparison of brain genetics has also revealed very few differences between chimpanzees and humans, and yet the human brain is three times the size of our primate ancestor. However, the most human gene transcripts (76%) are expressed in the brain and have a variety of mechanisms available for differential regulation. The most recent version of the human genome, ENCODE 2012, has revealed multiple tiers of gene regulatory networks which, if it could be printed out, would stretch some 30 kilometers and 16 meters high. Among its 3 billion nucleotide letters, the regions that code for proteins represent 1% of the genome (20,000 genes); the rest contains an unprecedented number of functional regulatory elements, including enhancers, promoters, silencers, insulators, and locus control regions with 2.9 million regions that provide for chromatin accessibility. There is certainly potential for error but, surprisingly, development usually gets it right, albeit introducing considerable individual variability. This variability is what characterizes the brain, as no two brains are identical, even when the genomes are identical in monozygotic twins. Brains are undeniably adaptable, but it is essential to constrain this adaptability along the pathway to peace for the well-being of all (Ecker et al. 2012).

6

Group Identity as an Obstacle and Catalyst of Peace

Douglas P. Fry

Abstract

Social identity is not only an obstacle to peace; it can also be engaged to advance peace, such as when children are raised to develop multiple and cross-cutting forms of identification. This chapter considers the evidence that nomadic forager band social organization is not particularly conducive to the formation of hostile "us versus them" social identities and that, consequently, "us versus them" distinctions have only become strongly manifested with the development of more complex forms of social organization (e.g., tribes, kingdoms, nations) within the last 12,500 years or so. Such a proposition highlights the malleability of the concept of identity and contradicts the school of thought that sees "us versus them" identity formation as a long-standing innate tendency. This chapter will also consider how social identity can contribute to peace when it is employed in inclusive and unifying ways, in contrast to exclusionary and dehumanizing ways. This occurs, for example, within non-warring peace systems, when additional overarching identities are developed in the service of peace. In terms of promoting peace and inclusive social identities during childhood, it is suggested that explicitly teaching global citizenship can contribute to raising a peaceful world.

Introduction

Group identification does not, in and of itself, lead to war. However, in times of conflict, the psychological states that accompany group identity can feed hostility and facilitate intergroup violence. Once conflict intensifies, a group can come to hold an increasingly negative image of another group, eventually dehumanizing its members and excluding them from the realm of moral obligation (Deutsch 2006b; Konner 2006; Staub 1989). These processes can provide a justification for violence (Staub 1989). Indigenous peoples, for example, have often been delegitimized and dehumanized as "savages" in order to rationalize brutality toward them (Miklikowska and Fry 2010).

Some scholars (e.g., Haidt 2012; Konner 2006) assume that this divisive, hostility-promoting aspect of identification constitutes a natural human tendency. Whether or not humans have a natural tendency to form hostile "us versus them" distinctions is a topic that undoubtedly will be debated for some time to come. In this chapter, I draw upon anthropological knowledge to raise questions and to question assumptions about identity and conflict:

- Has the "us versus them" view of human identity been overemphasized?
- Do anthropological data support the proposition that "us versus them" mentality reflects, as often assumed, an innate tendency?
- From a cross-cultural perspective, how might social organization affect social identity and its relation to conflict?
- Can social identity be developed to promote unity and peace?

First I will examine social identity and conflict in relation to different types of social organization. The overall conclusion is that the oldest form of human social organization, nomadic forager band society, is not particularly conducive to the formation of hostile "us versus them" social identities. Based on ethnographic analogy (Fry 2006; Marlowe 2010) this suggests that "us versus them" distinctions may well have arisen later in the social evolutionary sequence of humanity; that is, along with a host of changes that accompanied a worldwide shift within the last 12,500 years toward more complex forms of society, such as chiefdoms, kingdoms, and states. Such a proposition highlights the malleability of the concept of identity and contradicts the school of thought that sees "us versus them" identity formation as an innate tendency in humans. It highlights, instead, that the oldest form of social organization, the nomadic forager band, has dramatically different effects on identity formation and manifestation than does more recent social organizational forms.

Thereafter I turn to how social identity can be utilized to promote peace by examining peace systems. The cases to be considered suggest again that social identity is malleable and, furthermore, that humans are capable of simultaneously holding multiple identities. Social identity can contribute to peace when it is employed in inclusive and unifying ways, in contrast to exclusionary and dehumanizing ways. The development of an overarching *human identity* or *global citizenship identity* also holds potential for contributing to peace. How, then, can global citizenship be fomented over the course of formative child development?

Comparative Social Organization Opens a New Perspective

Haidt (2012) has proposed that intergroup competition and hostility during human evolution has led to cohesiveness within the group (in-group loyalty). In humans, suggests Haidt (2012:370), group loyalty constitutes an evolved moral foundation: "Our minds were designed for groupish righteousness."

Wrangham and Glowacki (2012) display a similar "us versus them" orientation when they propose that humans and their precursors evolved innate tendencies to attack the members of other groups whenever the risks to the attackers were low. Wrangham and Glowacki (2012) argue that hostility toward and inclinations to attack neighboring groups constitute evolved psychological mechanisms. As another instance of innate-tendency hypothesizing, Konner (2006:21) writes that "whether in large or small groups, a common manifestation of mass psychology is the identification and destruction of enemies."

Such statements about the universality of psychological mechanisms, moral foundations, and mass psychology do not rest on relevant empirical findings. In fact, such propositions can be seen as culturally biased in that they project onto all humanity the type of "groupishness" or "us versus them" mentality that a consideration of human social organization—based on data from archaeology and comparative ethnography—suggests has developed along with other aspects of social complexity only over the most recent millennia of social evolution. Whereas there are bountiful examples of the "us versus them" phenomenon from history, contemporary ethnography, sociology, and political science and how it sometimes facilitates the most barbaric atrocities against members of other groups, such contemporary examples do not prove that humans have an *innate* or *natural tendency* to divide the social world into "us versus them" identities or to evoke social identity in the name of violence and cruelty. In actuality, such natural tendency assumptions are contradicted by a relevant and important source of data: ethnographic material on the oldest form of human social organization, nomadic forager band social organization.

From one society to the next, the types of violence and approaches to conflict management vary in relation to social organization. Service (1962) proposes four basic categories of human social organization (bands, tribes, chiefdoms, and states), which although constituting a simplified typology nonetheless has heuristic value. Bands are the oldest and simplest social form, extending back over the evolutionary history of the species; other more complex societies arose only over the last 12,500 years (Haas 1996:1360; Kelly 2000; Knauft 1991). Therefore, if one is going to propose certain behaviors to be evolved human tendencies, it is important to consider nomadic forager social organization.

A number of cross-cultural studies comparing different types of societies suggest that warfare correlates positively with degree of sociopolitical complexity (Johnson and Earle 1987; Leavitt 1977; Malinowski 1941; Reyna 1994). After reviewing the cross-cultural studies, van der Dennen (1995:142) states that "one of the most consistent and robust findings is the correlation between "primitivity" and absence of war or low-level warfare, or in other words, the correlation between war and civilization." Reading the trends in the worldwide archaeological record, Haas (2001:343) correspondingly concludes that "the level, intensity, and impact of warfare tend to increase as cultural systems become more complex."

Most studies of social identity have been based on hierarchical, complex forms of social organization. Until about 12,500 years ago, however, all members of the genus *Homo* lived as nomadic foragers; that is, in a very simple form of egalitarian social organization compared to the more complex types of societies that would develop subsequently. An examination of egalitarian nomadic forager social organization may provide some new insights about the relationships between identity and conflict (Fry and Souillac 2013). Data on nomadic forager social organization does not support the assumption that humans are naturally inclined toward "us versus them" hostility and violence.

First, what exactly is a group? Nomadic forager group composition is not static, but shifts over time via fission-fusion dynamics that characterize this type of society (Fry 2006; Fry and Söderberg 2013). Enduring and clearly delineated group membership is a prerequisite to the development of strong within-group loyalties. In other words, group loyalties cannot exist in the absence of clearly defined groups. The recurring pattern of group fission-fusion and the existence of idiosyncratic individual-based relationship networks in nomadic band societies are potent obstacles to the formation of strong group identities. Under such conditions, groups are ephemeral. The persons living in a nomadic forager society are interconnected to relatives and friends, based on individual ties that crisscross groups, not on the basis of group residence or membership in a particular corporate or residential group, as is common in other types of society. It is noteworthy that ethnographies on nomadic foragers have virtually nothing to say about "group loyalty," whereas they wax long about fluctuating group composition and individual-based social connections, the so-called "flex and flux" of the nomadic band (Apicella et al. 2012; Barnard 1983; Lee and DeVore 1968).

Second, social ties that span social space are typical in nomadic forager societies. The recurring pattern is for persons who are camped together, at any given point in time, to have simultaneously friends and family in neighboring bands with whom they regularly interact, thus reflecting how cooperation, sharing, exchange, and friendship do not cease beyond the edge of a group (Apicella et al. 2012; Fry 2006; Tonkinson 1974). Moreover, band societies tend not to emphasize exclusively either matrilineal or patrilineal kinship segments, but to attend to both maternal and paternal descent lines (Knauft 1991; Marlowe 2010). In practice, this means that each member of a nomadic forager society thinks in terms of his or her own unique set of kin ties, rather than in terms of common corporate kin-group-based identity (e.g., a patrilineage). Of course, the kin networks of individuals may overlap, but even two brothers in all likelihood will have different sets of in-laws (Fry 2006). With only a few exceptions, such as the Tiwi of Australia (Fry and Söderberg 2013), nearly all nomadic foragers live in a social world constructed upon individually oriented, idiosyncratic relations (rather than corporate group membership). Importantly, this form of social organization discourages intergroup hostility and aggression as well as the domination of strong in-group identities and loyalties.

Third, in nomadic forager societies, generally, there is a paucity of factors that would drive intergroup competition: resources are widely spread out over the landscape and thus indefensible; surpluses and material property are lacking; slavery is absent; and disputes tend to be over personal matters, not corporate complaints (Fry 2006; Fry and Söderberg 2013; Kelly 1995; Kelly 2000; Meggitt 1965). As Malinowski (1941:538; see also Reyna 1994) observes:

> Under conditions where portable wealth does not exist; where food is too perishable and too clumsy to be accumulated and transported; where slavery is of no value because every individual consumes exactly as much as he produces—force is a useless implement for the transfer of wealth.

All of these characteristics dictate against the development of intergroup hostility and "us versus them" mentality at this nomadic forager level of social organization.

Additionally, Fry (2006) and Fry and Söderberg (2013) have shown, using a sample of 21 nomadic foragers in the Standard Cross-Cultural Sample (a systematically assembled worldwide sample of societies), that nomadic foragers tend not to be warlike. Moreover, feuding, which pits kin group against kin group, is not typical of foraging bands for the simple reason that most band societies lack corporate kin organizations (Fry 2006; Fry and Söderberg 2013; Knauft 1991). In other words, nomadic foraging bands are typically unsegmented or only weakly segmented compared to societies that have clear subunits such as lineages or clans (Kelly 2000). Kelly (2000:47) points out that when a society is unsegmented, "a homicide is consequently likely to be perceived and experienced as an individual loss shared with some kin rather than as an injury to a group." An offshoot of this individual-familial perception is that, in unsegmented nomadic band societies, justice is often realized when a killer, in turn, is killed by the victim's family. The payback killing can balance the score and restore the peace within the unsegmented social system of the nomadic band (Fry 2006; Kelly 2000).

However, in more complex and segmented forms of social organization, a homicide can easily be perceived not only as a wrong inflicted against one family but also more generally against a corporate patrilineage, subclan, clan, and so on (Reyna 1994). Therefore, the victim's corporate kin group may target for revenge any member of the killer's social segment. Kelly (2000) refers to this phenomenon as *social substitutability*. In segmented societies, such as tribes or chiefdoms, retaliatory violence may alternate back and forth between feuding clans or lineages (Fry 2006). Social substitutability can facilitate feuding. Among nation states, social substitutability can facilitate war, wherein an act of violence (e.g., a terrorist attack) provokes retaliation not merely against the actual perpetrators, but against persons who simply have the same national or religious identity as the original attackers (Fry 2006). Clearly, Kelly's (2000) observations about social substitutability have relevance for understanding some kinds of intergroup violence in today's world.

In conclusion, the frequently voiced proposition (e.g., Haidt 2012; Konner 2006; Wrangham and Glowacki 2012) that "us versus them" identity results from and contributes to intergroup hostility and violence as an evolved tendency in humans is not supported by the nomadic forager data. Consequently, in response to authors such as Haidt (2012), who discusses chimpanzee coalition formation, team sports in contemporary societies, and modern warfare to argue that the "us versus them" conceptualization represents a fundamental "moral foundation" for humanity, I suggest that we are seeing a cultural bias wherein current-day circumstances are projected onto the past and overgeneralized to all societies. Meanwhile, the various types of nomadic forager data, which contradict the proposition that humans have a natural tendency to be hostile to members of other groups, goes unnoticed or ignored.

Clearly, the "us versus them" group loyalty and war-supporting value constellations have developed throughout human history. The point is that such features are very recent developments, archaeologically speaking, that have accompanied the emergence of more complex forms of social organization. They postdate the adoption of agriculture, sedentism, social hierarchy, and other associated changes in human social evolution within the last 12,500 years or so, as opposed to having evolved as a behavioral tendency over the course of the Pleistocene. Humans can and do develop "us versus them" orientations under some social conditions. However, the nomadic forager data suggest that this is a behavioral *capacity* of humans in some circumstances rather than a *tendency* across all social conditions.

As Kelly (2000:2) points out:

> In the relatively brief span of 4,500 years, a global condition of warlessness that had persisted for several million years thus gives way to chronic warfare that arises initially in the Near East and subsequently in other regions where a similar sequence of transformative events is reduplicated.

This is an evidence-based conclusion. The archaeological evidence for war before 10,000 years ago anywhere on Earth is negligible, whereas the evidence for the multiple origins of war in different regions, always within the last ten millennia, is unambiguous (Ferguson 2013; Fry 2006; Haas 1996; Haas and Piscitelli 2013; Kelly 2000). Thus archaeological findings on the recent origins of war are in agreement with the nomadic forager data in contradicting the assumption that "us versus them" identifications have played significant roles in intergroup violence over the long expanse of evolutionary time.

Identity and Peace Promotion: Expanding the "Us" to Include the "Them"

Anthropology provides information about successfully operating peace systems from different world regions, which have various psychosocial mechanisms, to counter "us versus them" identification by creating inclusive overarching social identities (Fry 2006, 2009; see also Dovidio et al. 2000, 2009). Peace systems consist of neighboring societies that do not engage in war against each other, and sometimes not with outsiders either. Examples of peace systems include the peoples of the Upper Xingu River basin in Brazil, the Western Desert Aborigines of Australia, the Iroquois Confederacy of North America, and the European Union (Fry 2006, 2009, 2012; Miklikowska and Fry 2010).

The ten tribes of the Upper Xingu River peace system, for instance, representing four different language groups, have converted divisive "us versus them" perceptions of each other into a unified vision of their broader social system by expanding the "us" to include the "them" (Fry 2006, 2009). These horticultural peoples still have their own tribal identities, but they also see their tribes as belonging to something greater. Frequent intermarriage, shared ceremonies, and trade relationships that crisscross tribal boundaries reinforce that each individual, from whatever tribe, is also a member of a larger, peaceful social system. Children being raised in this social setting adopt multiple levels of identity that include identification with one or more particular tribe as well as with the peaceful Xingu social sphere as a whole. It is noteworthy that the tribes specialize in the production of particular trade items—such as pottery, hardwood bows, or salt—and this economic specialization contributes to material interdependencies among these tribes.

Likewise, the nomadic foragers of the vast Australia Western Desert region are interconnected by overlapping networks, which, like the tribes comprising the Upper Xingu peace system, transcend local band membership and language dialect (Myers 1986). The Western Desert peoples view themselves as "one country," for they see the land as boundary-less, as reflected by their inclusion of all inhabitants of this region within an overarching kinship system (Myers 1986; Tonkinson 2004). Thus children of each generation are socialized into this view of an inclusive social world, which encompasses peoples from many small groups spread over an extensive area. The Western Desert groups constitute "a vast interlocking network of persons" (Myers 1986:27). Berndt (1972:183) observes that the Western Desert peoples do not limit their travels to particular areas but, in fact, interact with Aborigines from different language dialects as they crisscross extensive areas of the region. As Myers (1986:93) explains, territories are "flexible, if not insignificant." As in the Upper Xingu peace system, creation of a larger, inclusive "us" identity across social subunits contributes to peace as it prevents "us versus them" perceptions from crystallizing into hostile intergroup relations. After studying in detail one Western Desert society, the Mardu, Tonkinson (2004) explains that in this arid environment of sporadic and unpredictable rainfall, open borders permit resource-sharing among groups as they forage in a nonhostile social atmosphere. Tonkinson (2004:92–93) explains:

To permit intergroup conflict or feuding to harden social and territorial boundaries would be literally suicidal, since no group can expect the existing water
and food resources of its territory to tide it over until the next rains; peaceful
intergroup relations are imperative for long-term survival....It is not surprising,
then, that the Mardu have no word for either "feud" or "warfare" and there is no
evidence for the kinds of longstanding intergroup animosity one associates with
feuding.

The Mardu and their Western Desert neighbors recognize their mutual reliance on each other and employ creative ways of maintaining peaceful relations through kinship, friendship, and spirituality. The friendly relations among
bands in the Western Desert area are maintained through intermarriage and
joint ceremonies conducted at periodic "big meetings," at which time people
from different groups "exchange weapons, ochre, pearl shells, sacred boards
and other objects and, importantly, resolve disputes to maintain links of friendship and shared religion among the groups present" (Tonkinson 1974:97).

The Iroquois Confederacy provides us with another example of a peace
system that constructed unifying, identity-expanding social institutions. The
peace system probably dates from the beginning of the sixteenth century and
effectively maintained the internal peace for over 300 years. The Iroquois
Confederacy consisted initially of the Cayuga, Mohawk, Oneida, Onondaga,
and Seneca and was subsequently enlarged when the Tuscarora joined the
union. Dennis (1993:77) writes:

Initiating new rituals and practices, and inventing new social and political institutions, the prophet Deganawidah and those who followed his teachings found
ways to assure domestic concord, to extend the harmony within longhouses, lineages, and clans to wider domains, and to confront the ever-present threats to
stability, reason, and peace.

With the creation of their confederacy, the Iroquois within this new social system put an end to the feuding and warring among them. Internal peace and security were both the driving objective and the remarkable result of the Iroquois
adding a new level of governance and social identity. In this way, these former
enemies actively transformed themselves into relatives and neighbors "who
found shelter, security, and strength under the branches of the Great Tree of
Peace" (Dennis 1993:109).

The formation of the Iroquois Confederacy included not only a shift in values toward peace, but also an expansion of identity and an elaboration of kin
relations to include members of other groups. It created new inclusive rituals, ceremonies, and symbols to galvanize unity, a higher-level identity and
peaceful interaction, and a new governing body, the Great Council, which
consisted of fifty chiefs that assembled regularly as a newly created political
entity (Dennis 1993). One concrete shift in Iroquois judicial philosophy was
the forbearance of blood revenge in favor of the payment of compensation for
any acts of violence that did occur. In this way, the Iroquois *expanded* the "us"

to include the "them" *within their legal system*: The law of force, as previously reflected in war and blood vengeance, was replaced by the force of law, as typified by the payment of compensation (Fry 2006, 2012).

On a final note, I suggest that a new overarching European identity is in the process of emerging within the European Union—not as a substitute for national identities, but rather as an added level of European identification. Concrete signs of a developing pan-European identity include the issuance of EU passports, expanding use of the Euro currency (now legal tender in most member states), the opening of borders to permit free movement of people, the creation of a European Parliament, an EU flag, and so on (Fry 2009, 2012; Bellier and Wilson 2000). The trend across Europe involves the progressive development of a new regional identity that parallels how the Upper Xingu peoples, the Western Desert Aborigines, and the Iroquois created unifying overarching social identities. Such higher levels of identification, in concert with other social features and institutions, can play a role in the creation and maintenance of peaceful relations.

Identity, Interdependence, and Cooperation

A threat from outside a society can facilitate internal unity and cooperation as well as strengthen the sense of common identity (Deutsch 1973; Rubin et al. 1994). Alliance and cooperation can also develop in situations that involve no common enemy but which do necessitate cooperation to accomplish an important task effectively. In Australia's Western Desert, it would seem that a harsh environment with unpredictable rainfall creates mutual dependence among different groups. This interdependence, in turn, facilitates peaceful intergroup relations that encourage the desert-dwellers to cooperate, offer assistance to each other in times of need, reciprocally share resources, and behave kindly toward others within and beyond the immediate group. Rather than the development of a hostile "us versus them" system, over time a common identity and an ethic of sharing and cooperation have emerged. This observation parallels how Sherif et al. (1961), in the final stage of their classic naturalistic experiment, orchestrated the emergence of cooperation by artificially creating conditions of interdependence between two teams of hostile boys, nicknamed the Eagles and the Rattlers, at a summer camp in Oklahoma. To accomplish important superordinate goals, such as towing a "broken" truck needed to deliver their lunches or working together to find and repair the leak in their camp water supply, the Eagles and Rattlers had to cooperate.

There is a parable here. Many of the challenges facing humanity today can be similarly conceptualized as occurring under conditions of mutual dependence because they can only be solved through cooperative approaches. Global warming and other environmental threats (e.g., oceanic pollution, overexploitation of the world's fisheries, deforestation and desertification, loss of species biodiversity) are common to all of humanity and observe no national boundaries. When it comes to effectively addressing these serious threats to our human existence, the peoples and nations of the world are interdependent; paralleling the Eagles and the Rattlers, the only way for humanity to tackle common threats is to work together. Under conditions of interdependence, it is first and foremost necessary that the parties involved realize that they will either sink or swim together, that their fates are inextricably intertwined in what Deutsch (2006a) calls *positive interdependence*.

There are many cases of "Rattlers" and "Eagles" arriving at the realization that unless they pull together, nobody is going to eat lunch or quench their thirst. However, when faced with conditions of positive interdependence, people sometimes fail to realize that the shared problem cannot be solved unilaterally and therefore requires a cooperative solution (Deutsch 1973). Psychologists Kagan and Madsen (1971) put children into an experimental game situation in which cooperation could lead to the greatest rewards. They found that some children could not shift from a habitual competitive response to a cooperative orientation that would have benefited both players. Moreover, Kagan and Madsen (1971) showed that cultural factors had a noteworthy influence: Mexican children acted more cooperatively than California-dwelling Mexican-American children who, in turn, demonstrated more cooperative responses than did Anglo-American children. One implication of these findings, as well as much other research that documents the impact of cultural factors on cooperation/competition (Kohn 1986), is that in parallel to the children in the experiment (who got "stuck" using only competitive responses in situations where cooperation would have paid more dividends), decision makers on the international stage, it would seem, often do not grasp that cooperation is necessary under conditions of positive interdependence, such as a planet facing drastic climate change. As Sachs (2008:3, emphasis in original) points out:

> The defining challenge of the twenty-first century will be to face the reality that humanity shares *a common fate on a crowded planet*. That common fate will require new forms of global cooperation, a fundamental point of blinding simplicity that many world leaders have yet to understand or embrace.

Stepping back from the current nation-state system and surveying the types of human societies that exist and have existed permits us to see that humanity has spent the overwhelming majority of its tenure on the planet living in nomadic forager bands. An emphasis on cooperation, a social system based on multiple individual-idiosyncratic social networks, a fission-fusion group dynamic that results in porous and malleable membership, and an emphasis, in ethos and practice, on egalitarianism are hallmarks of this original form of human social organization, meaning that they are reported with great consistency in nomadic forager ethnography (Apicella et al. 2012; Barnard 1983; Fry 2006; Fry and Söderberg 2013; Fry and Souillac 2013; Kelly 1995; Knauft 1991; Lee and DeVore 1968; Marlowe 2010). The absence of social segmentation, the presence of group fluctuations in membership and composition, and the patchwork of cross-cutting social ties in nomadic forager societies all work to counter the development of strong "us versus them" identifications.

Only within the last 12,500 years or so has humanity made a sociopolitical shift toward centralized leadership and authority with the rise of the first chiefdoms (Fry 2006). The subsequent development of the first ancient civilizations—a mere 5,000 to 6,000 years ago—gave birth to the state as a new form of social organization. Chiefdoms, ancient civilizations, kingdoms, and modern nation-states have social hierarchies with rulers at the top who hold positions of authority and leadership. In these stages of society, we see also the development and elaboration of social identities.

Despite the fact that a global system consisting of nation-states is largely taken as a fact of life in the twenty-first century, humanity's very first states, appearing in the form of ancient civilizations, are only several millennia old, whereas the modern version of the state, the nation-state, is only a few hundred years old. Thus politically speaking and in terms of social identification, it has not always been this way. Despite regular assertions to the contrary, a social lens that encompasses a broader view of human history and prehistory, including variations in human social structure and behavior, reveals that there is nothing inherently natural or normal about nation-states, national identities, or nationally patriotic "us versus them" conceptualizations of the social world. New forms of governance (e.g., with new supranational layers of identity) can be conceptualized as additives or alternatives to the taken-for-granted naturalness of the nation-state model. An anthropological perspective that surveys social systems over time and geographical distance broadens the view. One principle of central importance is that the unification of disparate social units with the concomitant development of a common, overarching social identity helps to reduce bias and hostilities as it simultaneously enhances cooperation and positive attitudes among the social groups (Dovidio et al. 2000, 2009).

Expanding the "Us": Creating the Human Identity of Global Citizenship

Mahatma Gandhi championed expanding the "us" to include the "them," as illustrated by his reply when asked if he were a Hindu: "Yes I am. I am also a Christian, a Muslim, a Buddhist and a Jew."[1] Darwin (1871/1998:126–127) also reflected on how social identity is malleable and expandable:

> As man advances in civilization, and small tribes are united into larger communities, the simplest reason would tell each individual that he ought to extend his social instincts and sympathies to all the other members of the same nation, though personally unknown to him. This point being once reached, there is only

---

[1]   http://en.wikipedia.org/wiki/Gandhism (accessed March 9, 2014).

an artificial barrier to prevent his sympathies extending to the men of all nations and races.

The Upper Xingu River basin tribes, the Aboriginal bands of the Western Desert, the Iroquois, and other such examples demonstrate that *it is possible for neighboring societies to expand the "us" to include the "them"* and create new common identities within peace systems (Fry 2009, 2012; Miklikowska and Fry 2010).

In respect to raising children for a peaceful world, the teaching and learning of a new social identity, called *global citizen*, holds potential for contributing to peace. But what exactly is the global citizen identity?

One answer to this question could highlight values that are taught to the young during socialization and reinforced by society among its citizenry of all ages. Values vary across cultures. They can support and promote war and violence, or, to the contrary, values can foster nonviolence. Specifically, certain values can reinforce a global citizenship identity. Such values might include, for instance, *tolerance* of religious, ethnic, and cultural differences, *respect* for all people everywhere, *social equality* in and among our societies, *nonviolence* in both ethos and practice, and *democracy, human rights, and justice* manifested in social institutions—all of which can be seen as elements important to the development and maintenance of peace (Souillac 2011, 2012).

Another path for teaching global citizenship, as a new social identity, could place human rights in a central position. Formal education across grade levels could include, for example, discussions of United Nations declarations that emphasize the rights of children, women, and indigenous peoples as well as consider carefully the implications of the Universal Declaration of Human Rights. A serious consideration of human rights, as an important component of the global citizenship identity, loops back to the centrality of values such as equality, respect, justice, and participatory democracy as well as the social institutions and practices that support them (Souillac 2012).

A third approach for the teaching of global citizenship to future generations could take the eight elements of the "culture of peace" as a starting point (Fry and Miklikowska 2012; see also the Foreword, this volume): education; sustainable development; human rights; gender equality; democratic participation; the advancement of understanding, tolerance, and solidarity; communication and information sharing; and peace and security. Some of these components directly relate to global citizenship, such as the promotion of peace and security, the values dimensions (equality, tolerance, and so on), and an emphasis on democracy. Most of the components interrelate with a conceptualization and enactment of a positive peace. Thus, the culture of peace components could be used as a bridge between the creation of peace and an expansion of the "us" to include the "them" that is inherent in a global citizen identity.

Anthropological and psychological studies show that there are many ways to expand the "us" and create overarching common social identities. First, interlinking ties can be developed among different groups through augmentation of exchange relationships, intermarriage, intergroup friendships, and participation in common rituals and ceremonies (Rubin et al. 1994; Sherif et al. 1961). For example, individuals from each Upper Xingu tribe nurture trade partnerships across tribal boundaries and this practice helps to expand the "us" identification across all ten tribes (Fry 2006, 2009). The potential contribution that intermarriage holds for expanding the "us" is seen in the description of an Upper Xingu man with parents from different tribes, who gestured from head-to-toe along the midline of his body and said: "This side…Mehinaku. That side is Waurá" (Gregor and Robarchek 1996:173).

Second, recognizing interdependence and then cooperating to attain superordinate goals can facilitate a higher-level social identification (Sherif et al. 1961). Furthermore, psychological studies demonstrate that engaging in cooperative activities across group lines can enhance trust, friendship, positive relations, and a common identity (Aronson et al. 1978; Deutsch 2006a, b; Dovidio et al. 2009; Sherif et al. 1961). Some additional methods that seem to facilitate expanding the "us" include empathy training, socialization to care about people beyond one's own immediate group, and the teaching of nonviolent conflict resolution strategies (Deutsch 2006a, b). Thus, social identity is not only an obstacle to peace; it can also be used to advance peace. Educating toward a new pan-humanity global citizenship identity can contribute to bringing the peoples of Earth closer to achieving peace (Fry 2012; Souillac 2012).

Future Research Questions

1. What features of childhood or of child rearing in nomadic forager band societies contribute to peacefulness? Clearly, there is variation in levels of aggressiveness-peacefulness across nomadic forager societies (as across societies, in general): Do some particular features of childhood or child rearing correlate with peacefulness?

2. Is there an association between types of caregiving and peacefulness across nomadic forager societies or in general?

3. Across societies, do particular value constellations contribute to raising peaceful children as opposed to raising more aggressive children?

4. Regarding social identity, how can "expanding the "us" processes be augmented during child development? How can "us versus them" processes be minimized during child development?

5. Are there some fundamental processes involved in the successful *creation* of non-warring peace systems? In what ways do non-warring peace systems *maintain* the peace within the system?

Acknowledgment

I am grateful to an anonymous reviewer, Ingrida Grigaitytė, and Patrik Söderberg for commenting on a draft of this chapter. I am also grateful to Geneviève Souillac and the Ernst Strüngmann Forum "Group 1" colleagues—Sue Carter, Markus Heinrichs, Barry Keverne, Iris-Tatjana Kolassa, Robert Kumsta, James Leckman, Barak Morgan, David Olds, and Diane Sunar—for fruitful discussions about ideas considered in this chapter.

First column (top to bottom): Barak Morgan, Diane Sunar, Doug Fry,
group discussion, Barry Keverne, Barak Morgan, Robert Kumsta
Second column: Sue Carter, Barry Keverne, Robert Kumsta, informal discussion,
Sue Carter, Jim Leckman, Iris-Tatjana Kolassa
Third column: Jim Leckman, Iris-Tatjana Kolassa, David Olds, Doug Fry,
David Olds, Diane Sunar

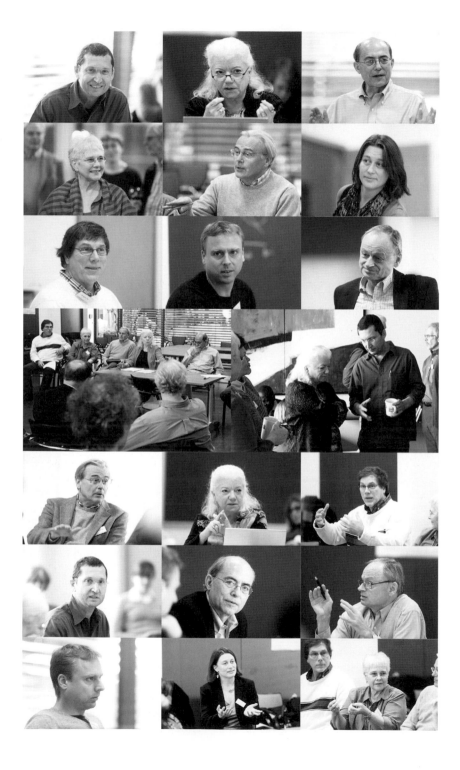

7

Human Biological Development and Peace

Genes, Brains, Safety, and Justice

Barak Morgan, Diane Sunar, C. Sue Carter,
James F. Leckman, Douglas P. Fry, Eric B. Keverne,
Iris-Tatjana Kolassa, Robert Kumsta, and David Olds

Abstract

This chapter examines the concept of peace from a biopsychosocial perspective. It reviews available knowledge concerning gene-environment regulatory interactions and their consequences for neurodevelopment, particularly during sensitive periods early in life. The hypothesis is explored that efforts on the part of parents to protect, nurture, and stimulate their children can lead to physically, psychologically, and socially healthier developmental trajectories and support the emergence of more peaceful families and communities. It is clear, however, that adverse environments, as in the context of structural violence, may result in lower parental investment in child rearing and negative outcomes for social harmony and health over the course of life. More research is thus needed to understand more fully the potential positive impact that interventions aimed at encouraging families to increase their investment in early child development will have on societal peace. The role of groups in shaping human behavior toward conflict or conflict resolution and peace is examined. Further research is needed to increase current understanding on the neurobiology of groups. In addition, steps need to be taken across multiple sectors of society to reduce all forms of direct and structural violence, as this will surely lead to "better" parenting behaviors, "better" childhood trajectories, and a model of fairness to guide interactions between groups.

Introduction

Peace can be defined as a positive, dynamic participatory process or a condition in which every person has the opportunity to develop to his or her fullest potential (Kagitcibasi and Britto, this volume). It can also be defined as a condition of *safety* for individuals or groups. Its opposite may be conceived as *threat*, which can take the form of direct conflict and violence or of structural violence (i.e., deprivation or social inequality and injustice), which can interfere with equal opportunities for human development.

In this chapter, we refer to the process of reducing direct violence as peacemaking and the process of reducing structural violence as peacebuilding. Peacemaking most frequently occurs at, and refers to, the individual and family levels, whereas peacebuilding generally refers to activities taken at broader levels (e.g., the community or nation).

When we use the term peace, we are generally referring to an emotional sense of safety. Threat and fear are also emotional constructs. The mammalian nervous system is exquisitely sensitive to states of threat and danger as well as to a sense of safety. Experiences of safety or danger are transduced into changes in gene expression, which can influence neural development, including structures and functions mediated by neurotransmitters and neurohormones (e.g., steroid hormones such as cortisol and neuropeptides such as oxytocin). The primate nervous system is a social organ that not only requires close attunement with other members of their species for normal development, it also produces behavior which constitutes relationships of various kinds. These relationships, in turn, are potentially peaceful or nonpeaceful. This is all the more so for humans who are ultrasocial primates.

Neurodevelopment comprises the unfolding and interweaving of a complex array of processes, all of which require genetic templates. However, the ways in which these genetic templates are used during neurodevelopment—both pre- and postnatally—are entirely dependent upon the environment as mediated[1] by epigenetic mechanisms. Epigenetics is where genes and environment ultimately (and physically) meet.

Violence

At first glance, "structural violence" may seem like a misnomer, for inequality and injustice may characterize very stable social structures in which there is little if any open conflict or physical violence (see Christie et al., this volume). In terms of their effects on genes, brains, development of potential, relationships and capacity for peaceful and productive living, direct and structural violence are nearly identical, differing mainly in their time frames. Direct violence can inflict trauma in a short space of time, whereas structural violence is persistent and insidious in wreaking its damage.

---

[1]   When discussing neural structures and functions, the term "mediate" is preferred to other terms like "regulate" or "based upon," which often imply a sense of causal origin or causal direction. "Mediated" is causally neutral, thus emphasizing the "circular causality" of organism-environment interactions.

In today's world, structural violence most often takes the form of poverty, the causes of which generate socioeconomic and health inequality. In recent years, interest in the impact of environmental adversity—especially low socioeconomic status (SES)—on the development of biological substrates of cognitive, behavioral, motivational, and social functions in humans has surged (Boyce et al. 2012b), driven in large part by momentous advances in understanding its impact on early biological development in animals (Cameron et al. 2005; Champagne and Meaney 2006; Hackman et al. 2010; Plotsky et al. 2005). The import of these advances lies in the ways whereby environmental conditions during early development become embedded in biology in largely irreversible ways, for better or worse (Gruenewald and Karlamangla 2012; Johnson et al. 2013; McEwen 2012; Shonkoff 2010).

However, both peace and violence are *relational*: they are conditions which are obtained between and among individuals or groups. This requires us to understand types of relationships and their implications for peace and violence. Both peace and violence are also *functional* in specifiable environments. Finally, violence is often regarded by the actor (person or group) as morally justified. Each of these points encompasses biological elements and has developmental implications.

Environment Becomes Epigenetically Embedded in Biology, Regulating Gene Expression

Environment Regulates Built-In Intelligence

Throughout the life cycle, organisms and environment work together as an inseparable whole. Even DNA functions only as part of a loop that always includes the environment. A particular trait, for example, may manifest under certain environmental conditions, but under other conditions it may not. Knowing under which genetic and environmental conditions a given trait will manifest is especially relevant vis-à-vis the developmental biology of formative childhoods.

Living systems possess built-in intelligence that "works the environment" for adaptive ends. Built-in intelligence means intelligence that is learned, where "learned" refers to inborn intelligence acquired through natural selection encoded in DNA as well as intelligence acquired through life experience encoded in epigenetics. Working the environment means that organisms use the environment to regulate this built-in intelligence in adaptive ways so as to promote survival and reproduction.[2]

Alone, built-in intelligence is entirely useless. Organisms absolutely depend on environmental information to "close a regulatory loop." Only the

---

[2] Evolutionists use the term "reproductive survival" to denote what organisms must ultimately do to avoid extinction: it is not enough simply to survive; one must survive *and* reproduce.

This is not synonymous with the old "blank slate" version of environmental determinism (cf. Pinker 2003). Rather, it recognizes that each of these types of behavior reflects built-in intelligence which has been selected over the course of evolution as adaptive in particular environmental settings and will therefore manifest (i.e., be regulated for) whenever these settings prevail.

Threat and Stress in Brain Development

The Stress Response

The profound relevance of developmental neuroscience to the great social questions of peace and violence lies in newly discovered epigenetic details that address exactly how environment and genes interact. The stress response denotes physiological and psychological changes that occur in response to a stressor and is comprised of two systems: (a) the sympathetic nervous system (SNS) and (b) the hypothalamic-pituitary-adrenal (HPA) axis (Figure 7.1). Both systems are activated by stress via corticotrophin release factor neurons in the amygdala and hypothalamus, respectively (Cameron et al. 2005; Gunnar and Quevedo 2007). The SNS responds rapidly, causing the release of epinephrine and norepinephrine from chromafin cells in the adrenal glands; this prepares the body (increased heart rate, blood pressure, respiration) and focuses the mind to respond appropriately to the stressor. If the stressor poses an imminent threat, the SNS will trigger a fight, flight, or freeze response accompanied by feelings and sensations of rage or panic. If the stressor does not pose an imminent threat, the SNS will keep the body and cerebral cortex in a state of anxious readiness, which orients cognition toward an assessment of the overall situation (what might happen next and what will be the best response).

If the stressor passes, the SNS response will die down, bodily functions will return to normal, and the mind will relax. If the stressor persists, the HPA axis begins to activate and releases glucocorticoids (CORT), also from the adrenal glands. The HPA stress response serves to provide the SNS response with energy (i.e., it increases blood glucose levels) needed to sustain increased heart rate, blood pressure, respiration as well as any strenuous physical activity associated with a potential fight or flight response. As is the case for the SNS, once a stressor passes, the HPA axis will be switched off and blood glucose levels will return to normal.

So what does the stress response have to do with gene-environment interactions, epigenetic marks, and *once-off* canalization in early childhood? To answer this question, we turn to the proverbial lab rat, where it was discovered that rat pups raised by mothers who lick and groom (LG) them more (the high LG group) become more resilient to stress (show normal HPA stress responses), whereas pups raised by low LG mothers exhibit exaggerated HPA stress responses and are susceptible to the toxic effects of stress. This is true

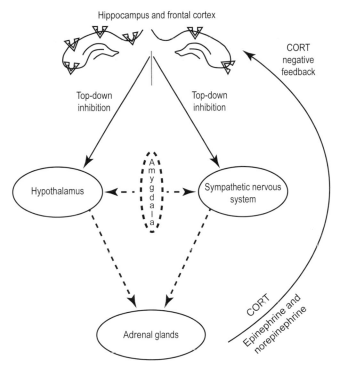

Figure 7.1 Overview of the neuroendocrine response to stress involving the cortex (hippocampus and frontal), subcortex (hypothalamus, amygdala, and sympathetic nervous system), and adrenal glands. In the absence of stress (solid arrows), the hippocampus inhibits the hypothalamic-pituitary-adrenal (HPA) axis stress response, while the frontal cortex inhibits the sympathetic nervous system (SNS) stress response. When significant stress is present (dashed arrows), the amygdala overrides top-down frontal cortex inhibitory control and activates the SNS to release epinephrine and norepinephrine. If stress passes, the SNS response subsides and the system returns to normal. If stress persists, hippocampal top-down inhibition is overcome and the HPA axis is activated causing glucocorticoids (CORT) to be released to provide the SNS response with energy. When CORT reaches the hippocampus via the bloodstream, it binds to CORT receptors (vee shapes, top of figure) like a key fitting into a lock. Opening this lock boosts top-down inhibition to the hypothalamus, thereby switching the HPA axis stress response off once again (negative feedback). If the number of CORT receptor locks in the hippocampus is low, as depicted on the top right-hand side of the hippocampus, there will be more CORT keys than there are CORT receptor locks to open and the hippocampus will be less able to switch off the HPA axis in a top-down fashion. As a result, the CORT stress response will be abnormally exaggerated. Crucially, the number of CORT receptor locks on hippocampal cells is epigenetically set for life in a once-off manner very early in life. After Meaney and Szyf (2005).

irrespective of the biological mother: pups born to a high LG mother but raised by a low LG mother will develop an exaggerated HPA stress response and vice versa (Claessens et al. 2011). Thus maternal environment (high or low LG) rather than genetic differences influence how the HPA system is "set up."

As shown in Figure 7.1, in the presence of stress, as CORT does its work around the body to increase blood glucose levels, CORT also reaches the hippocampus where it binds to CORT receptors like a key fitting into a lock. Opening this lock boosts the top-down inhibitory powers of the hippocampus on the hypothalamus, thereby switching the HPA axis off again (negative feedback).

If the number of CORT receptor locks in the hippocampus is low (Figure 7.1, top right-hand side of the hippocampus), the efficacy of negative feedback will be low; that is, there will be more keys than there are locks to open and the hippocampus will be less able to switch off the HPA axis. As a result, the CORT stress response will be abnormally high and prolonged. Importantly, *during the first few days after birth, the number of CORT receptor locks is under environmental control.*

For a newborn mammal, environment means mother.[3] For rats, the intensity of maternal licking and grooming behavior during the first six days of life regulates the level of gene expression of the CORT receptor gene in a *once-off* fashion *for life*. Pups raised by high LG mothers have fewer marks on this gene, resulting in greater gene expression; this, in turn, results in more hippocampal locks, more effective CORT key negative feedback, more inhibition of the hypothalamus, and hence more effective termination of the HPA stress response. Conversely, pups raised by low LG mothers have more epigenetic marks on this gene, resulting in less gene expression; this, in turn, results in less hippocampal locks, less negative feedback, and an exaggerated and prolonged HPA stress response. *Differences in maternal licking and grooming behavior disappear after the sixth day of postnatal life, whereafter the number of epigenetic marks that have been affixed in the hippocampus does not change. In other words, the HPA stress response is once-off epigenetically set (canalized) for life during a very brief and well-defined sensitive period (0 to 6 days of life)* (Meaney and Szyf 2005).

The same mechanism seems to apply to humans (Suderman et al. 2012). For example, one study found that early childhood adversity (i.e., parental loss, childhood maltreatment, and/or inadequate parental care) was associated with increased epigenetic marking of the CORT receptor gene, which in turn was associated with weakened negative feedback of the HPA axis (Tyrka et al. 2012). Others have found significantly more epigenetic marks on the CORT receptor gene and, as would be expected, significantly lower levels of CORT receptor numbers in the hippocampus, in brains of individuals with a history of early childhood abuse (McGowan et al. 2009), as well as in peripheral tissues such as blood cells in children exposed to (a) maltreatment and reduced nurturing (Perroud et al. 2011), (b) maternal anxiety and depression in pregnancy

---

[3] "Mother" refers to primary caregiver (i.e., the person who takes primary responsibility for the care of another individual who cannot fully care for themselves) and may not be biologically related to the child.

(Oberlander et al. 2008), and (c) in 10- to 19-year-olds whose mothers experienced intimate partner violence during pregnancy (Radtke et al. 2011). All of these studies connect early adversity associated with impaired parenting, both prenatally and postnatally, with once-off hypermethylation of the CORT receptor gene and, in some cases, with hippocampal-HPA changes consistent with impaired negative feedback. In addition, epidemiological studies have found differences in epigenetic marks on hundreds of genes in individuals whose childhood was spent in the lowest socioeconomic strata, irrespective of adulthood SES (Labonté 2012; McGuinness et al. 2012).

In sum, early-life experience has a profound and enduring once-off canalizing impact on gene expression patterns throughout life. This is true for the CORT receptor gene, which codes for hippocampal CORT receptor locks, as well as for the genome as a whole.

"Top-Down" and "Bottom Up" Brain Processes: Self-Regulation

Mammal brains, especially human brains, are characterized by a large cortex that overlies subcortical structures. Very roughly, psychological functions of the frontal cortex include conscious thought, attention, working memory, planning, and self-processes (e.g., self-control, judgment, and physical movement). Processes governed by the subcortical structures include emotional arousal, physical urges, vigilance, relaxation, and control of the autonomic nervous system. Infants are born with a well-developed subcortical system, but the cortex undergoes major development after birth, particularly in the first two years. Top-down regulation means that cortical structures inhibit bottom-up physiological and emotional responses so as to integrate instead a wide range of information needed to make more sophisticated assessments than the subcortex can. Bottom-up regulation means that the subcortex overrides top-down cortical control in situations where there is no time to ponder different options and one or more of a limited number of automatic built-in stereotyped fight, flight, or freeze stress or appetitive action responses are urgently needed.[4]

In general, top-down (cortical) regulation of the subcortex is voluntary, effortful, and relatively slow. In contrast, bottom-up (subcortical) activity is involuntary, effortless, and nearly instantaneous. Because top-down regulation is generally voluntary and often mentally challenging, it is also called self-regulation or "effortful control"; a healthy balance between top-down and bottom-up activity is important for personal and social well-being. Healthy balance means knowing when to remain calm and when to react. Not surprisingly, self-regulation has a profound influence on lifetime achievement and physical and

---

[4] Bottom-up activity encompasses much more than just the fight, flight, or freeze stress response and also includes appetitive reward-seeking motivations and other emotionally positive and negative states of mind.

mental health. In two large longstanding longitudinal studies conducted in the United Kingdom and New Zealand, Moffitt et al. (2011) found that children with poor self-regulation capacities at 3, 5, 7, 9, and 11 years of age had, at 32 years of age, significantly higher rates of substance dependence, criminality, financial problems, and single parenthood; they also had significantly lower income, less financial planning skills, lower SES and reduced physical health.

Self-Regulation and Socioeconomic Status

Diminished top-down self-regulation is strongly related to low SES, especially during the earliest postnatal years; thereafter, with each year spent in poverty, SES diminishes even further (Blair and Raver 2012b). Several studies in older subjects report similar relations between top-down self-regulatory capacities and SES. Parental SES predicted cognitive function (performance on a learning task) and prefrontal cortex fMRI activation in 8- to 12-year-old children, and this relationship was mediated by CORT stress response (Sheridan et al. 2012a). In a sample of nearly 1,300 children studied at 2 and 48 months of age, CORT levels were higher and decreased more slowly in children with greater cumulative years in poverty and with greater cumulative household poverty (Blair et al. 2013). Similarly, in a sample of sixty children (mean age 11.4 years), lower SES correlated with smaller hippocampal and larger amygdala volumes, suggestive of weaker top-down control and stronger bottom-up reactivity, respectively (Noble et al. 2012). Another study found that lower childhood SES predicted smaller hippocampal volumes 50 years later (Staff et al. 2012). Finally, the prefrontal cortex of 24-year-olds from lower childhood SES backgrounds was less able to inhibit amygdala activity during an effortful negative emotion regulation experiment independent of adult SES and chronic childhood stressor levels mediated this effect (Kim et al. 2013). All of this evidence suggests that socioeconomic adversity may steer brain development in early childhood toward brains characterized by diminished powers of top-down regulation. How does this occur?

From Maternal Regulation to Self-Regulation:
The Maternal Mediation Hypothesis

Moffitt et al. (2011) found that although lower SES in childhood correlated with poorer self-regulation, their main findings (see above) that poor self-regulation predicted a wide range of normatively negative adult outcomes still held after controlling for childhood SES. In many cases, poor childhood self-regulation was a stronger predictor of poor outcomes in adulthood than SES (Moffitt et al. 2011). This suggests that socioeconomic adversity per se does not canalize brain development along a trajectory biased toward greater bottom-up versus top-down modes of brain function. Something else must be mediating the links between early socioeconomic adversity and compromised top-down neuroanatomical, neurofunctional, neurocognitive powers, and HPA axis hyper-responsiveness—all evidence of diminished top-down self-regulation. What could this be?

Part of the answer is that SES *impacts on early self-regulation via the filter of parental care*. This is clearly illustrated in a study of working memory in a sample of youth from a low SES community. Doan and Evans (2011) found that working memory ability (a measure of top-down cortical self-regulation) varied with increasing allostatic load (a composite score of bottom-up physiological measures reflecting of HPA and SNS stress reactivity), according to maternal care. That is, youth with mothers high in maternal responsiveness showed no change in working memory as allostatic load increased. On the other hand, youth with mothers low in maternal responsiveness showed sharply diminishing working memory capacities as allostatic load increased. The influence of maternal care is not, however, limited to socioeconomic adversity. A prospective study of children between 6 and 12 years of age from nondeprived backgrounds found a significant correlation between maternal support and hippocampal volumes (Luby et al. 2012), highlighting the mediating role of early parental care in all SES circumstances.

These results indicate how maternal care serves to *buffer* or *not buffer* an adverse environment. In short, parental care mediates the effect of the environment on early brain development. This is what is called the maternal mediation hypothesis. Starting from birth, an infant has very limited powers of self-regulation because the immature cortex cannot integrate complex information or assert top-down inhibition. As described above for the HPA axis in rats and humans, the acquisition of top-down control is highly sensitive to parental investment in early life. In both species the quality of early parental care literally sculpts and canalizes the self-regulatory powers of the maturing cortex via once-off lifelong epigenetic marks that determine the density of CORT receptors on hippocampal cells. The same applies to the expression of many other genes in the brain (Blair et al. 2013; Blair and Raver 2012b; Cameron 2011; Gudsnuk and Champagne 2012; Monk et al. 2012; Provençal et al. 2012).

During development, CORT, epinephrine, and norepinephrine act on the brain as part of the bottom-up stress response. At moderate levels these hormones enhance synaptic activity in prefrontal cortex areas that subserve attention, working memory, and top-down emotion regulation. However at high levels, prefrontal cortex is shut down and subcortical systems dominate (Arnsten and Li 2005; Blair and Raver 2012a). Since attention, working memory, and emotion regulation are critical components of self-regulation as well as for processing and learning complex information, over time these hormones sculpt the firing and wiring pathways of the brain in ways that canalize brain development along either strong top-down, "reflective" or strong bottom-up, "reactive" stress response trajectories, according to the amount of environmental stress and the nature of maternal/parental care (Blair et al. 2013; Blair and Raver 2012b; Rinaman et al. 2011; Wiggins and Monk 2013).

Several studies (Knudsen et al. 2006; Moffitt et al. 2011; Raver et al. 2012) show that the differences in self-regulation which make a difference later in life are already forged during the first five years of life. Exactly how devastatingly once-off and irreversible early canalization of childhood development can be is tragically evident in studies of Romanian orphans adopted into Canadian and British families. At eight years of age, the social skills of Romanian children who were initially placed in severely deprived institutional conditions soon after birth differed dramatically according to age of adoption into nurturing foster families in Canada. Social skills in orphans adopted prior to 20 months of age closely approximated Canadian children raised in their own families, whereas orphans adopted after 20 months of age closely approximated their orphan peers who remained institutionalized in Romania (Almas et al. 2012). Identical findings were observed for self-regulation abilities in Romanian orphans adopted into British families (O'Connor et al. 2000).

In sum, because a baby is born with a well-developed subcortex but relatively undeveloped cortex, any distress it experiences triggers a powerful stress response which it has no means to curtail; there are no, or very few, CORT receptors in the hippocampus as yet and the child has no cognitive powers to self-regulate. Instead, the child must rely on maternal comfort to regulate its feelings. Even if maternal comfort is not entirely or immediately successful, the mother's mere presence and deeply caring attention results (similarly to high LG rat mothers) in fewer epigenetic marks on the CORT receptor gene and other genes important for top-down control. Strong top-down self-regulation is acquired from the environment, which for infants is predominantly the mother or caregiver.[5]

A further, crucially important dimension to the maternal mediation hypothesis is that while maternal behavior/investment (e.g., maternal responsiveness) mediates the impact of environment on offspring development, the environment also regulates maternal behavior/investment itself. Evidence that maternal investment style is sensitive to environmental adversity is available in both rats and humans. In rats, gestational stress decreases licking and grooming behavior in high but not low LG mothers. Under stressful conditions, once pups were born, LG behavior in the previously high LG mothers was no different from the low LG mothers and the offspring of both groups developed stress response profiles and maternal licking and grooming styles in accordance with having experienced low LG maternal care (Cameron 2011). Although LG behavior exhibits plasticity during gestation (change from high to low LG),

---

[5] Importantly, strong top-down self-regulation does not mean suppression of all emotional responses. Nonjudgmental tolerant and empathic parenting allows an infant to first safely express and later verbalize, and thereby self-regulate subcortically generated distress or excitement such as hurt, anxiety, fear, anger, and desires.

this plasticity does not persist. Initially high (as observed in their first pregnancy) LG rats, who switched to low LG when stressed during their second pregnancy, continued to exhibit low LG behavior toward the progeny of their third pregnancy even though they were not subjected to any further gestational stress. In other words, stress experienced during their second pregnancy served to embed and canalize maternal behavior along a low LG trajectory.

An extensive literature documents the disruptive impact of poverty on normatively positive maternal care in humans (Cameron et al. 2005 and references therein), particularly when mediated by maternal anxiety and depression (Murray et al. 2010). Maternal anxiety undermines maternal buffering capacity and is the biggest factor contributing to a mother's feelings toward her newborn (Cameron et al. 2011). Depressed and anxious mothers are less able to feel positive toward their baby (Cameron et al. 2005). Furthermore, poor maternal-infant bonding correlates with increased SNS and HPA stress responses; adult victims of child abuse also show increased HPA and SNS responses to stress (Cameron et al. 2005). Lower maternal SES also correlates with elevated maternal cortisol in pregnancy and elevated infant cortisol response to vaccination stress at six weeks of age (Thayer and Kuzawa 2014). Lastly, human maternal investment styles transmit across generations, with child abuse being more common in families where parents were themselves abused as children (Cameron 2011).

These findings suggest that the maternal mediation hypothesis is applicable to humans as well. Indeed, in humans as in rats, lower parental investment (including abusive parenting) is associated with greater epigenetic marking of not only the CORT receptor gene but of many genes across the entire genome. Some of these other genes are known to be involved in top-down and bottom-up regulation of the stress response as well as other relevant behaviors, including sexual and caregiving reproductive styles (Cameron 2011; Champagne et al. 2001; Feldman et al. 2012; Kumsta et al. 2013; Wang et al. 2014). Gonzalez et al. (2012) found that early-life adversity predicted decreased maternal sensitivity and that this relationship was mediated by increased HPA axis activity and decreased working memory abilities (i.e., diminished top-down control). Consequently, by regulating for decreased maternal investment, environmental adversity biases early brain development toward less efficient top-down inhibitory control, making spontaneous bottom-up activity more likely. The maternal mediation hypothesis is also supported by studies which show that controlling for parenting behaviors nullifies the association between SES and developmental outcomes (Cameron et al. 2005) as well as studies which show that parental investment in children as well as in resources for children, positive parenting, and decreased material hardship and stress are the major mediators of positive correlations between family income and child outcomes (Yoshikawa et al. 2012).

Strategic Life Histories

Why should low LG mothering in rats and its low parental investment human equivalent result in an overly sensitive stress response and poor top-down self-regulation to predispose an individual to normatively poor physical, psychological, and social outcomes later in life? How does this make evolutionary sense?

There is mounting evidence to support the idea that once-off canalization of the stress response, according to the quality of parental care early in life, serves to prepare offspring for the adult environment (Blair and Raver 2012b; Bugental 2012; Ellis et al. 2011; Ellis and Del Giudice 2014). In a relatively safe, bountiful environment where there is less maternal stress, mothers invest more resources in caring for their offspring. These offspring consequently develop strong top-down regulation of the stress response. Conversely, mothers who inhabit a relatively unsafe, impoverished environment invest fewer resources in maternal care, resulting in offspring that have a more readily activated and exaggerated stress response. This is understandable from an evolutionary perspective because impoverished environments are associated with nutritional deprivation, violence, and infection; weaker top-down control of the stress response provides enhanced protection against all three conditions. For example, weaker top-down control promotes greater anxiety, fear, caution, avoidance, defensive hostility, inflammation, immune reactivity, and mobilization of stored energy: all adaptive responses to a high-risk, resource-scarce environment (Blair and Raver 2012b; Cameron et al. 2005; Matthews and Phillips 2012).

This evolutionary perspective on early development constitutes a fundamental shift from a "rational top-down vs. irrational bottom-up," "healthy vs. pathological," "adaptive vs. maladaptive," or "well-regulated vs. dysregulated" normative framework (where rational, healthy, adaptive, and well-regulated are good and their opposites are bad) to an evolutionary framework in which environmental conditions steer development along canalized trajectories that make strategic sense under those conditions. In this light, irrational, pathological, maladaptive and dysregulated may indeed entail undesirable elements, but this negative aspect is understood as the cost of an early adverse environment regulating, in a once-off canalized fashion, for a strategic developmental trajectory that makes the best of a bad situation (Ellis and Bjorklund 2012). "The best" may still constitute a high-risk strategy that jeopardizes the person's health and survival (Ellis et al. 2012).

This view coheres with a wide range of evidence drawn from organisms as diverse as microorganisms, plants, insects, fishes, amphibians, reptiles, and mammals pertaining to the general notion of life history strategies (Bruton 1989) and, in particular, to the notion of psychosocial acceleration (Belsky et al. 1991; Ellis and Bjorklund 2012; Ellis et al. 2009). Psychosocial acceleration entails early maturation and a suite of behaviors that are diametrically opposed to development under benign conditions: early sexual debut, sexual

promiscuity, early first birth, unstable pair bonds, and limited parental investment in many closely spaced offspring (Ellis and Del Giudice 2014; Ellis et al.
2009). The strategic sense in such a trajectory is described as follows (Belsky
and Pluess 2013:1246):

> [F]rom the standpoint of reproductive fitness, it is better to "live fast and die
> young," having offspring along the way, than to die (or become disabled) before
> getting the chance to reproduce. Thus, adolescents who, for example, respond to
> dangerous environments by developing insecure attachments, adopting oppor-
> tunistic, advantage-taking interpersonal orientations, engaging in externalizing
> behavior, discounting the future, and experiencing early sexual debut are no less
> functional or even less regulated than are those responding to a well-resourced
> and supportive social environment by developing the opposing characteristics
> and orientations.

Animal evidence in support of psychosocial acceleration is found in the offspring of low LG rat mothers who demonstrate accelerated sexual maturation,
increased sexual behavior, and reduced parental investment (low LG behavior) (Cameron et al. 2005). In this light, limited parental investment serves
as a regulatory signal whereby parents forecast the prevailing environmental
conditions their newly born offspring are likely to encounter (for details of the
mechanisms undergirding fast versus slow life history strategies in rats, see
Cameron et al. 2011; Cameron 2011).

There is considerable evidence consistent with the idea that environmental
conditions regulate parental behavior to shape stress responsiveness, reproductive strategy, and other behaviors in human offspring. For example, adverse socioeconomic conditions are stressful and engender parental anxiety
and depression. These, in turn, undermine maternal buffering capacity and
reduce responsiveness toward newborns, infants, and children (Cameron et
al. 2005; Cameron et al. 2011; Murray et al. 2010). Similarly, environmental
adversity (e.g., low SES, father absence, maternal depression) disturbs parent-
child interactions and is associated with developmental trajectory differences
in life history styles (e.g., early menarche, early sexual debut, greater promiscuity) in human females (Belsky et al. 1991). For example, in a study of 958
American youth, household unpredictability and economic harshness—mediated by maternal depression (all measured from 0–5 years old) and maternal
sensitivity (measured at ±6–8 years)—all predicted psychosocial acceleration
as indexed by sexual behavior at the age of 15 years (Belsky et al. 2012).
Similarly, Simpson et al. (2012) studied a sample of 162 males and females
born into low SES characterized by varying levels of instability and stress.
Individuals who experienced greater unpredictability (measured by changes
in maternal employment, residence, and cohabiting male partners) and more
rapid environmental change during the first five years of life demonstrated
features of a faster life history strategy at 23 years of age. These features (more
sexual partners, more aggressive and delinquent behaviors) are consistent with

diminished top-down self-regulation. Notably, these features were unrelated to environmental adversity experienced between 6 and 16 years of age, again evidence of once-off canalization during a sensitive period early in life.

The potential costs of psychosocial acceleration characterized by features such as exaggerated stress responses, precocious sexual debut, sexual promiscuity, early menarche, unstable pair bonds, early reproduction, decreased parental investment, impulsivity, aggressive social attitudes, etc. are significant. Nevertheless, while the increased personal risks associated with the prevalence of these traits under conditions of socioeconomic adversity are normatively undesirable, they should not be seen primarily as pathology, dysregulation, dysfunction, or maladaptative. From the evolutionary perspective of life history theory, these social maladies are being regulated for as unavoidable costs of strategies evolved to make the best of adverse conditions. In other words, these traits are no less functional than their normatively positive opposites (Belsky and Pluess 2013; Ellis and Bjorklund 2012; Ellis and Del Giudice 2014; Ellis et al. 2011; Ellis et al. 2012), and trying to cure these social "maladies" without addressing the environmental context that regulates for them will be of limited value (Cameron et al. 2005).

For Better or For Worse: Individual Differences in Sensitivity to the Environment

A powerful, unifying biopsychosocial understanding of childhood development centered on relations between environmental adversity, caregiving behaviors, stress-response systems, genetics/epigenetics, neurodevelopmental canalization, and self-regulation is currently emerging (Blair and Raver 2012a; Garner and Shonkoff 2012). A comprehensive account of many other important dimensions flowing from and into this core biopsychosocial framework is, however, beyond the present scope. Here we wish to highlight some dimensions that are pertinent to the issue of peacebuilding.

First, not all offspring follow the same developmental trajectory in response to the same environmental conditions. In some individuals, adverse conditions may yield normatively negative, below average outcomes, whereas enriched conditions may yield normatively positive, above average outcomes for the same individuals. This is known as the "for better or for worse" model, where "better" and "worse" are relative to the case where yet other individuals follow average (or "middle of the road") trajectories *irrespective of whether they experience adverse or enriched rearing conditions.* The former type of individual is known as an "orchid" (i.e., a spectacular plant which either flourishes or withers according to the right or wrong conditions), whereas the latter are known as "dandelions" (a nondescript plant which grows equally well under a wide range of conditions) (Ellis et al. 2011). Thus, adverse conditions associated with structural violence not only blight communities with normatively negative human capital ("for worse" orchid outcomes), they also simultaneously rob such communities of their brightest prospects ("for worse" orchids hold the highest "for better" potential, including the potential for peacebuilding) (Ellis et al. 2011).

Second, transgenerational inheritance of canalized developmental trajectories can occur in various ways. As for the HPA axis, maternal licking and grooming behavior also determines epigenetic marking of the estrogen receptor alpha gene in the hypothalamus of female rodent pups. When they become pregnant themselves, estrogen receptor alpha influences the sensitivity of these hypothalamic cells to estrogen. This sensitivity, in turn, predicts the quality of maternal care that these second generation mothers render to their offspring, who later pass the same traits onto female offspring of the third generation (Gudsnuk and Champagne 2012). Thus gene expression profiles of both the CORT receptor gene and the estrogen receptor alpha gene (which determine the HPA stress response and maternal LG behavior, respectively) can be inherited over at least three generations, not via genetic information but via successive parental behavior to epigenetic marks cycles. Maternal style in humans is also passed from one generation to the next; similar neuroendocrine (Gonzalez et al. 2012) and epigenetic mechanisms are also likely involved (Cameron 2011).

Parental *experience* can also be transmitted *without* the mediation of parental *behavior*. To illustrate, we cite two possibilities: one via fathers, the other via mothers. In male mice conditioned to associate a fearful event (electric shock to the feet) with a specific odor, Dias and Ressler (2014) report that this fear-odor association was transferred to male offspring (who had never experienced the electric shock themselves) by means of epigenetic methylation differences in sperm DNA, involving the gene for the olfactory protein responsible for detecting the odor in question. This epigenetic information was also coded into the sperm of the second generation. Similarly, Gapp et al. (2014) found that early trauma resulted in changes to sperm RNA, which were inherited by the next generation.

Increasing numbers of studies are relating prenatal maternal mental health to neurobehavioral outcomes of offspring (Graignic-Philippe et al. 2014), and epigenetic mechanisms have been found to play a role (Keverne 2014) as does the placenta. The placenta serves as an interface between the developing fetal brain and the adult maternal brain as well as a conduit whereby external conditions can influence fetal development (Broad and Keverne 2011). The fetus controls its own destiny, but only if the mother can respond optimally. Thus the placenta produces hormones which suppress maternal fertility, reduce maternal anxiety, and increase maternal food intake in advance of fetal demands. Placental hormones also ensure production and postpartum delivery of milk, time of parturition, and priming of the maternal brain for maternal care.

These intergenerational adaptive events require coadaptation across fetal and maternal genomes. This is facilitated by co-expression of genes in both the developing hypothalamus and developing placenta; at the same time, the placenta is instructing the maternal hypothalamus. Critical periods for regulation of the developing fetal brain and developing placenta are co-adaptively co-regulated by the same epigenetically regulated genes (Keverne 2014). Under beneficent environmental conditions, therefore, offspring which receive normatively "optimal" gestational nourishment and maternal care will themselves develop a brain that is epigenetically predisposed to gestation, mothering, and general health trajectories that are normatively "optimal" and adaptive (for these conditions). Equally, however, environmental sources of stress and trauma to the mother transmit to the next generation predispositions toward gestational, maternal care, and general health trajectory consequences that are normatively "suboptimal" (but nevertheless adaptive for these adverse conditions), as described above. In other words, environmental regulation for different strategic life history trajectories begins in the womb, and the maternal stress response to adverse environmental conditions mediates the regulatory impact of the greater environment on fetal development.

To the extent that such mechanisms of transgenerational transmission of developmental trajectories occurs in humans, their significance lies in just how deeply structural violence and structural peace become embedded in a population across multiple generations. This, again, underlines the limitations of transient peacemaking in the absence of peacebuilding that endures for multiple generations.

Environmental Regulation of Threat-Related Built-In Intelligence

Here we examine in greater detail top-down and bottom-up modes of built-in intelligence for dealing with threat and their regulation. Humans, like most mammals, are highly dependent on others. Individual and close interpersonal relationships including parent-infant dyads and adult pair bonds are critical to both survival and reproduction. In this context, neuropeptide hormones synthesized in the brain, including oxytocin and vasopressin, have emerged as critical players in the body's management of both social behavior and reactions to both threat and safety. Other essential elements, largely outside the current focus, include sensory inputs, salience, reward, and threat detection pathways, the hypothalamic-pituitary-gonadal axis, and the hypothalamic-pituitary-adrenal stress response axis.

The Neurobiology of Responses to Threat, Stressors, and Trauma

The mammalian body thrives and reproduces most successfully under conditions of safety. However, evolved features of the human nervous system also exist to support survival and reproduction in the face of danger or threat. The physiological and behavioral management of threats depends on neural and endocrine systems that evolved from reptilian ancestors with modifications that are specifically mammalian and which over the course of evolution were adaptive (Porges 2011). In humans, the most complex defense strategies rely on cognitive strategies. These strategies may include elaborate physical or ritualized systems which, although primarily cognitive in implementation, may be motivated by more ancient physiological processes. Many of the apparently irrational behaviors shown by humans may be best understood in the context of attempts to provide physical and emotional safety for ourselves or for those to whom we feel attached.

Examples in humans of cognitive responses to a potential danger might range from simple avoidance of threatening situations to the development of weapons of mass destruction. However, more primitive strategies, based on older brain structures, also provide substrates for our responses to environmental and social demands or threats. Understanding the nature of ancient coping strategies and physical and emotional mechanisms associated with these strategies helps to demystify the human response to stress and trauma.

The sequence of physiological and behavioral responses that follow a stressful or traumatic experience may be considered to be adaptive coping and can follow several patterns, including cognitive planning as well as active or passive coping patterns that are dependent on this more primitive survival-based system. Complicating our understanding of the most ancient coping mechanisms is the fact that this system evolved before the modern neocortex and operates largely below the level of cognitive control. Moreover, when emotional feelings can be detected, they are often diffuse and difficult for the cortex to interpret.

In general, active coping is associated with physical mobilization (e.g., fight or flight) and in some cases emotional anxiety (mental mobilization). Passive coping is characterized by immobility (freeze) and behavioral and psychological depression. Individuals may show consistent and chronic coping responses or may shift from one state to another, in some cases due to changes in the external environment or in response to mental states. Oxytocin and vasopressin are powerful hormones/neuromodulators that have the capacity to modulate emotional states and traits and may help in the understanding of the developmental consequences of stressful or traumatizing experiences (Carter 2005; Carter et al. 2009; Carter and Porges, this volume). For example, the presence of high levels of oxytocin may be capable of creating a sense of safety, allowing both social engagement and refined forms of top-down cognition. Oxytocin may also have the capacity to regulate its own receptor, especially in early life. Vasopressin, in contrast, is a hypothalamic component of the HPA axis, often working in conjunction with corticotropin-releasing hormone. Vasopressin contributes to bottom-up self-regulatory biological states associated with vigilance, hyperarousal, and reactive aggression (Carter and Porges 2013). The actions of vasopressin on the central and autonomic nervous systems may help to explain several of the consequences of early adversity. At present, however, the nature of the dynamic interaction between oxytocin and vasopressin is poorly understood.

In mammals, including humans, the response to severe threat or traumatic experiences depends on the intensity and chronicity of the experience, as well as the history, age, gender, and health status of the individual. Clues to the body's response to traumatic experiences can be extracted from awareness of the evolution of the nervous system and the hierarchical nature of responses to stress or challenge. According to the polyvagal theory (Porges 2011), in the face of an acute mild stress and in the relative absence of a history of trauma, top-down self-regulatory cognitive responses and social engagement may be sufficient to allow adaptation and coping. More severe stressors may trigger active coping responses, such as increases in heart rate (sympathetic nervous system activation) and a relative reduction in vagal (parasympathetic) activity. These responses would facilitate bottom-up self-regulatory mobilization and if necessary defensive attack or escape. In response to an extreme stressor, and especially after repeated or chronic stress, the body may show even more primitive bottom-up parasympathetic (vagal) mental and physical shut-down responses. Shut-down responses, and other forms of passive bottom-up self-regulatory coping, are marked by reductions in heart rate and blood pressure, sometimes including difficulties in accessing cognition, dissociative states, and even loss of consciousness and fainting.

Exposure to chronic stresses, including circumstances that lead to flashbacks and the reliving of traumatic events, may over time create symptoms which are lumped together under the clinical diagnosis of PTSD. Such responses would be adaptive in protecting vital functions, such as breathing and blood flow to the heart or brainstem, but are incompatible with active forms of social engagement behaviors and higher cognitive functions. PTSD is sometimes characterized by mobilization, but may also include vacillations between hyperarousal and shutdown responses. Under these conditions it is possible for individuals to have a reduced capacity for top-down behavioral inhibition, and states of reactive aggression or rage may appear.

The vulnerability to shifting into either hypermobilized states or hypomobilized behavioral and autonomic shutdown appears to depend in part on brainstem and autonomic pathways that are shared among mammals. These pathways may have evolved in the evolutionary transition from reptiles to mammals (Porges 2011). The enlargement of the neocortex which characterizes primates is supported by modifications in the autonomic nervous system, including a more elaborate parasympathetic system, comprising a myelinated vagus nerve which makes for more efficient top-down self-regulatory control. The myelinated vagus originates in brainstem nuclei that are partly regulated by mammalian neuropeptides, including vasopressin and oxytocin.

The presence of the myelinated vagus normally helps to keep the cortex and hence top-down self-regulation online. However, as described above, newer components of this system may be withdrawn under stress, thereby bringing bottom-up self-regulatory systems online, allowing for more primitive fight, flight, or freeze survival functions, including supplying oxygen and nutrients to tissues.

Safety in the Brain: The Role of Others

Barring immediate physical dangers and privations, "the environment" for young children (and indeed all humans) consists of other people. For a child, this means close associations with others such as parents, other caretakers, and immediate relatives. In other words the environment is a social one, and the infant's brain comes prepared to socialize from the very beginning (Siegel 2012). Thus the neural substrates that subserve responses to both threat (as detailed above) and safety are regulated, with exquisite sensitivity, by social interaction.

At birth, humans as well as some of the simplest mammals demonstrate complex built-in social intelligence. Research in highly social rodents, such as prairie voles, provides evidence of the capacity of comparatively simple nervous systems to develop lasting social bonds and other complex patterns of sociality, and to use social support to modulate reactivity to environmental challenges (Carter 1998). This form of social intelligence depends, at least in part, on primitive components of the nervous system, which have been in existence long before the evolution of human behavior. An understanding of these older systems is shedding new light onto the deeper biology of human social behaviors.

Causal mechanisms of social (sometimes called prosocial) behaviors are often hard to identify and thus have sometimes been assumed to be simply the absence of aggression. Increasing evidence indicates, however, that social stimuli can induce a cascade of endocrine and autonomic events that may facilitate sociality. For example, male prairie voles are highly social, even prior to reproductive experience, and show parental behavior within seconds of first exposure to an unrelated infant (Kenkel et al. 2012b). The high level of male parenting behavior seen in this species is partly mediated by a unique cocktail of hormones, which include social neuropeptides implicated in other forms of social behavior (Carter and Porges, this volume). Even the presence of an unrelated infant induces (regulates) a transient release of oxytocin and vasopressin in male prairie voles, resulting in both nurturant and protective behaviors toward the infant. The physiological state associated with alloparental behavior in prairie voles also includes activation of both the sympathetic and parasympathetic nervous system; this allows males to show high levels of nurture toward offspring while retaining a capacity for defensive behavior, which may be necessary to protect the young from potential threats (Kenkel et al. 2013).

During interactions between a human mother and child, the nervous systems of both engage in a coordinated interplay of neuronal activation as well as production of neurotransmitters, hormones, and neuropeptides. Cues from one partner (e.g., eye gaze, smiling, vocalizing) are met by the other with rhythmic, contingent alternation or reciprocation at the behavioral level, while at the brain level these activities are accompanied by increased levels of oxytocin in both partners. In moments of extreme behavioral synchrony during a face-to-face interaction, physiological synchrony increases between mothers and their infants so that they share virtually identical heart rhythms within lags of less than one second (Feldman et al. 2012).

Based on information reviewed in the preceding sections, it can be hypothesized that the primal experience of safety for an infant is one which combines synchrony with another person, augmented levels of oxytocin, and activation of the myelinated vagus and the parasympathetic nervous system. *Social interactions permit not only adaptive responses critical in the face of threats but also the use of cues associated with safety to allow growth, restoration, and development of critical social skills and social affiliations.*

Childhood Adversity and Life-Time Trauma Exposure

Adequate nurturance in early life may predispose an individual to deal more effectively, in a top-down fashion, with subsequent experiences of trauma. Conversely, neglect or abuse in early life may sensitize an individual to bottom-up overreacting in later life. The following account of PTSD exemplifies the downsides of bottom-up self-regulation.

Several studies have repeatedly shown that the number of different traumatic event types experienced influences not only risk for PTSD, but also the severity of PTSD symptoms as well as the likelihood of spontaneous remission (Kolassa et al. 2010b; Mollica et al. 1998; Neugebauer et al. 2009; Neuner et al. 2004). It appears that there is no such thing as ultimate resilience for the development of psychopathology in the face of trauma. If traumatic load is extremely high, the risk for PTSD approaches asymptotically to 100% (Kolassa et al. 2010b).

Genetic factors seem to play a role in the individual risk for PTSD, particularly genetic factors which influence processes of memory formation (Wilker et al. 2014), such as fear conditioning, fear extinction, emotional memory formation, and long-term memory formation (Kolassa et al. 2010a, b; de Quervain et al. 2007; de Quervain et al. 2012; Wilker et al. 2013). Thus, something which might be assumed to be evolutionarily adaptive—good fear conditioning, good (emotional) and long-term memory formation—can become maladaptive in the case of trauma, leading to more (built-in, but not so intelligent!) suffering (de Quervain et al. 2012). In other words, PTSD appears to be a case of an adaptive mechanism being pushed by the environment beyond its regulatory limits, from one embedded canal into another, from which it is unable to return even after the environmental threat has gone.

Parental Mediation in Traumatic Stress

In war-torn societies such as Sri Lanka and Afghanistan, it has been shown that mass trauma has an impact on children and their families. The domestic violence present in these and other war-plagued countries puts additional traumatic load on these children. In Afghanistan, family size, child labor, and poverty predicted domestic violence, whereas in Sri Lanka, fathers' drug abuse predicted child maltreatment (Catani et al. 2008; Panter-Brick et al. 2009, 2011). It is likely that parental substance abuse increases as a means of coping with trauma in war-torn societies. Children of mothers with PTSD have an increased risk for child maltreatment (De Bellis et al. 2001; Chemtob et al. 2013). Children of substance-abusing parents are more likely to be exposed to family violence (Dube et al. 2001b). Traumatized parents are persistently unable to experience positive emotions (e.g., loving feelings, psychic numbing) and show a marked alteration in arousal and reactivity. As predicted by the hierarchical organization of the nervous system (Porges 2011), traumatized parents are more likely to exhibit hypervigilance, irritability, aggression, reckless, or self-destructive behavior. All of these can severely impact the parent-child relationship and thus the child's mental and physical health via alterations in systems underlying parent-child attachment (such as altered oxytocin and vasopressin levels). Under severe conditions these may alter epigenetic imprinting, with broad consequences for developmental trajectories and adult outcomes, possibly crossing several generations.

Distinct Relational Models Regulate Built-In Intelligence Differently

Relational Models in Early Development

Given the relational nature of peace and violence, it is not possible to understand causes or triggers of violence, or the perceived nature of injustice or normative expectations, without reference to the possible types of relationships and the nature of groups. From the earliest dyadic interaction of a newborn infant with the mother, to participation in ever-widening circles of family, friendships, and myriad group affiliations and alienations established over a lifetime, humans engage in relationships, in and through groups.

Fiske (1992, 2004) proposes that humans construct their relations in essentially four models, based on communalism, authority/hierarchy, equality, or equity (proportionality). Each of the models entails a different set of norms, expectations, and responses to deviation. Each entails a different understanding of justice and morality (Sunar 2009; Rai and Fiske 2011). And each holds the potential to contribute to either violence or peace, depending on circumstances. Predispositions to construe relations in these four models appear early in life: first as love and attachment plus sensitivity to helpful versus harmful actors (communal sharing), sensitivity to and understanding of dominance and hierarchy (authority ranking), demands for and proclivities toward equal sharing, turn-taking and reciprocity (equality matching), and somewhat later as demands for proportional fairness (market pricing).

It is a well-established finding that infants show signs of strong attachment to their caretakers before the end of the first year of life, and that security of the attachment predicts positive development into later childhood, with better social skills, self-regulation and resilience found in children with secure attachment histories compared to those with insecure attachment histories. Like other built-in intelligence, attachment is seen to be regulated by environmental factors such as caretaker sensitivity to the infant's needs or through "the dyadic regulation of emotion" (Sroufe 1996). It can also be a canalizing factor that influences adult experiences of romantic love (Hazan and Shaver 1987).

Other early developments which serve to bond baby and caretaker were reviewed above (see discussion on social neuropeptides). Through interactions with the caretaker(s), the infant repeatedly experiences closeness, safety, need satisfaction, and trust in concert with the operation and regulation of these neuropeptides and other brain mechanisms, including the resonance of shared brain states and synchronized behavior. All these experiences set the stage for full participation in the communal sharing relational model, with its defined boundaries, ethic of mutual help, and frequent induction of shared brain states through such modalities as music, rhythm, and food sharing. It is likely that this is the first relational model constructed by the infant mind, and the one in which most people continue to feel most comfortable, even in adult life. As with attachment processes, failure to experience basic trust in infancy can be a canalizing factor that leads to great difficulties in establishing and maintaining satisfactory relationships in later life.

Although infant sensitivity to dominance relations and hierarchy has been little studied, very recent investigations have found that dominance relations can be recognized as early as 10 months of age (Thomsen et al. 2011). Mascaro and Csibra (2014) found further that at 15 months, infants were able to learn linear (hierarchical) dominance structures more easily than circular structures. These findings suggest that very young children are prepared to notice and mentally represent dominance and hierarchies even before they are able to walk, and long before they can engage in the rough-and-tumble play of the preschool years (age three to four years), in which they establish their own dominance relations (Smith and Connolly 1980). According to Boyce et al. (2012a), dominance hierarchies are well-established in kindergarten classrooms (at age five to six years). These findings suggest strongly that children have an early-developing propensity to recognize dominance, to make sense of it (e.g., as linear hierarchies), to participate in dominance contests, and to accept their own place in the hierarchy. Even though dominance hierarchies would appear to be nearly ubiquitous in the modern world, Boyce et al.'s findings suggest that subordination, even at the age of five years in the relatively benign context of a kindergarten classroom, may have negative effects on children's development; this may be a clue to the pernicious effects of structural violence as manifested in status, class, or subjugation in the larger society.

The chief concern of the equality matching model is fairness, defined in terms of equality and reciprocity, supported by at least a rudimentary conception of rules or normativeness governing rights and obligations. Recent studies have begun to show that this concern has also very deep developmental, probably evolutionary roots (for a discussion on on reciprocal altruism, see Trivers 1971). For example, Rakoczy and Schmidt (2013) reviewed evidence for the "early ontogeny of social norms," showing that children as young as two years of age not only understand that social activities are governed by norms but they also enforce norms on third parties. There is considerable evidence that children from early in their second year onward look longer at unequal distributions or otherwise indicate that equal distributions are expected or approved (Geraci and Surian 2011; Schmidt and Sommerville 2011; Sommerville et al. 2013). When making distributions themselves, 3 1/2-year-olds allocated items to figures who had previously shared, showing awareness of the principle of reciprocity (Olson and Spelke 2008). Three-year-olds also shared the rewards from a joint task equally (Warneken et al. 2011). From these findings we can infer that children are prepared, from an early age, to judge the normative appropriateness of distributions, approving of equal distributions and disapproving of unequal distributions, and to require others to follow the norms of equality and reciprocity. These norms can be applied within a group (e.g., among siblings or in a classroom) or they can be applied to relations with new acquaintances or between groups.

It is very likely that the proportionality rule and the concept of common currency are not cognitively accessible to children until somewhat older ages. However, soon after starting school they must master the idea of "marks" or "grades," which is a system based on proportionality and readily incorporated into the general notion of "fairness."

These models are by no means mutually exclusive; they coexist in nested and/or partially overlapping configurations. We can see then that use of various relational models, with their potentials for different forms of peace and order as well as for conflict and violence, begins to manifest itself very early in life. Let us look briefly at some of the implications for peace and violence.

A communal group is characterized by the equivalence of its members, who are defined as members by clear group boundaries. Members are to be helped, when in need, protected, and trusted; however, there is no such obligation to outside individuals or groups. Indeed, when De Dreu et al. (2012) administered oxytocin intranasally to participants in a competitive game, they found that protection and trust of in-group members increased while defensive aggression toward competing groups increased. They concluded that "oxytocin appears pivotal in up-regulating the human response to (arbitrary) in-group/out-group distinctions, shifting the focus from protecting and promoting oneself toward protecting and promoting members of the in-group. This effect of oxytocin may also be seen at the individual level, for example in mothers' protection of their infants from strangers (Mah et al. 2014) and in social selectivity and exclusion in a wide variety of group-living mammals (Anacker and Beery 2013). It may appear paradoxical that the relational model which appears most intrinsically harmonious and peaceable is also intrinsically susceptible to suspicion and aggression toward out-groups, but inclusion *ipso facto* requires exclusion (for a discussion on parochial altruism, see Bernhard et al. 2006).

Communal and authority-based relational models provide members with no tools to deal with other groups other than competition. This can easily lead to hostility (Sherif et al. 1954/1961) or avoidance, neither of which offers a peaceable option in a crowded world.

In contrast, the "equality matching" model can be used both within and between groups. Within a group, equality matching leads to a demand for justice and rights which can be satisfied by equal exchanges and distributions, reciprocity, turn-taking, and other forms of procedural justice. This model can be seen as deriving from the evolutionarily selected tendency to "reciprocal altruism," as conceptualized by Trivers (1971; see also Sunar 2009). These methods of ensuring justice can also be used by groups in their relations with other groups (e.g., in trading relationships, agreements, and treaties).

By "pricing" not only commodities but behaviors (e.g., labor) in a "common currency," it becomes possible to apply an equality principle to proportions rather than to actual quantities: the principle of equity (outcomes should be proportional to inputs). Legal-rational systems of law as well as corporations and markets make use of this model, allocating everything from salaries to jail terms on the principle of equity. Like equality matching, market pricing also provides groups (including companies, governments, and international entities) with reciprocity-based tools for establishing exchange and agreements.

Unlike the communal and authority-based relational models, equality matching and proportional pricing are not defined by closeness, sharing, or care, nor do they require sharply defined boundaries (except for the case of distribution). They represent concerns for justice, rights, and reciprocity, which are conducive to both peacemaking (as violence reduction) and peacebuilding (as violence prevention).

The logic of this analysis of different varieties of human relating suggests that the conditions which regulate for peaceful versus aggressive behaviors may vary widely, depending on the relational model in which people are operating. It is important to keep in mind that changes in relational models themselves are regulated by environmental conditions, including environments the models themselves engender. Similarly, each model may be challenged by different circumstances or behaviors so that normal peaceful relations turn conflictual and possibly violent. Punishment, revenge, and rebellion are common responses to norm violation, harm-doing, failures of reciprocity, and exploitation. The use of the various relational models, with their potentials for different forms of peace and order as well as for conflict and violence, begins to manifest itself very early in life.

Altruism in Early Childhood and Evolution

The theoretical position outlined at the beginning of this chapter maintains that nature and nurture are inseparable, that what we need to conceptualize and study is how the environment regulates the built-in genetic intelligence potential. This stance, however, does not obviate the need to determine what the range of expression of that genetic potential is.

It is unnecessary to document the obvious propensity of human beings, from earliest infancy, to behave in selfish ways. However, it is important to document the opposite: the motivation for and performance of altruistic acts (acts that benefit another at some cost to the self) in young children. Evolutionary theorists have shown that kin selection (Hamilton 1964) and reciprocal altruism (Trivers 1971) are plausible products of evolution, leading to a large literature supporting these sources of prosocial (albeit ultimately adaptive) behavior. Recent studies have also shown that altruistic behavior is not contingent on kinship and that reciprocity begins to appear in infancy and early childhood. Sensitivity to whether others behave in helpful or harmful ways can be seen in the first year of life (Hamlin et al. 2007; Thompson and Newton 2013), along with approval for helping and disapproval for hindering or harming. Empathetic/sympathetic behaviors are also seen very early (Hoffman 1975, 2000). Sharing (sometimes solicited, sometimes unsolicited) can be observed by at least the third year (Dunfield et al. 2011; Warneken et al. 2011; Sunar et al., under review) and under normal conditions becomes a predominant response by six to seven years of age (Brownell et al. 2009; Fehr et al. 2008).

Helping also appears early, sometime in the second year, consonant with infants' approval of helping agents (De Bellis et al. 2001; Dunfield and Kuhlmeier 2013; Warneken and Tomasello 2009b). Supporting the idea of an evolved tendency to help, human infants as well as young chimpanzees show some degree of spontaneous help toward a human trying to achieve a goal, without expecting any reward. This suggests the presence of built-in intelligence expressed as altruistically motivated help in the context of a fellow primate's goal-oriented efforts (Warneken et al. 2007; Warneken and Tomasello 2006). The important lesson to draw from these studies of the early developmental and evolutionary emergence of altruism is that helping and sharing behaviors are spontaneous in everyday social circumstances in the absence of any expectation of reward or reciprocation. Children possess built-in intelligence which, all else being equal, inclines them to initiate behavior in support of reciprocal exchanges. Indeed, prosocial behaviors appear to be the default response (i.e., a neutral environment regulates for prosocial as opposed to selfish behaviors in human infants) (Warneken and Tomasello 2006).

It is imperative not to essentialize, reify, or romaticize spontaneous prosocial behavior. However, it is useful to understand from a social evolutionary perspective that cooperation can pay such huge dividends that humans are ever alert to opportunities for cooperation and for making themselves as appealing as possible to others as potential cooperators. Sometimes cooperation yields a win-win result where both parties enjoy immediate rewards, but often one party (individual or group) helps another party without deriving any immediate benefit, but with the expectation that the favor will be returned at a later time. Dynamics like these probably drove the evolution of prosocial motivations and behaviors such as altruism, loyalty, honesty, fairness, and rule-following. While these are normatively upheld as noble qualities, they may have sprung from evolutionary self-interest and may still function in these ways, manifesting and vanishing according to what is perceived as most advantageous under a given circumstance. Thus, cooperation (especially within a group) or competition (often toward "out-group" members) may be adaptive and may coexist.

Although the signs and early forms of use of relational models as well as altruistic behavior are striking, they are far from mature and may require ingenious experimental designs to allow detection. Development of these capacities and tendencies requires not only maturation of cognitive and affective abilities (such as perspective-taking, empathy, and various aspects of self-regulation), but also exposure to and socialization into the specific ways of the surrounding culture. In other words, their development depends heavily on the social environment; to discover the extent to which canalization may belong to the "one-off" variety will require further work.

Groups: Environments of Social Development

Whenever the opportunity is there, children enter into relationships with other young children, from earliest toddlerhood, to form rudimentary groups for play (Sheridan et al. 2011; Whiting and Whiting 1975). The brain is exquisitely tuned to information from the group, so much so that reality itself can be defined by group opinion (e.g., Sherif 1936; Festinger 1954). Group acceptance and status within groups are vital matters for each individual.

In turn, individuals accept group identities with an astonishing alacrity (Tajfel 1982), showing in-group favoritism even in minimal groups. Children as young as three years of age show in-group bias, and by age 6 they begin to derogate out-groups (Buttelmann and Böhm 2014). Within groups, norms shape relational models and govern individual action; their internalization by members results in attitudes, stereotypes, and prejudices, which are also detectable by school age (McKown and Weinstein 2003). Thus some of the most basic elements in human conflict and violence—in-group vs. out-group distinctions as well as competition, stereotypes, and prejudice—are part of typically developing minds of children, experienced during the course of becoming members of a group. At the same time, they are acquiring the benefits of group living: cooperation, sharing, empathy, forgiveness, loyalty, and obedience.

Neurobiology of Groups and Shared States

Key unresolved questions remain concerning the interplay of the central and peripheral components of groups as complex biobehavioral systems that dynamically engage brain and body over the course of development (Gordon et al. 2011). Research is progressively showing that participation in groups involves an animal's genetic makeup, neuroanatomy, and neurophysiology. All group-living species, but especially primates and the large-brained sea mammals, provide remarkable examples (Connor 2010). Complexity of social groups is associated with brain size, leading to the hypothesis that the human cortex evolved to its current size and intelligence emerged, at least partially, in response to the cognitive demands of complex group environments (Dunbar 2008; see also Cummins 2005). Social neuroscience has produced much information about brain activity of individuals in various social situations. Relevant to our discussion is the finding that the brain reacts to rejection by a group with virtually the same pattern of activation seen in physical pain (Eisenberger et al. 2003). Similarly, loss of status frequently leads to depression, especially in males (Tiffin et al. 2005). Tabibnia and Lieberman (2007) found that fair compared to unfair distributions aroused distinctive patterns of brain activation, with fair distributions leading to activation of reward pathways.

Brain imaging studies are also showing that interconnectedness is not only a feature within one brain; it may also exist across brains. When we listen to music, it appears that there are many similarities in brain activation across individuals, even though the personal listening experience is idiosyncratic (Abrams et al. 2013). Humans engage in neurobehavioral synchrony during singing, chanting, dancing, or other rhythmic activities that foster affiliative relationships within groups. Similarly, when focusing on the same stimulus (be it a film, a speaker, or an athletic performance), certain brain networks exhibit a high degree of synchronization between individuals (Hasson et al. 2004). Findings regarding synchrony between infant and mother are also relevant here. Oxytocin, which is fundamental to child-adult interactions, may have evolved to facilitate both intra- and interindividual synchrony (Carter 2014).

Groups define us, but perhaps even more importantly, group discussion and action has the potential to bring about change (Lewin 1951). Because group processes are so powerful and so fundamental to the pressing issues of peace, it is thus imperative to study shared neurobiological processes beyond the individual or dyad. Advances in measuring real-time behavior in concurrence with ambulatory measures of neurophysiological activity (whether autonomic activity or the peripheral concentration of biomarkers, such as oxytocin or vasopressin) opens the way toward more advanced experimental paradigms tailor-made for investigating group processes (Gordon et al. 2014).

Can Formative Childhoods Be a Path to Peace?

To our knowledge, there is no evidence to suggest that amelioration of environmental stress for individual children or families will automatically reduce structural violence or lead to greater social harmony at the community or national levels. The evidence and theory reviewed herein indicate two extremely serious hurdles in the path between experience in early childhood and peacebuilding. Both can be best understood as paradoxes that make sense in light of the distinction between peacemaking and peacebuilding.

The first paradox, set out in detail in the foregoing sections, stems from the ultimate dependence of development on the environment, which, combined with parental mediation, canalizes and embeds neurodevelopmental trajectories characterized by greater top-down or bottom-up modes of brain function. These opposing modes of brain function are the embodiment of greater or lesser top-down self-regulatory capacities and slower versus faster life history strategies, respectively. In other words, adverse environments regulate for lower parental investment. This, in turn, regulates evolved built-in intelligence in offspring to manifest in deeply embedded, strongly canalized bottom-up accelerated developmental trajectories characterized by impulsiveness, diminished empathy, defensive hostility, short-term thinking, precocious sexuality, and diminished investment in more offspring—traits which favor reproductive survival under adverse conditions (Belsky and Pluess 2013; Ellis and Del Giudice 2014). Taken alone, this suggests that interventions aimed at supporting a high level of maternal investment would be effective in regulating for individuals with the opposite slowed developmental trajectories characterized by strong top-down inhibitory capacities, better capacities for empathy, conflict resolution and long-term thinking, delayed sexuality, and higher investment in fewer offspring. In other words, individuals adapt to make the most of favorable environmental conditions wherein reproductive survival is better served by reasoned peacemaking than by impulsive aggressive violence, which is both counterproductive and entails significant risks. However, in a context of structural violence, harsh environmental conditions can lead to reduced parental investment in offspring (both pre- and postnatally). This, in turn, will regulate bottom-up built-in intelligence for accelerated developmental trajectories. Thus, unless structural violence is also addressed, interventions which aim directly to change parenting behavior so as to steer childhood development along a "better" trajectory will be going against the grain of evolution, which cares nothing for health, morality, or peace. To the extent that structural violence persists in the environment, efforts to improve the capacity for peacemaking may often be overwhelmed by failures in peacebuilding.

The second paradox stems from the relative independence of the relational models from one another, with the result that peacemaking inclinations and abilities that are supported or useful in one model may be irrelevant or even counterproductive in others. The built-in intelligence that directs individuals to care for others in their in-group simultaneously directs them, depending on the circumstances, to ignore, compete with, exploit, or try to destroy the out-group and its members. Interventions designed to support parents in caring for their children and in preventing neglect and maltreatment are certainly beneficial to children and in fact to all family members; benefits can be expected to extend to participation in other in-groups characterized by norms of mutual help and sharing. However, the attitudes, values, and skills that serve peacemaking within the family may have only limited usefulness in intergroup relations. Favorable early experience, including experiences of bonding and trust accompanied by production of neuroactive substances (e.g., oxytocin) cannot alone prevent—and may under some circumstances actually help set the stage for—hostile attitudes and direct violence between groups.

Dealings with larger groups and with out-groups may activate entirely different relational models. Competition and its resultant victory or defeat engage the attitudes and values of authority ranking, while issues of exchange and distribution engage the relational models of equality matching or market pricing, where the basic issue is not care but rather fairness or justice. And it is justice that is the *sine qua non* for both peacemaking and peacebuilding.

Part of the reason for these potential discontinuities is the mutual independence of relational models; another part is that (direct) violence—like life history strategies—is not simply a dysfunctional, expressive response to difficult circumstances. In a very large proportion of cases, whether of individual or group violence, there is a sense in which violence, in the minds of those who engage in it, has a rationale or justification, such as self-defense, punishment, or the restoration of justice. Very rarely is it a matter of striking out blindly or without purpose. Rather, it is most often seen as a response to injustice or to violations of normative expectations in a relationship, or as instrumental in bringing about a desired change (Boehm 2012; Pinker 2011). These subjective justifications may depend strongly on construals of the immediate situation, including the relevant relational model as well as the group norms governing regulation of relationships defined by these models.

For this reason, we cannot assume that amelioration of environmental stress for individual children or families (peacemaking) will automatically reduce structural violence (peacebuilding) or lead to greater social harmony at community or national levels. Conversely, existing evidence and theory described in this chapter support the hypothesis that the reduction of structural violence (peacebuilding) will have far greater positive impact on early childhood development than the protection of early childhood development (peacemaking) can ever have on reducing direct and structural violence. Obviously, portraying these two intervention models as mutually countervailing hypotheses is an oversimplification; they must always be taken in context. Nevertheless, as a starting point, it is fundamentally necessary to separate them first and only then address any "gray" areas whenever and wherever they arise, not least because there are strong biological grounds for doing so (Cameron et al. 2005). Since reality is never black and white, much further research is vitally necessary, at multiple biopsychosocial levels, to delineate, evaluate, contrast, and better comprehend the strengths, weaknesses, and social meanings of peacemaking and peacebuilding interventions across diverse societal contexts as well as across varying time frames.

Basic Motivations and Capacities That Can Be Mobilized by Interventions

Throughout this chapter, evidence for the thesis that structural violence may overwhelm peacemaking has been advanced. Nevertheless there is evidence that social policies and a wide variety of interventions, short of wide-scale social change, can bring about some degree of real benefit to the individuals and groups. Humans have a basic capacity and motivations which allow them (as individuals and groups) to respond to and utilize these benefits for the improvement of their own and their children's lives. At this level, peacemaking and peacebuilding can be seen as overlapping to a certain extent.

According to anthropologists and primatologists (e.g., Fry, this volume; Fry and Szala 2013; de Waal 1996, 2009), tendencies that contribute to peacemaking potentials (e.g., restrained agonism, reconciliation after disputes, and continuation of social relations after reconciliation) are common throughout the class of mammals but especially among primates. Likewise, skills in negotiation and other nonviolent means of conflict resolution can be taught and learned by humans as well as other primates (Sapolsky 2013) reinforcing the assumption that such capacities can be brought to the fore by relevant social ecologies (another example of environmental regulation).

The extremely wide variation in social organization that can be observed in human societies—from egalitarian, generally peaceful foraging bands with shifting memberships to rigidly stratified caste societies, to highly mobile market economies, to aggressively militarized societies—is testimony to the malleability of *Homo sapiens*. To the extent that national and other entities are able to write their own constitutions, literally or figuratively, the creation and maintenance of more benign environments is within the realm of possibility. Indeed, legal systems, which both provide protection from criminal predation and offer procedural justice, are hypothesized to be a major factor in the reduction of direct violence (Elias 1939/2000; Pinker 2011). Other social mechanisms include a variety of methods to reduce exclusive in-group identifications and stereotyping of other groups: cross-cutting memberships and a focus on superordinate goals with benefits for both/all sides (interdependence); coalition formation, although, being formed implicitly or explicitly as defense against other groups, coalitions carry an inherent danger of conflict.

In keeping with the finding that controlling for parenting behaviors nullifies the association between SES and developmental outcomes, early intervention programs that fail to change parental behavior have been found to be of limited value (Cameron et al. 2005). Conversely, interventions that do change parental behavior can be effective, not least because they harness parents' deep desire to nurture and protect their children, a trait consistently observed across mammalian species. This primal built-in strategic motivation can be counted on across cultures and contexts, as a driving force needed to nurture children over the long periods of development required for them to develop the capacities required for self-sufficiency. Effective programs for parents build a sense of collaboration aligned with up-regulating this instinctual drive. While this is not the only motivational factor required for effective interventions (others include self or community efficacy), conscious alignment of interventions with built-in motivations increase their likelihood of success (Ellis and Bjorklund 2012).

Programs that target parents as well as those that directly target children may produce beneficial effects. Carré et al. (2014) found that young men who had received an intervention in childhood designed to reduce negative attributions in conflict situations had reduced testosterone reactivity and, in turn, lower levels of aggression in a conflict-inducing game compared with men who had not received the intervention. This reinforces the idea that experience canalizes brain processes, in this case including hormone secretion.

Another example comes from programs which target preschool and early school experiences (Killen and Turiel 1991). Since even very young children are attuned to issues of equality and equity, early age interventions that teach constructive responses to conflicts over unfairness and intergroup negotiation skills may have potential for strengthening top-down self-regulation. This, in turn, might enable more peaceful behavior in later life.

Acknowledging the potential power of group processes, one can also ask whether mothers or fathers from diverse backgrounds might form groups that transcend the usual cultural, ethnical, and religious boundaries. In their work with father support groups, this phenomena has been observed by the Mother Child Education Foundation (AÇEV): in father support groups composed of men from diverse backgrounds, united only by their concern for their children's positive development, friendships between men from different backgrounds emerged and continued past completion of the program (Koçak, pers. comm.). Here is another potential entry point for formative childhoods to support the development of more peaceful communities and societies.

The Way Forward

For many people around the world, structural violence (poverty, adversity, injustice) contributes to an adverse environment. During sensitive periods early in life, such adversity can lead to a loss of children's developmental potential and the diminishment of their mental and physical health. Helping parents invest in their children may well increase the well-being, health, and resilience of future generations. More research is needed to explore this question in both human populations as well as in animal model systems.

Initial findings in human populations are already shifting social policies at national and international levels toward greater investment in early childhood development (Shonkoff and Fisher 2013; Shonkoff and Levitt 2010; Kagitcibasi and Britto, this volume). Based on persuasive biological and related evidence, policy makers are realizing that to improve developmental outcomes, it is necessary to do more than intervene early, based on the rationale that this is the most sensitive period during which canalization occurs. Also required are long-term social policies that reduce structural violence (peacebuilding) across the life span in order to regulate for higher caregiver investment and hence for "better" developmental trajectories. High-quality, long-term peacemaking efforts at the family level that are applied across whole communities will overcome the above obstacles precisely because, and to the extent that, these efforts reduce structural violence.

More research is also needed to better understand the neurobiology of groups and how best to encourage groups to view the "other" in a more compassionate fashion (Gordon et al. 2014). Here, studies in humans and primates will be instructive, but the development of intersectorial partnerships at every level of society will be crucial if peace is to be achieved.

Early Childhood Events
and Relationships

8

Comparative and Evolutionary Perspectives

Dario Maestripieri

Abstract

Any effort to understand or shape human behavior must take into consideration the notion that there are universal tendencies to behave in particular ways, which are shared by all human beings, as well as differences in the extent to which these tendencies are expressed in particular individuals. Taking a comparative and an evolutionary perspective can help us understand the universal aspects of human aggressive and peaceful tendencies as well as their variation among individuals. Human aggressiveness has a biological basis, but it is neither necessary nor inevitable. Aggressive competition is common in some animal species but uncommon in others, depending on the ratio between the benefits of aggression (obtaining resources or status) and its costs (physical, physiological, psychological, or social). Humans have a high potential for aggression, but aggressive tendencies can be suppressed in particular environmental circumstances. Individuals living in different environments adopt slow or fast life history strategies that make them adapted to those environments. The quality of the early environment, including social experience, is a key determinant of life history strategies. Selfish, exploitative, and aggressive tendencies are more common in individuals with fast life histories who are exposed to early stress, violence, harsh parenting, or unpredictable changes in their environment.

Comparative research on animal behavior can provide the theoretical framework for understanding the effects of early experience on the development of aggressiveness and peacefulness as well as elucidate some of the physiological or social mechanisms underlying these effects. Rhesus macaque females exposed to harsh and abusive parenting in the first few months of life show anxiety, impulsiveness, and abusive parenting in adulthood. They also reach puberty earlier, are more interested in infants, and tend to be more fertile but die at a younger age than other females. Rhesus macaques raised by nurturing mothers who provide emotional and social support, but also encourage their independence, show normal maternal behavior in adulthood and greater resilience in response to stressful challenges. Even species-typical aggressive tendencies can be reduced through manipulation of the early social environment. Young rhesus macaques with high propensities for aggression can acquire effective skills for peaceful conflict resolution after cohabitation with young stumptail macaques, a species in which peaceful conflict management and resolution are more common. The findings of comparative research are therefore consistent with those of research in developmental psychology in indicating that a supportive family[1] environment and positive experiences acquired during child development are important prerequisites for the creation of peaceful and resilient adults.

Introduction

Drawing from evolutionary theory and data from comparative research with nonhuman animals, this chapter examines (a) human tendencies for aggressiveness and peacefulness in relation to other animal species, (b) individual differences in aggressive or peaceful tendencies, and (c) the role that events and relationships early in life play in the development of aggressive and peaceful tendencies. An evolutionary perspective helps us understand aggressiveness and peacefulness from a functional perspective (see also van IJzendoorn and Bakermans-Kranenburg, this volume); comparative animal research can highlight some general principles governing human development and shed light on the possible biological and environmental mechanisms underlying the effects of early experience on the expression of aggressiveness and peacefulness later in life (see also Carter and Porges; Keverne; Morgan et al.; and Fox et al., all this volume).

Aggressiveness and Peacefulness in Humans and Other Animals

Violent crimes have been reported in every human society, and wars and gen ocide have occurred repeatedly throughout human history (Pinker 2011). According to the Austrian ethologist Konrad Lorenz (1966), aggression is a necessary and inevitable aspect of human nature. He conjectured that impulses to act aggressively build up in our bodies, like fluid filling a tank. Every now and then, before the tank becomes full and the fluid overflows, our aggressive impulses need to be released, preferably channeled into nonviolent competitive activities such as sports.

Not many contemporary behavioral biologists share Lorenz's views on aggression. Human aggression is neither necessary nor inevitable, and there is no fluid filling up our tank. Human beings clearly have the ability to live peacefully in close proximity to millions of other people, as it happens in many cities around the world. Many people are fortunate not to be the victims of violent aggression ever in their lives and are exposed to violence only through television and the movies.

---

[1] Note: the term "family" is used to describe a group of people bound together by kinship, roles in caring for each other, cultural traditions, or close affiliation.

It is clear that human beings have a high potential for aggression, but it is also clear that the realization of this potential depends on many factors, most notably the environment. Other animal species have a lower potential for aggression than humans and, as a result, live in societies in which aggression and violence are rare or nonexistent. Thus, a comparative study of human and animal behavior from an evolutionary perspective can help us understand why human beings have a relatively high potential for violent aggression, and under what circumstances these aggressive tendencies are expressed or suppressed (see Georgiev et al. 2013).

From a functional perspective, aggression can be viewed as an expression of competition (see Steele et al., this volume). There are different ways in which organisms can compete for resources, however, and competitive strategies do not necessarily involve aggression. Organisms in any given species will use a particular competitive strategy only when its benefits outweigh the costs. If different competitive strategies are available, organisms will tend to use the strategy with the highest benefit-cost ratio. Thus, in some animal species, aggression is rare because individuals would not gain much from being aggressive, and therefore it is simply not worth it. In other species, aggression is rare because although individuals would gain something from it, they would have to pay a high price for it. When the benefits of aggression are high and costs are low, then a species has a high potential for aggression (Georgiev et al. 2013). But what are these benefits and costs of aggression, exactly?

Whenever aggression reflects competition for resources (e.g., food, space, mates), the benefit of aggression is obtaining those resources. Variation in the potential benefits of aggression generally depends on the characteristics of the resource: its value, abundance, spatial distribution, and extent to which it can be effectively monopolized by individuals or groups. The costs of aggression include risk of injury or death, physiological or psychological stress, energy expenditure, increased risk of attracting predators, and damage to social relationships. Generally, variation in the potential costs of aggression depends on the characteristics of the organisms and the kind of aggressive behavior they use, particularly whether they are equipped with dangerous weapons (e.g., antlers, fangs, and claws) and the extent to which they can hurt each other when they use them. In summary, the benefits of aggression depend on what animals fight about, while the costs depend on how they fight (Georgiev et al. 2013).

During our early evolutionary history, it is likely that competition for food, space, and mates played a key role in shaping human nature. Meat, fruit, and other highly caloric foods have probably been central to the human diet. The benefits of aggressive competition over valuable food that can be effectively monopolized by individuals or groups were probably high throughout the early history of *Homo sapiens* and that of our most recent hominid and nonhuman primate ancestors. Insofar as valuable food was localized in areas that could be effectively defended, aggressive competition for space was also highly beneficial. Fertile females are also a relatively rare, highly valuable, and monopolizable resource for human males, making aggression over mating highly beneficial. Whether aggressive competition is over food, territories, mates, or the social status that enhances access to these valuable resources, it is safe to conclude that ours is a species in which interindividual competition can be very intense and in which aggressive competitive strategies can be highly beneficial, especially for males (Georgiev et al. 2013).

Relative to some other mammals, humans are not particularly large and strong, they also do not come equipped with dangerous weapons, such as large and sharp canine teeth, claws, horns, or antlers. Before humans started using objects and tools as weapons, physical combat depended on hits inflicted with hands or feet and scratches or bites. Risk of injury or death from this type of fighting, however, is relatively low. Therefore, the physical costs of aggression in humans were relatively low compared to some other species. The energetic costs of human aggression are also probably lower for humans than for other, larger-bodied animals. The psychological, physiological, and social costs of aggression in humans are probably comparable to those in other social species. However, these psychosocial costs of aggression are expected to be significant mainly with regard to aggression between family members or friends and allies. These costs may be much lower if aggression is directed toward individuals from other groups, particularly enemies (see Fry, this volume). Human beings have opportunities to interact with many unrelated individuals from other groups to a much greater extent than other animals. If damage to valuable social relationships is considered one of the main social costs of aggression, then aggression toward individuals in other groups has low social costs because relationships with them are nonexistent.

The invention and elaboration of projectile weapons and the consequent ability to hit, injure, and kill other individuals from a distance have significantly reduced all the costs of aggression. Killing someone from a distance by launching a spear or firing a gun has virtually eliminated the risk of physical injury for the aggressor. In addition, the energy expenditure involved in the use of weapons is minimal. Finally, the psychological, physiological, and social costs of aggression through projectile weapons are also low, because this type of aggression allows one to attack individuals (or groups) that are not seen or known, with whom there are no social relationships of any kind, and without being exposed to the direct consequences of the violence.

With some exceptions, competition through violent aggression generally has a high benefit-cost ratio for humans (Pinker 2011; Georgiev et al. 2013). Consider, for example, the situation of the European colonial armies that first encountered the local populations in America, Africa, Asia, or Australia. The benefits of using violent aggression against the indigenous populations were enormous: taking away their land, their possessions, and even their people to use as slaves. The costs of the colonists' aggression were minimal: armed with rifles, they could quickly kill large numbers of indigenous individuals at little or no physical risk to themselves. Moreover, the indigenous populations looked different and spoke a different language, making it quite easy for the colonists to find a psychological, political, historical, or religious justification for their violence, without suffering any consequences. These unusual high benefit-cost ratios for violent aggression against people from other countries are rare or nonexistent in animals, which may explain why large-scale aggression toward conspecifics is absent in animals, with the possible exception of chimpanzees and some species of ants and termites which stage wars against other colonies, destroying or taking away their resources and enslaving the workers.

When the benefit-cost ratio of violent aggression is lowered (e.g., by punishing aggressive individuals or imposing sanctions on belligerent countries), humans do become less aggressive. Changes in the benefit-cost ratio of aggression through the history of Western civilization can also account for a historical trend in a general reduction in human violent aggression (Pinker 2011). The benefits and costs of human violent aggression may vary not only over historical time but also in relation to geographic location, culture, education, intelligence, religion, availability of resources, and many other factors (see Fry, this volume). Experience acquired interacting with one's environment early in life is a particularly powerful determinant of aggressiveness or peacefulness later in life (see also Steele et al., this volume). Evolutionary biology provides theoretical reasons to indicate why this should be the case, and comparative research with animals illustrates some of the mechanisms underlying these effects.

Early Environment and Individual Differences in Aggressiveness and Peacefulness: Life History Theory

Life history theory is a branch of evolutionary biology (mainly derived from research in animal behavioral ecology) that addresses the way organisms allocate time and energy to the various activities that comprise their life cycle, such as growth, reproductive maturation, mating, and parenting (e.g., Kaplan and Gangestad 2005). Organisms have limited amounts of resources, such as energy and time, to devote to these activities, and if they invest heavily in one of them, they can invest less in others. In other words, there are trade-offs between activities. For example, young individuals who invest heavily in their own growth cannot invest as much in reproduction, so that in many cases reproduction is delayed until growth is almost completed. Similarly, adults that invest heavily in parenting cannot invest as much in mating and vice versa.

Life history theory postulates that within a population, there should be a great deal of interindividual variation in traits related to survival or reproduction because different individuals can find themselves in dramatically different environmental conditions. Different environments pose different problems: variable life history strategies usually represent adaptive solutions to these problems. In addition, life history strategies are, in part, genetically based.

Natural selection tends to maintain genetic variation when there are multiple ecological niches in the environment, and individuals are able to select the niche that best fits their genotype and phenotype. In these heterogeneous environments, natural selection may favor fixed alternative phenotypes (i.e., specialists), which can be based on DNA sequence variation (polymorphisms). In other cases, life history strategies develop early in life, on the basis of input provided by the environment (for a discussion of the role of gene-environment interactions in brain development, see Keverne, this volume). Typically, organisms acquire information about their environment early: in some cases, through environmental gestational effects before birth, but most commonly during infancy or childhood. Early environmental conditions can shape life history strategies through developmental plasticity (West-Eberhard 2003). In a population, one should expect a balance between genetic and environmental determination of life history strategies such that both "specialists" (fixed phenotypes) and "generalists" (plastic phenotypes) should be found (Wilson and Yoshimura 1994). Moreover, even among the generalists, children may show differential sensitivity to environmentally induced effects on behavioral, psychological, and physiological functioning (Belsky 1997; Belsky et al. 2007; Boyce and Ellis 2005).

The main aspects of the environment that affect the development of life history strategies are resource availability, extrinsic morbidity/mortality,[2] and unpredictability, as signaled by observable cues (e.g., Del Giudice et al. 2011). The availability of food in the environment is generally signaled by caloric intake. Energetic stress during prenatal or early postnatal life can cause the developing individual to adopt a slow life history strategy, characterized by slower growth, delayed sexual maturation, low gonadal steroid production, small adult body size, and low fecundity. Developmental responses to resource scarcity, therefore, include trade-offs that favor maintenance over growth, future over current reproduction (late age at first birth), and offspring quality over quantity (low offspring number) (e.g., Ellis 2004; Del Giudice 2009; Del Giudice et al. 2011). Fast life history strategies depend on adequate energetic resources to support growth and development. Once this energetic threshold is crossed, other environmental conditions become salient determinants of life history strategy: extrinsic morbidity/mortality and unpredictability (Chisholm 1993). When environmental factors cause high extrinsic morbidity/mortality, many adults in the population are likely to die at a relatively young age. Cues of high levels of extrinsic morbidity/mortality may involve infectious diseases and exposure to violence, psychosocial stress, dangerous ecological conditions, or harsh parenting styles. These environmental cues can cause individuals to adopt fast life history strategies: they mature and start mating early, mate frequently, and invest relatively little in relationships and children (Belsky et

---

[2] Extrinsic morbidity/mortality refers to the probability that an individual will die or get sick for environmental causes that are beyond the individual's control.

al. 1991). In general, high extrinsic morbidity/mortality favors quantity versus quality of offspring. Similar fast life history strategies can also result from environmental unpredictability.

Although life history strategies refer mainly to growth- and reproduction-related traits, such as maturation timing, age at first reproduction, fertility, and number of sexual partners, they can include a much broader range of traits and behaviors (Del Giudice 2009; Del Giudice et al. 2011). For example, human males adopting a fast life history strategy must compete intensely with other males and attract a high number of females. This is likely to involve status-seeking behavior and considerable investment in traits and displays that women find attractive in short-term mates, such as verbal and creative displays, competitive sports, or humor (Del Giudice et al. 2011). The cues of environmental risk that drive the choice of the strategy will also prompt higher risk-taking in other domains (e.g., exploration, fighting, and dangerous sexual displays), preference for immediate over delayed rewards, and impulsivity (Del Giudice et al. 2011). In general, life history strategies play a powerful role in the organization of behavior. Traits and behaviors that covary along life history dimensions form a broad, integrated cluster, which includes exploration/learning styles, mating and sexual strategies, pair bonding, parenting styles, status- and dominance-seeking, risk-taking, impulsivity, aggression, cooperation, and altruism. Correlations within this cluster have been documented both in humans and other animals (Del Giudice et al. 2011). Included in this are evolved physiological mechanisms (e.g., hormones of the hypothalamic-pituitary-adrenal (HPA) and the hypothalamic-pituitary-gonadal (HPG) axes, or neuropeptides such as oxytocin; see Carter and Porges, this volume) capable of coordinating the development of life history-related traits in an integrated, adaptive fashion (Del Giudice et al. 2011).

Although the general physical, ecological, and life history characteristics of our species are responsible for our high potential for violent aggression, according to life history theory there is enough genetic and environmental variation within our species to cause our aggressive tendencies to be expressed in some individuals but suppressed in others. This idea has stimulated a great deal of empirical research aimed at examining the effects of early environment, genes, and gene-environment interactions on the development of many aspects of behavior, including aggressiveness and peacefulness and their physiological substrates.

Empirical Research with Animal Models of Human Behavior and Development: Two Primate Examples

Comparative research with animals has historically been a source not only of general theories and testable hypotheses but also of empirical information that can be extrapolated to humans (for many examples of this, see Carter and

Porges; Keverne; and Morgan et al., this volume). Nonhuman primates are excellent animal models for research on human behavior and development. The primate species that are phylogenetically closest to humans, such as apes and Old World monkeys, are particularly good animal models because they are likely to share with humans not only homologies (similarities due to common descent) but also analogies (similarities due to adaptation to similar environments) in their behavioral and psychological functioning.

My collaborators and I have conducted research on the effects of early experience on development in rhesus macaques for over twenty years. In one project, we examined the intergenerational transmission of abusive parenting in a population of approximately 1,500 rhesus macaques at the Yerkes National Primate Research Center of Emory University. Previous studies had shown that 5–10% of adult females in this population abuse their offspring and that abusive parenting runs in families, being present in some matrilines for more than 6–7 generations while completely absent in others (Maestripieri et al. 1997; Maestripieri and Carroll 1998). In our project, the rhesus macaques were studied in their own social groups, where they had the opportunity to express naturally occurring variation in behavioral tendencies.

The project involved the longitudinal study of 16 females that were cross-fostered at birth between abusive and nonabusive mothers, along with 43 males and females that were born and raised by their biological mothers, half of which were abusive and half nonabusive. All infants raised by abusive mothers experienced maternal abuse in the first three months of life, while none of the infants raised by nonabusive mothers experienced any abuse. When our female subjects gave birth for the first time (at approximately four years of age), about half of the females who were abused by their mothers early in life (whether cross-fostered or not) exhibited abusive parenting, whereas none of the females reared by nonabusive mothers did (Maestripieri 2005a). This result underscores the importance of early experience for the intergenerational transmission of infant abuse.

In this project, we also reported that cross-fostered females reared by abusive mothers developed interest in other females' infants earlier in life and tended to conceive for the first time at an earlier age than other females, suggesting that these young females were on a fast life history track (Maestripieri 2005b). Consistent with this hypothesis, we noted that abusive females showed high fertility but died at younger ages than other females (Maestripieri, unpublished data). These findings parallel those of human studies which show that girls who are exposed to early psychosocial stress reach menarche earlier, engage in sexual activity and conceive earlier, and develop interest in infants earlier in life than other girls (Ellis 2004; Maestripieri et al. 2004; Del Giudice 2009). These effects have been hypothesized to be mediated by the quality of parenting (i.e., psychosocial stress is associated with harsh and inconsistent parenting style; Belsky et al. 1991), which is consistent with the results of our macaque study.

In our study, we elucidated some of the physiological mechanisms underlying the effects of early experience on abusive parenting and fast life history traits. We showed that abused females exhibited higher cortisol responses to environmental (novelty) and neuroendocrine challenges (a corticotropin-releasing hormone challenge) (Sanchez et al. 2010; Koch et al. 2014). Moreover, the abused females, both cross-fostered and non-cross-fostered, who became abusive mothers had lower cerebrospinal fluid concentrations of the serotonin metabolite 5-HIAA than the abused females who did not become abusive mothers (Maestripieri et al. 2006). Along with other behavioral data, our results suggest that experience-induced alterations in HPA function and serotonergic function resulted in elevated anxiety and impaired impulse control, and that high anxiety and impulsivity increased the probability of occurrence of abusive parenting; social learning, however, that resulted from direct experience of abuse early in life or observation of abusive parenting displayed by one's own mother with siblings was also important. Developmental interactions between hormones of the HPA and HPG axes probably accounted for the acceleration of reproductive maturation in the abused females.

Although some of the characteristics of individuals exposed to early stress are likely to be adaptations to a harsh or unpredictable environment, these individuals also exhibit maladaptive behavior (e.g., abusive parenting) and often transmit it to the next generation. Whether adaptive or maladaptive, early stressful experiences seem to increase the risk for aggressive or violent behaviors later in life. In our rhesus macaque study, the finding that none of the females born to abusive mothers, but raised by controls, exhibited abusive parenting in adulthood suggests that being raised by nurturing mothers in a supportive and predictable social environment may suppress or counteract any possible genetic predispositions for violent interpersonal interactions. In addition, experienced rhesus mothers use moderate rates of rejection to encourage competent social development in their offspring and enhance their resilience in response to stressful challenges later in life (Parker and Maestripieri 2011). Therefore, in both human and nonhuman primates, the quality of the early environment provided by the mother and her behavior can be crucial for the development of appropriate/peaceful or inappropriate/violent social behavior.

In both nonhuman primates and in humans, other aspects of the early social environment besides the mother and her behavior can play an important role in the development of aggressive or peaceful social behavior, and more generally, life history strategies (see also van IJzendoorn and Bakermans-Kranenburg, this volume). This is exemplified by the importance of interaction with peers and observation of other adults in the development of conflict management and conflict resolution skills. Most Old World monkeys and some apes live in stable social groups and are thought to derive benefits from group living such as protection from predators and increased competitive ability over neighboring groups. However, competition (for food, mates, or status) among members of the same group can be intense, and such competition is often expressed through fighting. This fighting can be frequent, especially between closely related and/or adjacently ranked monkeys, who generally spend a great deal of time in close proximity. Fighting with group members can be costly in terms of risk of injury but also for the damage it can cause to social relationships with valuable supporters and allies.

The increased dependence on others and the need for coexistence in social groups have promoted the evolution of conflict resolution strategies that are not costly to the individual (Judge 2003). In the many primate species in which close kin live in the same group, the benefits of effective conflict resolution are magnified. Even among nonkin, nurturing a valuable relationship with a partner through reciprocity and exchange increases an animal's competitive ability within its group. Such cooperative long-term relationships require competent conflict resolution skills.

A cognitive/developmental perspective emphasizes adaptive social functioning and the developmental changes that occur as individuals learn to adjust to conflict-producing situations (Judge 2003). Strategies develop as individuals learn the complexities of interpersonal interactions and acquire the competence to address them. For example, studies have found that children's conflict resolution strategies change as a function of their age (reviewed by Judge 2003). Young children (two to ten years old) tend to use coercive strategies designed to produce one-sided outcomes, whereas older children tend to use more negotiation to resolve conflicts. Some developmental changes in conflict resolution strategies are associated with the acquisition of linguistic skills and the development of abstract moral reasoning. The development of conflict resolution skills is also influenced by third parties, such as parents, peers, siblings, and teachers (see also IJzendoorn and Bakermans-Kranenburg, this volume).

Nonhuman primates, such as macaques, appear to acquire conflict resolution skills at young ages (Judge 2003). Young monkeys have been shown to change their conflict resolution behavior based on previous interactions with others as well as observation of third parties. The role of observing third parties has been demonstrated with an experiment that took advantage of interspecies variation in aggressiveness/peacefulness and in the tendency to engage in reconciliation after fighting. Among the 19 extant species of macaques, some species are inherently more antagonistic and more likely than others to use aggressive strategies of conflict resolution. Rhesus and stumptail macaques are an excellent example of this phenomenon (de Waal and Johanowicz 1993). The two species are closely related and sympatric, yet rhesus macaques have evolved a despotic and intolerant style of social interaction that includes strict enforcement of an established dominance hierarchy, while stumptail macaques have evolved a more egalitarian and tolerant mode of social existence. Accordingly, rhesus macaques are more likely than stumptail macaques to use coercive aggressive solutions during conflicts of interest and less likely to reconcile aggression.

In one experiment aimed at testing whether individuals of the aggressive species could learn the conflict resolution skills of their more peaceful cousins, juveniles of both species were housed in mixed groups for five months (de Waal and Johanowicz 1993). Following this manipulation, they were observed for six weeks with conspecifics only. This manipulation created a different social culture by producing rhesus monkeys with a three to four times higher conciliatory tendency than age mates that had never met the other species. Thus, young rhesus macaques housed with stumptail macaques appeared to adopt the stumptail macaques' characteristic tendency to resolve conflicts through friendly behavior. Peacemaking tendencies rose gradually during co-housing with the peaceful "tutor" species and remained high after its removal. This experiment demonstrates that reconciliation behavior of monkeys can be modified by social experience and that interactions with peers play an important role in this process. A combination of cognitive (e.g., observational learning) and physiological (e.g., alterations in emotion regulation and responsivity to social stimuli) mechanisms may be responsible for these developmental changes in behavior (see Morgan et al. as well as IJzendoorn and Bakermans-Kranenburg, this volume). These changes in behavior are probably adaptive and consistent with life history theory, which predicts adjustments in social and reproductive strategies in response to changes in environmental conditions.

Conclusions

Human beings are highly social animals, and competition and cooperation with others are fundamental aspects of human nature (see also Steele et al., this volume). Aggression and violence can be an adaptive expression of competition. Maladaptive aggression and violence can also result from competition-related stress or be transmitted between individuals through social learning. Whether aggression is adaptive or maladaptive, any efforts to reduce violence and create peaceful individuals and societies seem to require an understanding of competition and management of its intensity. Not all competitive strategies, however, necessarily involve violent aggression. Species and individuals resort to aggressive competition when the benefits of aggression are high and its costs are low. There are species and individuals with high and low potential for violent aggression, and such differences are in large part genetically based. However, the expression of aggressiveness and peacefulness is modulated by the environment. Developmental plasticity is especially high early in life, when young individuals are responsive to environmental cues that signal the quality of their future environment (see Keverne, this volume), particularly in terms of unpredictability and danger as well as risk of morbidity and mortality. The cues are processed through cognitive (e.g., learning) or physiological mechanisms (e.g., resetting of stress-sensitive endocrine and neurochemical systems). Individuals exposed to aggression and violence early in life, whether through the quality of parental care received, relationships with their peers, or observations of adults around them, tend to adopt fast life history strategies that are characterized by rapid growth and reproductive maturation, exploitative and unstable social relationships, use of aggression and violence to accomplish social goals, focus on short-term mating, and failure to provide adequate investment to their children. In some cases, individuals reproduce the cycle of violence that began with their own personal experience in childhood.

Many human and animal studies are consistent with the predictions of life history theories in showing what early environmental conditions can lead to the development of nonaggressive individuals, and how such individuals can then contribute to the establishment of peaceful relationships and societies. These early environmental conditions include consistent, nurturing, and supportive parental care, environmental stability and predictability, reduced exposure to danger or violence, and active teaching or modeling of management of negative emotions and competition, including effective conflict avoidance and conflict resolution skills (see Fox et al. as well as IJzendoorn and Bakermans-Kranenburg, this volume). Modern biological theories of behavior recognize the importance of genetic predispositions but also the important role of environment in the expression or suppression of behavioral tendencies (for a discussion of gene-environment interactions, see Keverne, this volume). Since many different psychological, behavioral, and physiological traits tend to occur in clusters that are stable over the life course, it is important to understand how early environment selects for different clusters of traits, such as those associated with slow and fast life history strategies. Comparative research on human and animal behavior can help develop the theories that guide research in this field as well as provide empirical evidence that elucidates how different traits are organized and the physiological and cognitive mechanisms that are responsible for their integration.

Although we have made tremendous progress in our understanding of the role of genetic and experiential factors in the evolution and development of aggressive and prosocial behavior, many issues remain unanswered:

- The importance of maternal epigenetic influences on different aspects of brain development (e.g., Provençal et al. 2012).
- The role of stochastic epigenetic variation as a driving force of behavioral evolution and adaptation (e.g., Feinberg and Irizarry 2010).
- The role of genomic imprinting in the inheritance and expression of behavioral traits (Reik and Walter 2001).
- The existence of genes that confer differential susceptibility to environmental influences (Belsky et al. 2007).
- The genetic and experiential characteristics that make some individuals more resilient to stress than others (Parker and Maestripieri 2011).
- The extent to which an evolutionary life history perspective can be useful in understanding, preventing, and treating psychological and behavioral disorders (Del Giudice 2014).

One important limitation of comparative and evolutionary approaches to human development is that they do not directly address the role played by language, and by social, moral, and religious norms in the shaping of adult beliefs and behavior. Furthermore, although research in biology and psychology has made important contributions to our understanding of the universality of human behavior as well as of individual differences in behavior, anthropologists and sociologists have highlighted important variation among groups such as societies and cultures. Clearly, understanding and promoting peacefulness in human lives and human societies is a complex endeavor that requires contributions from individuals with broad and complementary kinds of expertise.

9

The Problem of Institutionalization of Young Children and Its Consequences for Efforts to Build Peaceful Societies

Nathan A. Fox, Charles A. Nelson, and Charles H. Zeanah

Abstract

Institutionalization of children is a worldwide problem. The consequences of these deprived early experiences have been known for some time. Indeed, neuroscientists have long been aware of the effects of early adverse experience, particularly profound deprivation, on the developing brain. However, the majority of work to date has focused on examining the effects of experience on brain and brain development in rodents and nonhuman primates. In a rigorous attempt to examine how profound early neglect impacts the course of *human* development, we designed the Bucharest Early Intervention Project. The Bucharest Early Intervention Project is the first randomized controlled trial of family care intervention on young children institutionalized in infancy. The study is unique in that it includes measures of brain structure and function. Results suggest that early psychosocial deprivation has profound effects on gray matter structure that do not appear to remediate, although subtle intervention effects were observed for white matter volume. EEG activity was significantly affected by early psychosocial deprivation, but there appeared to be remediation of this functioning by the time children were eight years old and had spent close to six or seven years in families. The data from this project argue for changes in the manner in which societies address abandoned children. An important step toward building just and peaceful societies is to provide family-type care for young children instead of institutional life, as being raised in a family[1] greatly

---

[1] Note: the term "family" is used to describe a group of people bound together by kinship, roles in caring for each other, cultural traditions, or close affiliation.

enhances a child's skills in emotion regulation. The link to peaceful societies is through these processes.

Introduction

UNICEF has estimated that over 8 million children live in some form of institutional care around the world. For many years, psychologists have known of deleterious effects on cognitive and social behavior in children who have undergone early institutional experience. Thus, the large number of children living in these circumstances reflects a worldwide public health problem. We know that the foundation for a successful society and the source of peace among communities is built in the period of early childhood (see Abu-Nimer and Nasser, this volume). The foundation of healthy child development results in educational achievement, economic productivity, responsible citizenship, and lifelong health. These attainments lead to the emergence of strong, peaceful communities with successful transmission of these values across generations. Therefore, addressing the dire conditions of children living in institutions is a critical need and an important step in creating a peaceful and just society.

Developmental psychologists have, for many years, argued that experiences early in life can have a profound effect upon the course of subsequent development. Studies of human infants demonstrate that learning takes place from a very early age and sets the course for trajectories of either adaptive or maladaptive behavior. Recent evidence suggests that there are certain periods during early development when experiences have a more significant effect than others. These periods, called sensitive periods, are thought of as windows of time during which certain types of experience have a foundational effect upon the development of skills or competencies (Fox et al. 2010; Zeanah et al. 2011).

Progress in understanding the effects of early experience on development has been facilitated by advances in neuroscience that describe the pattern of brain development during the early months and years of life as well as the role that experience has in shaping development. A number of neuroscientists (Huttenlocher and Dabholkar 1997; Granger et al. 1995) have illustrated changes in synaptic density, increases in neural connections, and the subsequent pruning or decreases in synaptic number that occur during the postnatal period. This blooming and pruning occurs in different brain areas at different times, particularly during postnatal development. These changes occur early in postnatal life in sensory and perceptual regions of the brain; later they occur in areas of the brain involved in higher cognition. The idea of exuberant overproduction is one linked to the notion of maximal plasticity being a function of overproduction of adaptive units followed by highly governed attrition. It is analogous to the principles of contextual learning in infancy and childhood proposed by Vygotsky and others. Maximal benefit is obtained by providing scaffolding during which time the infant or young child can move freely within their zone of comfort into new and unexplored areas. Once these new areas are mastered, the scaffolding can be removed. This comfort zone could be the result of an "open neural system" in which exuberant projections increase and are gradually pruned away. Data that support the effects of early experience on development have primarily been derived from studies in rodents and nonhuman primates. Because of obvious ethical considerations, it is not possible to assign infants randomly to conditions of significant deprivation, including those in which there is a lack or absence of experience, particularly experience-expectant stimulation. Thus research has relied on situations, medical and environmental, that provide the contexts in which examination of the effects of early experience can be made. For example, Maurer et al. (1999) examined the effects of visual deprivation in infants born with bilateral cataracts. Maurer followed these infants, who ranged in the age at which they had surgery to remove those cataracts, to determine if and how extensive the effects of early deprivation were. Similarly, Neville and Bevellier (1998) studied infants born deaf with regard to their language development, and Schorr et al. (2005) examined the effects that the age of acquiring a cochlear implant in young children born deaf had on their abilities to integrate auditory and visual information. In all of these cases, identifying populations of children who are deprived because of a medical or genetic condition of early experience provides researchers a window into the effects of deprivation and timing of remediation on behavioral outcomes. Until recently, examination of the effects of more general psychosocial deprivation and neglect in human infants has been missing from the research field. Children who are institutionalized in early infancy represent a "natural" condition in which examination of the effects of early experience can be studied.

Since the early part of the twentieth century, psychologists have recognized the detrimental effects of psychosocial deprivation (Bowlby 1952; Goldfarb 1945). Multiple reports on the effects of institutionalization on cognitive, motor, and social development have been published. More recently, neuroscientists have begun to study the impact of early experience on brain development and with that the impact of psychosocial deprivation. Studying the impact of experience on brain function and development, neuroscientists distinguished between experience-expectant and experience-dependent changes (Greenough et al. 1987). Experience-expectant changes are those that occur as a result of the "expectation" of certain experiences common to all members of the species (e.g., patterned light, complex sound, consistent caregiving). Psychologists in the 1960s enumerated the types of stimulation and experiences that they found important for typical infant and child learning, which included vestibular, kinesthetic, and tactile stimulation and contingent social interaction. Infants and young children in institutions develop in environments in which these experience-expectant stimuli are absent, hence creating a weak foundation for brain development in the first years of life.

Experience-dependent changes are also important in the context of institutional rearing. Not only does the lack of contingent stimulation and positive social experiences affect brain and behavior, adaptation to a chaotic environment does as well. For example, researchers have speculated that indiscriminate social behavior may be adaptive in settings of social deprivation where children may seek social contact wherever they can find it. In our view, early psychosocial deprivation violates both of these developmental principles: thus, experiences expected by all members of the species are absent (e.g., a caregiver to tend to the child's needs since the child cannot do so him/herself), as are experiences unique to that individual (e.g., exposure to limited language input, leading to poor language ability).

Knudsen (2004) has proposed three mechanisms by which sensitive periods are instantiated and ultimately closed in the brain. These include dendritic elaboration, synaptic pruning, and cell adhesion processes at the level of the synapse. Each or all of these may be operating during experience-expectant processes. However, the mechanisms of learning that take place during experience-dependent periods may be quite different. More recently, Hench (2005) has proposed the important role of parvalbumin positive cells in regulating the closure of sensitive periods.

The research presented in this chapter is drawn from the Bucharest Early Intervention Project. This project was designed to examine the effects of early psychosocial deprivation on social and cognitive development among young children living in institutions in Romania. The Bucharest Early Intervention Project is not the first study to examine the effects of early deprivation and institutionalization post Ceausescu. The English and Romanian Adoptee (ERA) study, directed by Michael Rutter with a group of investigators at the Institute for Psychiatry in London (Rutter et al. 2009), identified 144 children raised in Romanian institutions and later adopted into families living in the United Kingdom. All of the children in the ERA sample were adopted by the time a child was 42 months of age. Rutter and colleagues assessed these children as of four years of age, comparing them to infants born in the United Kingdom and adopted by U.K. parents. This study is admirable for its detailed longitudinal study of these children. However, it is possible that the children in this study were "selected" by the adoptive parents for certain characteristics. In addition, all assessments were done in the United Kingdom as these children adapted to their British lives. The Bucharest Early Intervention Project differed in two important ways from the Rutter ERA study. First, it was the first randomized controlled trial of a foster care intervention to examine its efficacy in remediating some of the negative effects of exposure to early psychosocial intervention. Second, infants were assessed while they still lived in the institutions and foster home placement took place in Bucharest. A large cohort of infants and young children living in institutions in Bucharest, Romania, were screened for genetic anomalies and gross sensory or physical handicaps. A final sample of 136 infants and young children were selected and assessed while they lived in their institutions. Subsequent to that, the sample was randomized to either remain in the institution (care as usual) or be placed into a foster care family home (foster care group). All children were subsequently followed up at 42, 54, and 96 months of age. Assessments were completed across a wide range of domains (see Zeanah et al. 2003). Here we focus on the effects of institutionalization on brain activity and the possible effects of intervention, as well as whether there are sensitive periods for the effectiveness of the intervention.

Ethics of the Bucharest Early Intervention Project

Before presenting data on the effects of institutionalization on brain activity and development, it is important to mention that the ethical issues of completing a project of this nature on a vulnerable population are complex and have received considerable attention. At the time that we started the study, there was a debate in Romania regarding the efficacy of institutionalization as an intervention for infant and child abandonment. Foster care had only recently been legalized, and very few foster homes were licensed in Bucharest when the study began in 2000. We were invited by the Minister for Child Protection to conduct a study that would compare a family-based intervention to institutional care. We negotiated an agreement with the Romanian government so that no child removed from an institution and placed into our intervention would go back to an institution at the completion of the trial. Instead, the local authorities took over support and supervision of the foster care network that we created. In addition, we maintained a policy of noninterference for both those children in foster care as well as those randomized to care as usual. This means that for children participating in the study, all decisions after randomization regarding their placements were made by Romanian child protection authorities; study participation and group assignment had no effect on those decisions. Thus, some children from both groups were adopted, and some were returned to their biological parents. Finally, once efficacy of our intervention was established, we organized a news conference, invited government ministers, and distributed findings from the study. While we did not have the funds to recruit and support additional foster homes, the Romanian government did later begin to expand foster care and began taking children out of institutions and placing them into government-supported foster homes. Subsequent legislation, passed in 2005, also banned institutionalization of any child under the age of two years. The study was reviewed and approved by three institutional review boards (University of Minnesota, University of Maryland, and Tulane University), and by an institutional review board at the Bucharest University. Our approach has been described in detail elsewhere (Nelson et al. 2014; Zeanah et al. 2012), and several ethical commentaries on the study have been published (see Millum and Emmanuel 2007; Miller 2009; Rid 2012).

Effects of Psychosocial Deprivation on the Brain

One approach to understanding the mechanisms by which institutionalization affects behavior is through an examination of the effects of early deprivation on brain structure and function. The Bucharest Early Intervention Project was the first study to assess brain functioning in institutionalized young children. There are, however, a number of studies that have examined post-institutionalized infant brain structure and function.

In one of the first studies to examine the effects of early institutionalization on brain development, Chugani et al. (2001) used PET scans to study ten children who had been adopted from a Romanian institution. At the time of the study, the average age of the children was eight years; nearly all of the children had been institutionalized before the age of 17 months and had lived in the institution an average of 38 months before being adopted. These children were compared with a group of healthy adults and a group of ten-year-old children with medically refractory epilepsy. Chugani et al. (2001) reported that the adoptees showed significantly reduced brain metabolism in select regions of the prefrontal cortex (i.e., orbitofrontal cortex) and the temporal lobe (the amygdala). These are regions typically associated with higher cognitive functions, memory, and emotion. Neuropsychological testing revealed that the adopted children suffered from mild neurocognitive impairments, including impulsivity, attention, and social deficits. One must be cautious in making too much of these findings, given that the sample size was small and highly selected (in who was allowed to leave the institution).

This same group of investigators conducted a follow-up study of the same sample of children, this time examining white matter connectivity using magnetic resonance imaging (MRI) (Eluvanthingal et al. 2006). This study examined structural effects of institutionalization rather than functional differences. They found that white matter connectivity was diminished in the uncinate fasciculus region of the brain in the early deprivation group compared with controls. The uncinate fasciculus provides a major pathway of communication between brain areas involved in higher cognitive and emotional function (e.g., amygdala and frontal lobe), leading the authors to conclude that connectivity between brain regions is significantly reduced by early institutionalization. Fewer connections may lead to deficits or delays in inhibitory control, emotion regulation, and other functions that are overseen by the connections between these brain areas.

In a third study, Chugani et al. (2001; Govindan et al. 2010) evaluated further white matter changes in children with a history of early deprivation, again using MRI as well as a highly sensitive neuroimaging analysis technique, Tract-Based Spatial Statistics (TBSS). Seventeen children with a history of institutional care since birth and subsequent adoption were compared with 15 typically developing nonadopted children. The children came from a diverse range of institutions, including in Eastern Europe and Southeast Asia. They were found to have reduced organization of portions of the bilateral uncinate and superior longitudinal fasiculi, with the magnitude of white matter disorganization significantly associated with duration of time spent in institutional care. Again, these were structural rather than functional differences between those with a history of institutionalization and those without such a history. The authors speculate that these findings may underlie the inattention/overactivity syndrome that was previously described by Rutter and colleagues as part of the institutional syndrome. Collectively, work by Chugani and colleagues suggests that children who experienced early institutionalization suffer from metabolic, structural, and connectivity deficits in the areas of the brain believed to be involved in higher cognition, emotion, and emotion regulation (Chugani et al. 2001; Govindan et al. 2010).

To date a number of studies have used MRI methods to examine children who were living in the United States after being adopted from institutions around the world. Bauer et al. (2009) completed a structural imaging study of 31 post-institutionalized children living with adopted families in the Midwest. The children were mainly from institutions in Eastern Europe (12 from Romania, 12 from Russia, 5 from China, and 2 from other European countries). Their average age at adoption was 31 months, and they were tested at a mean age of 11 years. The post-institutionalized children had smaller volumes of the superior-posterior cerebellar lobes, and poorer performance on memory and executive function tasks compared with typically developing children who served as controls. Structural differences in the cerebellum mediated the relation between institution history and cognitive performance. This is one of the few studies to identify the cerebellum as being affected by early experience and related to higher-order cognitive function. The cerebellum is a structure deep in the brain that is involved in motor control and basic learning processes. The fact that early experience of deprivation can affect this basic structure helps account for the deficits seen in post-institutionalized children in motor ability, learning, attention, and cognition.

Tottenham et al. (2010, 2011) published two imaging studies with post-institutionalized children from Asia and Eastern Europe, examining structural differences between these children and a typically developing control group. Findings from the first study showed no differences in cortical volume or gray matter between the different groups of children, though late-adopted children had larger amygdala volume compared with the early-adopted children and the typically developing controls. In their second study, they report finding greater amygdala activity in the post-institutionalized group in response to the fear stimuli, with amygdala activity mediating the relation between early institutional care and eye gaze pattern (post-institutionalized children showed less direct eye fixation on faces). Coupled with the first study's finding of enlarged amygdala in post-institutionalized children, these studies show the importance of this subcortical structure and its apparent sensitivity to deprivation experiences in children. Importantly, in both studies, the imaging took place years after the children had left the institution and were now adopted into stable families in the United States, thus emphasizing the effects of early experience on amygdala volume and activity.

Finally, Mehta et al. (2009) completed MRI studies of the children followed in Rutter's ERA study. Gray and white matter volume was measured and the researchers found significantly smaller white and gray matter volume in those adolescents adopted from Romania (previously institutionalized) compared to children who were never institutionalized but adopted. These researchers also report that previously institutionalized children had smaller hippocampal and amygdala volumes compared to controls.

What is the significance of these amygdala findings? The amygdala refers to bilateral, almond-shaped structures deep in the brain that are involved in the detection of threat and novelty. It helps in the processing of emotional information from others' faces, and particularly fear learning. The amygdala plays a role in the processing of emotionally salient information, both in terms of the formation of emotional memories and the guiding behavior based on emotional- or threat-related stimuli through the attentional modulation of other areas of the cortex (Adolphs and Spezio 2006). As a basic structure in the brain involved in fundamental responses to stimuli (novelty detection, approach-withdrawal), the amygdala plays a significant role in many social and cognitive behaviors. Hence, disturbances in amygdala activity and structure, as a function of early experience, have a significant impact on more mature and complex social and cognitive processes (Tottenham and Sheridan 2009).

A paper from the English Romanian Adoptees study (Mehta et al. 2009) used MRI to examine amygdala structure among post-institutionalized children. This study found that the adoptees had significantly reduced total gray and white matter volumes compared with the control group. After correcting for brain volume, adoptees had enlarged relative amygdala volumes compared with the control group, particularly in the right hemisphere. Left amygdala volume correlated significantly with the duration of institutional care, with longer stays in an institution correlated with a smaller left amygdala volume.

As can be seen from this brief overview of brain-imaging studies of post-institutionalized children, the findings are highly variable: some find increased amygdala size along with reduced gray and white matter volume, whereas others find an association between structural size or function and duration of institutionalization. The variability in findings is most likely a function of the heterogeneity of experiences, contexts, and durations of exposure to deprivation across the different samples, as well as the small sample sizes in any particular study. Nevertheless, the findings provide important guideposts for thinking about the effects of early experience on brain development and understanding the mechanisms by which early experience influences cognitive and social behavior.

In the Bucharest Early Intervention Project, we recorded brain waves using an electroencephalogram (EEG) before the children were randomized and while they all still lived in institutions. After randomization, we made EEG recordings at 30 months and 42 months of age, while the children were viewing an entertaining visual display: bingo balls rotating in a bingo cage (the goal was to engage the child's attention for a few minutes, standardizing attention to the wheel and minimizing movement).

The complex EEG signal comprises many different oscillatory processes that have specific frequencies and amplitudes, ranging from very slow high-amplitude activity, associated with sleep, to very fast low-amplitude activity, associated with complex information processing. These different oscillations can be broken down into individual frequency bands: alpha activity, which we associate with attention to sensory experience (e.g., eyes open, staring at bingo balls), beta activity, which we associate with complex cognitive activity, and theta activity, which may be stimulus-driven (responsive to memory tasks and some aspects of emotion) but when measured in the resting EEG is often associated with cognitive impairment and delta activity, associated with sleep.

Each of these frequency bands has a distinctive "signature." For example, we were interested in beta activity (13–20 Hz), alpha activity (6–9 Hz), theta activity (3–5 Hz), and delta bands (1–3 Hz). At rest these different frequency bands reflect the activity of brain areas, as they are involved in arousal and different states of consciousness. For example, the delta band (1–3 Hz) is found to predominate in sleep whereas the alpha band predominates in states of alertness and vigilance. Over the first three years of life, the resting EEG alpha and beta frequencies increasingly contribute to the EEG signal while theta decreases (Marshall et al. 2002). Changes in both the amplitude and the frequency distribution of the EEG with age are thought to reflect development of the structural integrity of white matter tracts, which again helps speed up the transmission of electrical activity. As white matter increases linearly across child development, so do alpha contributions to EEG signal. Increased alpha and beta frequency contributions, coupled with decreased theta contributions, have been associated with increased cortical maturity and greater control over attention (Barry et al. 2003). One can think of the EEG as a marker of the integrity of the connectivity of brain circuits and one way of tracking cortical maturation.

At baseline, we found large differences in resting EEG power at particular frequency bands between children living in institutions and the community controls. The children who lived in institutions had greater slow-frequency activity (theta) and less high-frequency (alpha and beta) activity relative to the community controls (Marshall et al. 2004). It was as if someone had turned down the dimmer switch on alpha and beta power in the institutionalized children (alpha and beta activity) and increased theta brain activity. This profile was maintained through the initial period of the intervention.

Figure 9.1 illustrates this pattern for alpha activity at baseline, comparing the children in the institutional group with those in the community sample. This figure represents the amount of brain activity using different colors to

Institutionalization and brain activity
Theta, 3–5 Hz

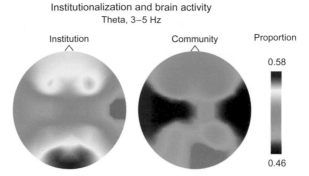

Figure 9.1   False color maps that illustrate the amount of EEG (EEG power) in the theta band in two groups of children. Top-down perspective: the front of the head appears at the top of each figure and the back at the bottom. Increases in EEG power are represented along the blue/green to red spectrum; red indicates higher power and blue/green less power. After Marshall, Fox, and the Bucharest Early Intervention Project Core Group (2004).

reflect different levels of activity. We can easily see how much more brain activity there is (particularly recorded from electrodes placed over the frontal lobe) among children in the community sample compared with the institutionalized children.

The topographic "maps" presented in Figure 9.1 illustrate the amount of EEG (EEG power) in the theta band in the two groups of children. To orient the reader, we are looking from the top down, such that the front of the head appears at the top of each figure and the back at the bottom. Increases in EEG power are represented along the blue/green to red spectrum, such that red indicates higher power, and blue/green less power. The institutionalized children show high power in the theta range, whereas the community children show low power across the scalp. These findings in the resting EEG of higher theta and lower alpha power have been identified in a number of populations that range in pathology. For example, this same pattern has been identified in low IQ children with attention deficit disorder (Clarke et al. 2005), in children with Fragile X Syndrome (Van der Molen and Van der Molen 2013), as well as in children with Down Syndrome (Bablioni et al. 2010). Hence this was a worrisome pattern to have identified in young children living in institutions.

Naturally, we recorded the EEG during the follow-up phase of our study. However, the intervention effects were initially relatively subtle. That is, although no differences were found between the foster care group (FCG) and the care as usual group (CAUG), we found a moderate correlation between the amount of electrical activity and the length of time the children had been placed in FCG (Marshall et al. 2008). By then, children in the FCG had been in their foster care families for around four years. At eight years of age, there was a strong intervention effect and a timing effect in the EEG data (Vanderwert et al. 2010). Children placed into our foster care intervention program before the age of two years displayed a pattern of brain activity that was indistinguishable from that of never-institutionalized children (see Figure 9.2). Children who were taken out of the institution before the age of two years showed a pattern of higher alpha activity and lower theta activity. Foster care children also had more significant high-frequency beta activity compared with children random-ized to the institution. Indeed, as with the alpha power finding, there was both an intervention and a timing effect for beta power at the age of eight years.

These eight-year data are plotted in a fashion similar to Figure 9.1. The data presented in the upper left panel, from the CAUG, are identical to the upper right panel, representing the data from children placed in foster care after 24 months. Similarly, the data from the lower right panel, from the never-institu-tionalized group (NIG), are identical to data from the children placed in foster care before 24 months (lower left panel).

These findings suggest two important conclusions. First, there may be a sensitive period for the development of neural structures underlying increased alpha power in the EEG signal, with amelioration of the environment before two years of age necessary for remediation to occur. Second, though this devel-opmental "catch-up" was made possible by placement into foster care before the age of two, it required years of exposure to foster care before it emerged.

Previously we recorded EEG at 30 and 42 months and found little change from baseline to 42 months. There was a hint at 42 months that the youngest children placed into foster care had higher alpha power. Of course, since the mean age of the children placed into foster care was 22 months, the average

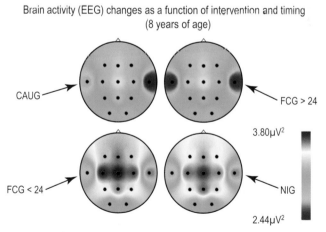

Figure 9.2 Pattern of EEG activation at the age of eight years. In the upper left panel, from the care as usual group (CAUG), EEG activation is identical to the upper right panel, representing data from children placed in foster care (FCG) after 24 months. Similarly, the pattern of EEG activation from the lower right panel, from the never institutionalized group (NIG), is identical to data from the children placed in foster care before 24 months (lower left panel). After Vanderwert et al. (2010).

duration of intervention at 30 months was only 8 months and at 42 months, 20 months. We thought that perhaps this was not long enough to affect brain activity. By eight years of age, children had experienced the intervention and other life events that may have facilitated brain changes, particularly among those who received the initial intervention. Thus, the intervention and timing effects could reflect a subtle combination of age of placement *and* duration of intervention. In other words, the initial period of intervention from a mean of 22 months to 54 months of age was sufficient to accelerate brain activity in the intervention group. However, as time passed and children began to spend more time out of institutional care (e.g., the child in the CAUG who is removed by child-protection authorities at age three and reunited with his family), the effects of current life experience began to contribute in addition to the effects of early-life experience. Understanding what our EEG findings mean has been perplexing since our initial observations at baseline. Over the years, we have entertained a number of possible interpretations of these data. For example, if smaller head size correlates with smaller brain size, what exactly is it about the brain of the institutionalized child that is smaller? Is it the loss of neurons, the loss of neuronal elements, such as axons and dendrites? Perhaps it is the loss of synapses. Might it be that the normal process of apoptosis (i.e., programmed cell death) has gone awry, such that there has been an excessive *pruning* of neurons, as would occur from underuse of circuits? Finally, might there be less white matter (i.e., the portions of neurons that contain myelin and which lead to short- and long-distance connections among neurons) which might contribute to our EEG and event-related potential (ERP) observations? In other words, might the brain be less well interconnected and, as a result, its electrical activity reduced?

When the children were between the ages of eight and ten we were finally in a position to test some of these hypotheses. We did so by performing structural MRI scans to examine brain structure in detail.

In collaboration with a neuroradiologist in Bucharest, we performed structural MRIs (using a Siemens 1.5 Tesla MRI scanner) on 78 randomly selected Bucharest Early Intervention Project children when they were approximately nine years old. Of these, 20 came from the NIG, 27 from the FCG, and 31 from the CAUG (Sheridan et al. 2012b). We set out with several very specific hypotheses:

1. Based on the head circumference, EEG, and ERP data, we expected to see an overall reduction in total cerebral volume among the CAUG. What we could not specify was whether this would be due to a reduction in gray matter, in white matter, or in both.

2. Based on both human and animal research, we anticipated that the CAUG would show a reduction in the size of the hippocampus. This hypothesis derived from the literature linking chronic stress exposure

to elevations in glucocorticoids, which in turn can be neurotoxic to the hippocampus, making it smaller.

3. We thought we might observe changes in the amygdala, though the literature is ambiguous as to the direction in which this change might occur—some have reported an enlarged amygdala and others no change (e.g., Tottenham et al. 2010; Mehta et al. 2009).

4. We expected to see some changes, most likely in reduced volume, in the corpus callosum (the large bundle of myelinated axons that connects the two hemispheres), possibly because the connections between the hemispheres are sensitive to experiential input.

5. Based on our EEG and ERP findings after placement in foster care, we thought we might see an increase in white matter among the FCG relative to no change among the CAUG or the NIG. This speculation is based on extensive data from rodents, which have consistently shown that increases in myelin can occur when rats are raised in complex (so-called enriched) environments (Huttenlocher 2009).

What we did observe was a reduction in total cortical volume among ever-institutionalized children (CAUG and FCG) compared with never-institutionalized children. We also observed a reduction in gray matter among both the CAUG and the FCG compared with the NIG; in other words, there was no intervention effect on gray matter. In terms of white matter, we observed a reduction in the CAUG compared with the FCG and the NIG, which did not differ from each other. Despite some regional variation, we saw a reduction in the volume of the corpus callosum in the CAUG compared with the other two groups (which do not differ from each other). These last two findings collectively suggest that the foster care intervention is having a beneficial effect on white matter volume but not on gray matter, consistent with the experience-dependent nature of white matter (which permits the inference that the CAUG may have fewer synapses). Finally, we did not see any differences across groups in either the hippocampus or the amygdala, and only very subtle changes in one or two regions of the basal ganglia.

These findings were examined to see whether they could explain the pattern of low-voltage EEG that we had seen since the early assessment points in our study. Using mediation analysis, we found that EEG power could be explained by differences among the children in white matter volume. Those children with low white matter volumes were more likely to have low EEG power, and, conversely, high white matter volume was related to typical EEG power. This is a critical finding for our research study, since EEG power is a strong predictor of maladaptive outcomes in the institutionalized children (including increased incidence of attention deficit hyperactivity disorder symptoms).

Overall, findings from the Bucharest Early Intervention Project suggest that early psychosocial deprivation has profound effects on brain structure and function. In addition, results from the study argue for the efficacy of intervention if that intervention occurs early in life (before the end of the first two years of life). It should be noted that while the intervention remediated EEG power, there were no intervention effects on brain structure. Thus, early deprivation has profound effects on brain development which no doubt affects both social and cognitive behaviors.

Unanswered Questions

Perhaps the most important question or area of future research concerns individual differences. While the findings from the Bucharest Early Intervention Project portray group differences in outcomes as a function of intervention and sensitive periods, there are individual differences in outcomes among children in both the intervention and the care as usual group. There appears to be a gradient in response to intervention, with some children benefiting more than others. Some children in the care as usual group, even though they remained in the institution, displayed resilience and positive adaptive outcomes. How are we to understand this individual variation?

One important avenue of exploration is by examining both genetic and epigenetic variation among our samples to understand the neurobiological processes underlying sensitive periods in brain development. These processes, discussed in detail by Keverne (this volume), most probably have a significant explanatory power for individual outcomes.

A second, unexplored area in our work is the effects of early-life experience on the development of the stress system and the role of neurohormones, like cortisol and oxytocin, in shaping brain circuitry early in life. Research, particularly with rodents, shows quite clearly that early deprivation affects the stress system and impacts the wiring of brain architecture. As illustrated by Carter and Porges (this volume), certain neurohormones, such as oxytocin, can in the presence of sensitive caregiving provide buffers against early-life stress.

A third area of important exploration and unanswered in the current study is exactly what aspects of caregiving are needed and necessary for the formation of healthy attachment relationships between a caregiver and child. The data from the Bucharest Early Intervention Project show clearly that attachment relationships are critical for adaptive outcomes later in childhood. Data from this study also demonstrate that if infants who have experienced neglect and psychosocial deprivation as a result of institutionalization early in life are removed before the age of two years, they are able to respond positively to the family situation and form secure attachment relationships (Zeanah et al. 2005). What we do not know is what aspects of the family environment are critical for this plasticity and recovery. Steele et al. (this volume) provide an important overview of the types of experiences that are important for the formation of secure attachment relationships and hence a window into what is missing in the institutional environment.

A fourth unanswered question must be addressed through further study of the sample in the Bucharest Early Intervention Project. That is, did the intervention that ended when children were 54 months old incur advantage to children as they enter adolescence and then adulthood? Are there effects that were not present in certain domains early in life that appear later in life and, conversely, are effects that were present early in childhood transitory? Do they disappear with development? Further research is needed to answer these questions.

Conclusions

The findings from the Bucharest Early Intervention Project have implications for the worldwide public health problem of institutionalized children. If we are to develop a peaceful and just society, we must acknowledge the importance of a foundation of healthy child development and the importance of developing adaptive skills in emotion regulation. The many attainments of healthy child development, including educational achievement and economic prosperity, can be derailed if children experience neglect and psychosocial deprivation early in life. It is important, therefore, to take the lessons of the Bucharest Early Intervention Project and use them to advocate for family-based care for abandoned infants and young children. Such contexts can strengthen communities and lead to a peaceful and just world.

10

Prosocial Development and Situational Morality

Neurobiological, Parental, and Contextual Factors

Marinus H. van IJzendoorn and
Marian J. Bakermans-Kranenburg

Abstract

Prosocial behavior is any (voluntary) behavior intended to benefit others, and it is one of the potential contributions that an individual can make toward a more peaceful world. In this chapter, neurobiological, parental, and situational factors that might shape the prosocial behavior of children are discussed and emerging prosocial and antisocial behavior in infancy is reviewed and the question posed whether prosociality is inborn or obtained through socialization by parents. Twin studies suggest a considerable genetic component in prosociality, but current molecular genetic studies fail to support this outcome. Studies on gene-environment interaction, in particular on differential susceptibility, might be more promising as the influence of the family[1] and wider social context on prosocial development seems undeniable. Hormonal influences on prosocial behavior have recently been studied using intranasal oxytocin administration, and some studies on prosociality related to neural activity and brain morphology in children have become available. This chapter ends with some thoughts and findings on situational morality. Environmental "nudges" might play a more important role than is currently acknowledged in child development research and theories of prosociality.

Introduction: Prosocial Behavior and Situational Morality

Do neurobiological, parental, and situational factors shape children's prosocial behavior, and, if so, how? Prosocial behavior can provisionally be defined as

---

[1] Note: the term "family" is used to describe a multigenerational group of people bound together by kinship, roles in caring for each other, cultural traditions, or close affiliation.

any (voluntary) behavior intended to benefit others, with or without costs for the agent. Prosociality may include at least the following four categories of behavior (derived from Warneken and Tomasello 2009a; Eisenberg and Fabes 1998):

1. Comforting: providing emotional support to others in distress or pain.
2. Sharing resources: giving food or objects to others.
3. Informing: providing useful information to others.
4. Instrumental helping: acting to enable others to reach their goals.

Depending on the ethical value of what others want to achieve, prosocial behavior could be used to affect completely opposite outcomes. However, in this chapter, we will use this working definition.

Prosocial behavior can be inspired by empathic concern as well as altruistic or other moral motivations. However, the reasons or motives behind prosocial behavior can be amoral or immoral ("I donate to keep children in the majority world dependent on our aid"), and motivations may be selfish instead of altruistic. The ambiguous nature of prosocial behavior is why most schools of ethics emphasize the intentions of an act or the feelings that accompany the act, instead of the act itself, and define morality as acting in line with morally good character traits (see Aristotle's *The Nicomachean Ethics*, translated by Ross and Brown 2009) or morally elevated levels of reasoning (Kohlberg 1984).

Having the right feelings, the right character traits, or correct moral reasons disconnected from actual behavior is, however, irrelevant for those situations in which moral choices really matter; for instance, helping victims of genocidal regimes to flee or to hide or discontinuing torturous treatment of prisoners when individuals in command insist on continuation (Zimbardo 2007). In our discussion here,[2] we focus, therefore, on prosocial behavior and its prerequisites, not (only or mainly) on morally adequate but abstract reasoning capacities, empathic feelings, or altruistic personality traits.

We begin with a discussion on some studies of signs of prosocial behavior in infancy as well as on emerging antisocial inclinations, in particular against members of out-groups, to address the issue of whether humans have inborn capacities to act in a prosocial way. Thereafter we turn to the role of parents and ask whether they are able to make a difference and socialize their children in a prosocial direction. Twin studies suggest a considerable genetic component in prosociality. However, can this genetic determination be identified on a molecular level, or do studies on gene-environment interaction (in particular, on differential susceptibility) explain more of the variation in prosocial behavior? In search of hormonal influences on prosocial behavior, we present work on intranasal oxytocin administration and how it might stimulate costly donating

---

[2]   This chapter is an update and extension of van IJzendoorn et al. (2010; van IJzendoorn and Bakermans-Kranenburg 2011) and builds on a presentation that we gave in 2011, "On situational and embodied morality," at the symposium on The Development of Character: The Aristotelian Tradition and Contemporary Developmental Psychology, Keble College, Oxford University, February 12–13, 2011.

behavior (see also Carter and Porges, this volume). Prosociality might become "embodied" in our brains, and we present the few studies on prosociality in relation to neural activity and brain morphology in children. We conclude with some thoughts and findings on situational morality, defined as prosocial behavior canalized by environmental "nudges," which might play a more forceful role than is currently acknowledged in child development research and theories of prosociality.

Early Signs of Prosocial and Antisocial Behavior: The First Two Years of Life

Human infants seem to be endowed with an inborn capacity to be empathic to distress and to favor morally good individuals over morally bad persons (for an extensive account, see van IJzendoorn et al. 2010; van IJzendoorn and Bakermans-Kranenburg 2011). The empathic baby is an appealing idea. In a pioneering study on empathic distress, Sagi and Hoffman (1976) exposed one-day-old infants to a newborn cry, a synthetic cry, or silence. Infants exposed to a real cry cried significantly more often than those exposed to a synthetic cry of the same intensity, or to silence. Although mimicry may be a viable alternative explanation, the authors suggest that this selective cry response in newborns may provide some evidence for an inborn empathic distress reaction.

Hamlin et al. (2007) showed that six- and ten-month-old infants already evaluate an individual on the basis of their hostile or helpful actions in computer-animated events. Astonishingly, most preverbal infants prefer an individual who helps another to one who hinders another, a helping individual to a neutral individual, and a neutral individual to a hindering individual—even if that "individual" is not more than a geometric figure in a computer animation. Hamlin et al. (2013) argue that the capacity of very young children to derive moral evaluations from simple actions may serve as the foundation for moral thought and action, and they suggest that its early emergence supports the view that morality is inborn.

In a series of experiments with 14- and 18-month-old children, Warneken and Tomasello (2006, 2009a) showed that children are inclined to help an adult who is unable to reach his or her goal without help. One of the settings the researchers created was the experimenter's use of a clothespin to hang towels on a line; after a few moments the experimenter dropped the clothespin by accident and was unable to pick it up. The large majority of children who observed the event were eager to help the experimenter by picking up the clothespin and handing it to the experimenter. This also occurred, to the same extent, when a child had to "pay" for helping the experimenter; that is, when the child had to interrupt playing with new and exciting toys in another corner of the room. Surprisingly, rewards did not increase helping behavior; on the contrary, when children were rewarded for helping, they were less inclined to help when the reward was stopped (Warneken and Tomasello 2009a).

In contrast to this optimistic view of human nature, another study by the same research team showed that at the age of 14 months, children prefer a helpful puppet to a neutral puppet, and a neutral puppet to a harmful puppet—but only if the puppet involved is similar to themselves (Hamlin et al. 2013). Similarity was established by food preference. The children first had to select their preferred food and, in a next phase, the puppets were presented as preferring the same food (similar) or choosing the nonpreferred food (dissimilar). When the 14-month-old children were then asked to choose between two other puppets that were either helpful or harmful to the target puppet, they preferred the helpful puppet when the target was similar to them in terms of food preference, and they chose the harmful puppet when the target was dissimilar to them. Here we might see the beginning of "parochial morality" (see also Fry, this volume); that is, empathic concern and prosocial behavior extended only to members of an in-group, and an active dislike and subsequent antisocial tendency to the out-group. At nine months of age, the findings were less clear-cut and in-group favoritism appeared to be less developed (Hamlin et al. 2013).

If the idea of the empathic baby were valid, somewhere during the early years this moral capacity must have been pruned quite drastically or, alternatively, kept in check by the social context. Lamb and Zakhireh (1997), for example, have documented a remarkable lack of empathic behavior in 45 toddlers (18 months of age) in the natural setting of a day-care center. These researchers observed 345 distress incidents during 20 hours of video recordings in the (average quality) centers, and registered how children in the group responded to this distress. Only unambiguous instances of prosocial responses to distress (e.g., offering a toy or patting a crying child) were coded; simple approaches or concerned looks were not. Of the 345 incidents, a meager 11 incidents were followed by a prosocial action from one of the peers. Prosocial response (whether or not the child had ever responded prosocially) was not related to age or gender. This study, of course, does not prove that young children would not have the disposition to be empathic; it demonstrates that in the day-care setting, children display indifferent behavior. The children may have the competence to act empathically, but their prosocial performance does not emerge in this specific situation.

Young children are not the innocent creatures we would like them to be (Rousseau 1762/1979). In the Generation R study (Tiemeier et al. 2012), we observed how often four-year-old children cheated in two game-like settings in the lab, and how many cheating children lied when asked afterward about their cheating behavior during the games (Zwirs et al., in preparation). These games were designed in such a way that when the children followed the rules they would certainly lose: in the "dart game," children had to throw the darts from too far a distance to be able to hit the target; in the "frog game," children were asked to find brown frogs under a tablecloth where only green frogs were hidden. In the first few demonstration trials, the games were made very easy to win, whereas after the experimenter had left the room, children could only lose in the real trials. The results were somewhat depressing. Almost 90% of the children (N = 460) cheated in one or both games; cheating was not associated with age or gender of the child, nor with socioeconomic status of the parents. Most children who cheated subsequently lied about the cheating when the experimenter asked what had happened in her absence and whether the rules of the game had been followed (Zwirs et al., in prep). Similar cheating and lying results were found in previous studies (Talwar et al. 2007; Lewis et al. 1989).

If infants are born with a preference for prosocial behavior, they certainly develop antisocial inclinations very quickly, triggered by their perception of the situation (membership of an out-group or competitive game). Tremblay's (2010) idea of children being born with the "original sin" that has to be socialized into a more prosocial direction might not be too far-fetched. Are parents able to make a difference and socialize their children into a more prosocial direction?

Prosocial Parenting: Attachment, Sensitivity, and Child Prosocial Behavior

More than 25 years ago, Hoffman (1984) suggested that parents play a role in promoting or hampering the development of prosocial behavior. He contended that if parents create a warm, sensitive atmosphere and, at the same time, consistently discipline child behavior that is damaging to others, a path would be paved for feelings of empathy to develop in their children. Non-empathic, authoritarian control combined with frequent threats and love withdrawal would, on the other hand, lead to compulsive compliance and a lack of moral internalization (van IJzendoorn 1997; Eisenberger et al. 2006). Sensitive parents who respond promptly and adequately to the distress and anxiety of their children stimulate a secure bond and, at the same time, provide a model of empathy and altruism (de Waal 2008; Hrdy 2009; Spiecker 1991; for a detailed account, see van IJzendoorn et al. 2010; van IJzendoorn and Bakermans-Kranenburg 2011).

In a study on the association between parental sensitivity and prosocial behavior in 24-month-old children, Brooker and Poulin-Dubois (2013) assessed parental sensitivity with a short version of the Maternal Behavior Q-set (MBQ) (Pederson and Moran 1995). Brooker and Poulin-Dubois used an adaptation of a helping task developed by Warneken and Tomasello (2009a) to measure instrumental helping behavior. The child saw the parent trying to reach a goal but was unable to accomplish this without help. In the "book task," the parent stacked three books on top of each other in front of the child, but the parent failed to stack the fourth book and expressed his or her disappointment, looking back and forth between the book and the child. More than half of the children helped the parent reach the goal. Most importantly, this study examined the association between parental sensitivity observed in a different setting with the MBQ and the level of helping behavior. No primary effect of sensitivity was found but gender played a role. For boys, parental sensitivity did not predict the level of helping, whereas for girls higher levels of parental sensitivity were associated with more helping behavior (Brooker and Poulin-Dubois 2013).

Whereas gender is taken into account in most studies on empathy and pro-social behavior, other constitutional and relational factors might also be important predictors or moderators. In particular, temperament and security of attachment have been considered to affect the development and expression of prosociality. The quality of the attachment relationship with the child has been shown to reflect the level of parental sensitivity. Thus it has been proposed that children with an insecure attachment relationship with their parent may be less inclined to act prosocially than children with a secure relationship (van IJzendoorn 1997). Mikulincer and Shaver (2008) present some experimental evidence for the role of attachment in adult helping behavior. They primed young adults with security-enhancing figures, such as their best friend, and observed more compassion with a woman in distress and more willingness to take over her disagreeable tasks after priming than in the control condition.

Temperamental fearfulness may moderate the effect of parenting on moral development (Kagan and Lamb 1990). Kochanska et al. (1995, 2007) found evidence for diverse pathways to moral internalization and prosocial behavior of children with different temperaments. For temperamentally fearful children, gentle maternal discipline predicted optimal moral internalization. For fear-less children, however, security of attachment was associated with internaliza-tion, and gentle discipline appeared less important. Attachment security and temperament emerged as complementary factors in the development of moral-ity. The moderating influence of temperament on the impact of parenting was restricted to assessments in the second year of life predicting preschoolers' prosocial behavior (Kochanska et al. 2007). It should be noted that tempera-ment may also play a role in the process of translating empathic distress into prosocial action. Fearful or emotionally reactive children might be more upset by another individual's pain and distress, and then incapacitated to take action (van IJzendoorn and Bakermans-Kranenburg 2012a).

In the Leiden Longitudinal Empathy Study we observed the development of empathy from infancy to middle childhood, examined its relation to donating to a charity, and searched for predictors of empathy: 87 middle-class Dutch mothers with a firstborn female infant were seen at 15, 18, and 89 months of age. Our sample included only girls to enhance the power of statistical analy-ses. Simulations of pain and sadness were used at 18 and 24 months (Van der Mark et al. 2002) and again at 89 months (Pannebakker 2007). The experi-menter pretended to hurt her finger or her knee, and mothers also pretended to hurt themselves; they also coughed as if they choked, several minutes after the other simulations. Mothers did not look at the child during these simulations to avoid extra stimulation of the child's reactions. Simulations were done during ongoing activities to minimize awareness of the pretend actions in the child.

Empathic concern toward the mother increased from 18 to 24 months and then decreased from 24 to 89 months. Empathic concern toward the experimenter decreased from 18 to 89 months. Contrary to the developmental model of Hoffman (2000) and others, growing older did not mean becoming more empathic. In line with evolutionary psychology, children showed more empathic concern toward their mother than toward an unrelated person. Women, especially, seem generally more inclined to help relatives than to help nonrelatives (Burnstein et al. 1994; Eagly and Crowley 1986). The associations across time were significant but disappointingly low and did not point to strong early childhood determination of a developmental pathway for empathic concern. The lack of associations between attachment, parental sensitivity, and temperament in early childhood, on the one hand, and empathic concern to stranger or mother in middle childhood, on the other, supports this conclusion. A lack of associations between empathy to mother and to the experimenter also throws doubt on the concept of general empathy, independent of the target. In fact, the (biological) relationship to or familiarity with the target might affect empathic concern rather substantially resonating the sharp in-group versus out-group differentiation by 14-month-old infants discussed above (for converging neural evidence in young adults, see Beckes et al. 2013).

Behavioral Genetics of Prosocial Behavior

To address the role of genetic factors in the explanation of individual differences in altruistic and prosocial behavior, studies with monozygotic and dizygotic twins have been conducted (e.g., Zahn-Waxler et al. 1992; for a detailed account, see van IJzendoorn et al. 2010; van IJzendoorn and Bakermans-Kranenburg 2011). Simply put, if correlations of moral behavior for monozygotic twins (100% genetically similar) are substantially higher than the correlations for dizygotic twins (on average 50% genetically similar), there is evidence for a genetic basis. One of the first twin studies on altruism included 573 adult twin pairs, who were asked to complete the Self-Report Altruism Scale: respondents were required to report the frequency with which they had engaged in twenty specific moral behaviors, such as "I have donated blood" (Rushton et al. 1986). More than 50% of the variance in self-reported prosocial behavior was found to be genetically based, whereas an almost equal percentage was explained by the unique environment component including measurement error. A tiny fraction, 2%, appeared to be due to common environmental factors, such as parenting, that make individuals within a family similar to each other.

Only two twin studies have been published on children's observed prosocial behavior (in particular, empathic helping behavior and concern for another person's pain and distress). Volbrecht et al. (2007) observed more than 200 twin pairs in the second year of life reacting to their primary caregiver, who pretended to have pinched her finger in a clipboard and feigned pain for a brief period. Helping behavior and empathic concern to distress did not show any genetic influence; both shared and unique environment explained the variation in these prosocial behaviors. In the second study, Knafo et al. (2008) observed more than 400 twin pairs longitudinally from 14 to 36 months of age in a similar empathic distress procedure, but one that also included a stranger simulating pain. At 14 months, no genetic effect was found on a composite measure of empathy, based on mother and experimenter simulations. By 24 months, a genetic effect, which accounted for about a 25% of the variance, emerged and this effect remained stable toward 36 months. With age, genetic effects on prosocial behavior and empathic concern appeared to increase, whereas shared environmental effects appeared to decrease (van IJzendoorn et al. 2010).

In our Leiden studies, high-cost donating behavior, without the expectation of any return, is usually measured by the amount of money (the number of €0.20 coins) a child donates in response to a videotaped call for donation to UNICEF. After an hour or more of performing various experimental tasks in one of our studies (Gilissen et al. 2008), the children received ten coins of €0.20 for their cooperation, in the absence of their mother. Their reactions showed that this was quite an amount of money for the young participants. They were then left alone and shown a two-minute UNICEF promotional film of a child in a "resource-limited," developing country. During the last fragments of the promotion, the voice-over asked for money donations, and a money box was prominently positioned next to the video screen. The money box was filled with several coins to enhance credibility. After one minute, the experimenter came back into the room and asked in a matter of fact manner whether the child would like to donate any money.

We used the donating paradigm in a study of 91 same-sex twin children who were seven years old (30 monozygotic, 61 dizygotic; 43 male, 48 female pairs) to examine whether individual differences in donating after being probed by the experimenter are genetically based, or whether at this age the (shared and unique) environment also affects donating behavior. The percentage of children that donated without being probed was too small to allow genetic modeling. This, of course, is a striking outcome in itself, indicating that completely voluntary high-cost prosocial behavior is not evident in the large majority of children in this age range.

As apparent from behavioral genetic analysis, 45% of the variance in donating was explained by shared environmental influences (e.g., similar parenting styles to both children in the family) and 55% of the variance by unique environment (e.g., uniquely different parental treatment of the twins or unique peer relationships) and measurement error (for statistical details, see van IJzendoorn et al. 2010; van IJzendoorn and Bakermans-Kranenburg 2011). Our results are in line with Volbrecht et al.'s (2007) finding of no genetic component in explaining differences in empathic concern. It should be noted, however, that the genetic component in the Knafo et al. (2008) study amounted to only about 25% of explained variance, and such percentages might go undetected in our small sample because of lack of statistical power. Most importantly, the absence of a main genetic effect is not incompatible with gene-environment interaction effects.

Gene-Environment Interactions and Differential Susceptibility: Family Environments and Experimental Tasks

We turned to molecular genetics to test whether experiences with parents might make a difference in children's donating behavior, depending on their genetic makeup (for a detailed report, see Bakermans-Kranenburg and van IJzendoorn 2011). Main effects within subgroups may be hidden in interactions (Bronfenbrenner 1979; Wachs and Plomin 1991), as children may be differentially susceptible to their environment (Belsky et al. 2007).

Differential susceptibility theory has emerged as an alternative to traditional cumulative risk or diathesis-stress models of human vulnerabilities (Ellis et al. 2011). Central to the diathesis-stress model is the postulate that some individuals are at heightened risk for psychiatric or behavioral disturbance when they encounter adversity, whereas others that lack such (genetic) vulnerability are not so affected when exposed to the same adversity. Seemingly "vulnerable" individuals may actually be more susceptible to the environment, for better *and* for worse. Dopamine-related genes (e.g., DRD4), which through their influence on attention and reward mechanisms have been shown to make children more vulnerable to negative parenting, also turned out to be susceptibility genes that promote optimal development in supportive family environments (Bakermans-Kranenburg and van IJzendoorn 2011).

In our donation study, we expected to find children who are securely attached to be more willing to donate money to a charity, since they may have experienced more often examples of sensitive empathic concern, and thus better moral exemplars from their parents. Children's attachment representations can be considered mental crystallizations of the degree to which their parents interacted with them in a sensitive way. In line with the differential susceptibility model, we expected the strongest association between attachment security and donating behavior in children with the DRD4 7-repeat allele.

We found, indeed, that for children without the DRD4 7-repeat allele, attachment security did not influence their donations. In the donating behavior of children with the DRD4 7-repeat allele, however, attachment security was important: secure children were inclined to donate more money *and* insecure children exhibited less donating behavior. This two-sided effect of DRD4 7-repeat, for better *and* for worse, supports the differential susceptibility theory (Bakermans-Kranenburg and van IJzendoorn 2006, 2007; Belsky et al. 2007).

Thus, both genetic and environmental determinants of prosocial donating be-havior appear important and should be considered in interaction. Since our study included only seven-year-old children, one should be careful in making generalizations to other age cohorts. Grunberg et al. (1985) found that donating to a charity is not linearly related to age. In their study of children aged 3–16 years, donating drops around seven years of age, as children have become more aware of the importance of individual ownership; this might be overgeneral-ized in a way analogous to young children who overapply rules of grammar.

Interaction effects are difficult to replicate because of lack of power, and this is certainly true for samples as small as ours in the previously discussed study. One of the few, rather exact replications has been conducted in Israel. Knafo et al. (2011) observed self-initiated prosocial behavior of 3.5-year-old twins in three settings in the Longitudinal Israeli Study of Twins. In the "help-ing task," the experimenter accidentally drops a box with pencils and is slow in picking them up, leaving space for the child to engage and help. The "empathic concern task" consists of the experimenter hurting her knee. In the "donating task," the experimenter and child each receive a box containing snacks; how-ever, the experimenter discovers to her disappointment that she has only a few snacks whereas the child finds many more in his or her box. Similar tasks were designed to assess the child's compliant prosocial behavior; that is, prosocial behavior on request from an adult.

Only a minority of the children showed self-initiated prosocial behavior, whereas a majority showed compliance, again evidence for the lack of spon-taneous altruism on the part of the children in this age range. The two types of prosocial behavior were not associated, which throws (again) doubt on a unitary concept of prosociality that ignores context and motivations. Only in monozygotic twins was prosocial behavior correlated, leading to the conclu-sion of a large genetic component in the absence of a shared environmental influence (Knafo et al. 2011). Mothers reported their parenting style to each of the twins, and no main effect on prosociality was found. DRD4 did not show main effects on prosociality either. However, parenting style, in particular the use of punishment, was related to prosocial behavior in the subgroup of chil-dren carrying the DRD4 7-repeat allele, whereas in the subgroup of children without the 7-repeat allele, no association was found. For children with the DRD4 7-repeat allele, self-initiated prosocial behavior was four times more frequent among children of mothers using punishment from time to time than among children of mothers low in punishment. In this subgroup the most pro-social as well as the least prosocial children were found, depending on their mother's parenting style; this demonstrates differential susceptibility albeit in an unexpected direction (Knafo et al. 2011). The meaning of punishment might differ depending on the parental context: if embedded in a warm relationship, punishment might express sensitive limit-setting that is needed, for example, in the case of overactive children (overrepresented in the group of carriers of DRD4 7-repeat alleles). Self-reported parenting styles may not reveal these subtle contextual qualifications. More robust molecular genetics findings may be expected from going beyond single candidate genes to genetic pathways, taking into account epigenetically regulated gene expression (Bakermans-Kranenburg and van IJzendoorn 2015; see also Keverne, this volume).

Hormonal Influences on Prosocial Behavior

Morality might not only be rooted in genetics but also in hormonal functioning. The first hint in the direction of oxytocin as a potentially important hormone came from a study on the oxytocin receptor (OXTR) gene that we found to be related to sensitive parenting (Bakermans-Kranenburg and van IJzendoorn 2008). The neuropeptide oxytocin has been called the "love hormone" and is increasingly used to study the influence of hormonal functioning on feelings, attitudes, behavior, and neural responses (see Carter and Porges, this volume). In particular, its positive role in parenting (Naber et al. 2012) and interpersonal trust and empathic concern (Baumgartner et al. 2008) has been documented in experiments using intranasal oxytocin administration, and these experiments seem to support the important role of oxytocin in prosociality (for a meta-analysis, see van IJzendoorn and Bakermans-Kranenburg 2012b).

Nevertheless, oxytocin might not be the panacea to promote love and to suppress aggression for all people under all circumstances (Bartz et al. 2010a, b). In a competitive game that triggered decisions with financial consequences to the subjects themselves, their in-group, and a competing out-group (De Dreu et al. 2010), oxytocin administration appeared to drive a "tend and defend" response in that it promoted in-group trust and cooperation, while enhancing defensive aggression toward competing or threatening out-groups. Similarly, only in the non-ostracism condition of the Cyberball computer game (see below) were individuals more inclined to play the social-interactive game again after oxytocin administration; when they were in the ostracism condition, where they felt as if they belonged to the rejected out-group, they did not wish to play (Alvares et al. 2010).

In a donation study of female undergraduate students aged 18–30 years, we examined in a double-blind experiment whether intranasal administration of oxytocin promoted the donation of money to UNICEF, and how this related to experienced parental caregiving. Participants were paid 50 Euros for participating in a series of experiments and then were asked to watch a video while the experimenter cleaned up in the other room. They were shown the 2-min UNICEF promotional film, after which a text appeared on the screen in which the participant was asked to donate money, and a money box had been positioned next to the video screen. Participants also reported whether they had experienced love withdrawal as a parental disciplinary strategy. Parental use of love withdrawal, involving withholding love and affection when a child misbehaves or fails at a task, has been associated with high concern over mistakes, low emotional well-being, and feelings of rejection and resentment toward the parents (e.g., Assor et al. 2004). These feelings may hinder empathic concern for others in distress and thus lead to lower levels of altruistic behavior (Koenig et al. 2004).

In our experiment, oxytocin appeared to increase participants' donations, but only in individuals who experienced low parental love withdrawal. In contrast, individuals with high love withdrawal experiences tended to donate even less when oxytocin was administered. Thus, oxytocin stimulates empathic, prosocial behavior, but not in everyone or across all contexts. Oxytocin makes some individuals more generous but its donagenic effect may be limited to those who feel accepted by their parents. We found similar differences in oxytocin effects, depending on the participants' experiences with parental love withdrawal in several other studies (handgrip, resting state: Bakermans-Kranenburg et al. 2012; Riem et al. 2013b). These findings lead us to suggest that oxytocin might not promote prosociality in individuals with unfavorable caregiving experiences. We speculate that such experiences might impact the oxytonergic system, for example, through hypermethylation of oxytonergic receptor genes that may downregulate the influence of exogenous oxytocin on the feedforward system of endogenous oxytocin production (Bakermans-Kranenburg and van IJzendoorn 2013).

Prosocial Cyberball

The virtual ball-tossing game called Cyberball (Williams and Jarvis 2006) has been most often used to study the effects of ostracism; that is, the experience of being rejected, which would feel like physical pain (Eisenberger and Lieberman 2004; Eisenberger et al. 2006). The original Cyberball consists of three players tossing a ball to each other. The participant is one of the players; the other two are virtual players programmed to begin after a while throwing balls only to each other, excluding the real player. We created a prosocial version of Cyberball consisting of four players, one of whom is the participant who observes how one of the players (known to the subject) at some point in time is consistently excluded by the two other virtual players. The question that was posed was whether the real player would compensate for this rejection by throwing more balls to the excluded player. Indeed, participants showed prosocial behavior by throwing on average almost twice as many balls to the excluded player. A sniff of oxytocin increased this prosocial behavior, but only in individuals who reported a childhood without many experiences of love withdrawal as a disciplinary strategy used by their parents (Riem et al. 2013a). It is unclear whether similar effects would have been found when the excluded player would be a complete stranger (or member of an out-group), and would not have been a person who was briefly introduced to the participant before the start of the game, thus associated perhaps with in-group membership.

Our findings are in line with previous research that shows, in individuals with harsh caregiving experiences, that beneficiary oxytocin effects are absent at the behavioral (Bakermans-Kranenburg et al. 2012) as well as at the neural level (Riem et al. 2013b). Fries et al. (2005) showed that children who experienced early adversity did not show a change in oxytocin levels after physical contact with their mother, whereas oxytocin levels were increased in children who were reared in a supportive family. Another study showed that subjects who experienced early parental separation exhibited attenuated cortisol decreases after intranasal oxytocin administration (versus placebo), compared to control subjects without early separation experiences (Meinlschmidt and Heim 2007). Furthermore, women who were exposed to child abuse or neglect exhibited lower oxytocin concentrations in cerebrospinal fluid (Heim et al. 2009).

Early adversity may lead to a dysregulation of the oxytocinergic system, possibly by influencing the level of methylation in genetic areas that regulate the oxytocinergic system (McGowan et al. 2009; van IJzendoorn et al. 2010; Bakermans-Kranenburg and van IJzendoorn 2013), which might lead to lower oxytocin levels and a decreased sensitivity to intranasal oxytocin. In a meta-analysis of 19 clinical trials with oxytocin sniffs, covering autism, social anxiety, postnatal depression, obsessive-compulsive problems, schizophrenia, borderline personality disorder, and posttraumatic stress, only studies on autism spectrum disorder showed a significant positive effect. For some of the other disorders, etiological factors rooted in negative childhood experiences may play a role in the diminished effectiveness of treatment with oxytocin (Bakermans-Kranenburg and van IJzendoorn 2013). Oxytocin sniffs and interventions aimed at elevating levels of endogenous oxytocin, such as massage, may not be very effective in promoting prosocial behavior and peace in those who need it most, and in preventing violence universally. Context and history must be taken into account.

Neural Activity and Prosocial Behavior

EEG Asymmetry

Can we identify neural correlates of individual differences in early prosociality? Because healthy infants are not allowed to be examined in an fMRI scanner with loud noises and restricted space, electroencephalogram (EEG) recordings are the preferred method to observe brain activation in relation to prosocial tendencies. Differences in power within the alpha band (8–12 Hz) of the EEG over left and right frontal areas are widely used to quantify asymmetric frontal brain activity (see also Fox et al., this volume). Asymmetric frontal brain activity has been implicated in reactions to emotional stimuli and is thought to reflect individual differences in approach-withdrawal motivation (Harmon-Jones et al. 2010). Paulus et al. (2013) recorded infant brain electrical activity, using 17 electrodes, and registered frontal activation asymmetries at 14 months of age. Instrumental helping was observed at 18 months using two procedures developed by Warneken and Tomasello (2009a), including the clothespin task discussed earlier. Prosocial comforting was assessed at 24 months in an episode in which the mother simulated to have hurt her finger. Infants' competent helping was associated with relative greater right than left cortical temporal activity. In contrast, comforting behavior was associated with relative greater left than right frontal activity (Paulus et al. 2013). This intriguing difference in cortical activity between two types of prosociality might be related to the difference in target individual: own mother versus unknown experimenter.

Interestingly, greater left to right frontal activity was found to be related to more donating to a charity in one of our studies on young adults (Huffmeijer et al. 2012). In our study on donating to UNICEF, we found that frontal alpha asymmetry and donating behavior were rather strongly associated ($r = .30$). More positive values, and thus greater relative left frontal activity, were related to larger donations to UNICEF. However, the situation became somewhat more complicated when the effects of intranasal administration of oxytocin and love-withdrawal were taken into account: low levels of parental love withdrawal predicted larger donations in the oxytocin condition for participants showing greater relative right frontal activity. We speculate that when approach motivation is high (reflected in greater relative left frontal activity), individuals are generally inclined to take action upon seeing someone in need, and thus to donate money and actively help. Only when approach motivation is low (reflected in less relative left and greater relative right activity) do empathic concerns affected by oxytocin and experiences of love withdrawal play an important part in deciding about donations (Huffmeijer et al. 2012). These results should be considered preliminary and need to be replicated in larger samples. The same is true for the Paulus et al. (2013) study discussed above. Research on EEG frontal asymmetry and prosocial behavior is still rare, primarily because EEG studies are extremely time-consuming and suffer from a high dropout rate, as young children are unable to sit still for the duration needed to record high-quality EEGs.

Functional MRI Approaches

If prosociality is inborn or becomes ingrained in the organism through development, altruism and empathic concern should be traceable in brain neural activity during events provoking prosociality. In addition to emerging associations with frontal asymmetry, there is growing evidence that empathy and prosocial behaviors can be located in specific areas of the brain, showing that individual differences in prosociality might be associated with individual differences in blood oxygenation level dependent (BOLD) signals registered by functional magnetic resonance imaging (fMRI) during an empathy or prosocial behavior task. It should be noted, however, that this area of research is still in its infancy, in particular with respect to prosociality in children and adolescents (see also van IJzendoorn et al. 2010; van IJzendoorn and Bakermans-Kranenburg 2011).

One of the first studies to use a donating task in the scanner was reported by Moll et al. (2006). Nineteen participants were asked to choose to endorse or oppose societal causes by donating or refraining from donating to real charitable organizations, with missions such as promoting children's rights or fighting the death penalty. Participants would receive $128 if they solely made egoistic choices. The amount of money decreased depending on how often they made (costly) prosocial choices. The results were striking. Not only did the mesolimbic reward system seem to be engaged in donations (suggesting the self-serving nature of donating behavior, or "feeling good"), so too was the orbitofrontal cortex, which is implicated in reward sensitivity. Most importantly, anterior parts of the prefrontal cortex (where higher cognitive and executive functions are located) were more active in costly choices between altruistic and selfish interests.

In one of the few fMRI studies on children, Masten et al. (2010) asked 13-year-olds to watch the original Cyberball with three players in the scanner. Children completed an empathy questionnaire a day before they were observed in the scanner, and after the fMRI procedure they were asked to write an email to the excluded player which was coded for the prosocial support and help for this player. During the observation of the social exclusion episodes, regions involved in mentalizing (i.e., dorsomedial and medial prefrontal cortex, precuneus and posterior superior temporal sulcus) were activated more strongly than when watching the inclusion episodes, particularly among highly empathic children. Children wrote more prosocial emails when they showed more activation in the anterior insula (as in previous studies linked to empathy for physical pain and social exclusion) during the observed ostracism in Cyberball; this suggests that they might have felt the pain of social exclusion stronger and thus expressed more supportive feelings in the email correspondence. In a similar study with young adults, the same research team found converging results, and, interestingly, they also found significant mediation by neural activation (in particular of the medial prefrontal cortex) of the link between more trait empathy (as measured prior to the scanning) and more prosocial emails (Masten et al. 2011).

In the Cyberball games presented thus far, Masten et al. (2011) used strangers as "players" in the game. An important question, from the perspective of differential treatment of in-group versus out-group members, is whether in Cyberball more empathic concern and prosociality is displayed toward a friend who is seemingly rejected as the third player, or toward a third player who is a stranger. In a study of native Chinese university students, Meyer et al. (2013) examined this difference in prosocial behavior as well as in neural activity, asking their subjects to bring their best friend to the lab. The participants were made to believe that in one version of Cyberball they watched their friend being ostracized and, in a second round of the game, an unknown person was ostracized. While observing the stranger version of Cyberball, previous results were replicated with activation in dorsal medial prefrontal cortex, precuneus, and temporal poles. In the friend version of Cyberball, increased activation of the dorsal anterior cingulate cortex, left insula, and medial prefrontal cortex in the exclusion trials compared to the inclusion trial were observed. In a functional connectivity analysis, the researchers only found increased connectivity between the medial prefrontal cortex and both the dorsal anterior cingulate cortex and insula in the friend version, not in the stranger version. Meyer et al. (2013) suggest that social exclusion of a friend triggers firsthand feelings of pain, whereas empathy for exclusion of a stranger may rely more heavily on mentalizing systems.

The previous studies may, however, be liable to an important drawback in some fMRI research; namely, the occurrence of impossibly high correlations (Vul et al. 2009; see van IJzendoorn et al. 2010). For example, the correlation of the BOLD signals in the prefrontal area during the donating task and self-reported engagement in real-life voluntary activities amounted to r = .87 in the Moll et al. study (2006). However, correlations as high as .87 or even .70 for any brain-behavior association may be too strong to be true. Analyzing 55 reports in social neuroscience using fMRI, Vul et al. (2009) showed that many published correlations are much higher than can be expected, given the limited reliability of both fMRI signals (test-retest of about .70) and prosociality measures (.80 at most). The maximum correlation between any two measures would be the square root of the product of the reliability figures of the two measures; in this case, .74 (Nunnally 1970; Vul et al. 2009). A nonindependence problem in preselecting significant voxels might be the reason for the implausible correlations (Vul et al. 2009). As in the study by Moll et al. (2006), associations between the three crucial variables in the Masten et al. (2011) study were exceptionally strong, although the sample was small and underpowered. The findings are nevertheless important, as they suggest directions into which future larger studies should explore associations between empathic traits, brain neural activity, and prosocial behavior.

Brain Morphology and Prosocial Behavior

Even more explorative are studies into the association between prosociality and brain morphology. Prosocial behavior tendencies have been speculated to be embodied in structural features of the brain, which would determine functional differences in neural transmission. Compared to functional imaging studies, structural imaging studies on prosocial behavior have been scarce. To our knowledge, only one study, including very preterm children, on the association between structural MRI and socioemotional development has been published (Rogers et al. 2012). This study reported a positive relation between bifrontal diameter and prosocial behavior in five-year-old boys (term-equivalent age). Since this study looked only at fetal brain metrics, the association between prosocial behavior and brain morphology at later ages is not yet clear. Furthermore, it is unclear how the results of Rogers et al. (2012) can be generalized to the association between brain morphology and prosocial behavior in children born at term.

In the Generation R study (Tiemeier et al. 2012), structural brain scans were conducted on 464 children, aged six to nine years (Thijssen et al., in prep). Their parents had completed the prosocial scale of the Strengths and Difficulties Questionnaire (Goodman 1997). The aim of the study was to examine the association between cortical thickness and prosociality, controlling for age, antisocial tendencies, IQ, socioeconomic status, and parental psychopathology. After Monte Carlo correction for multiple testing, the general linear model testing for the relationship between cortical thickness and prosocial behavior revealed one significant cluster covering part of the left superior frontal cortex and the rostral middle frontal cortex. A higher score for prosocial behavior was related to a thicker cortex in this cluster. The medial prefrontal cortex, which involves the anterior part of the superior frontal cortex, has previously been implicated in empathic concern in the Cyberball game as well as with prosocial behavior toward the excluded Cyberball player (Masten et al. 2010, 2011). The rostral middle frontal cortex has been linked to inhibitory control in both children and adults (Durston et al. 2002). Activation of the left dorsolateral prefrontal cortex, which involves the middle frontal cortex, has recently been reported in association with making costly donations (Telzer et al. 2011). Based on this finding, it may be suggested that inhibition of a selfish response precedes the performance of a prosocial act (Thijssen et al., in prep).

Associations between brain structure and behavior should be interpreted with caution, not only because they are weak (in our case only a small amount of variance in prosociality could be explained by brain morphology) but also because the direction of causal effects is not self-evident. The brain is a relay station between mind and body—not a homunculus that is the ultimate causative agent of moral behavior. Across the life span, brain morphology and activity can be affected by environmental input influencing epigenetic programming (McGowan et al. 2009), and recovery from extreme circumstances has been shown to change electrical activity permanently in the brain (Marshall et al. 2008; Fox et al., this volume). Brain morphology and activity may therefore be the "explanandum" as well as the "explanans"; that is, the end product as well as the starting point of moral behavior. One well-known example of behavior influencing morphology is the famous study of London taxi drivers, who showed an increase in the size of the hippocampus related to their memorization of the map of London (Maguire et al. 2000). Similarly, a recent study suggests that meditation is associated with greater cortical thickness in frontal regions, but reduced cortical thickness in regions more posterior in the brain (Kang et al. 2013).

Situational Morality

In view of the meager evidence for a trait-like interpretation of morality embodied in genes, brain, and hormones, prosocial and immoral behavior might better be considered as being shaped by the demand characteristics of specific situations (Hartshorne and May 1928/1932; Zimbardo 2007; Milgram 1963, 1974). We now turn to the influence of situational pressures on moral and immoral behavior, with an emphasis on research with children (see van IJzendoorn et al. 2010; van IJzendoorn and Bakermans-Kranenburg 2011).

Milgram Experiment with Children

To our surprise we discovered that in the 1970s, Milgram's original test of obedience had been replicated in children. Shanab and Yahya (1977) tested 192 Jordanian children (aged 6–8, 10–12, and 14–16 years) in two kinds of punishment instructions. Half of the children received instructions similar to the original Milgram experiment; namely, to administer electric shocks to learners each time the latter made a mistake in a paired-associate learning task and to increase the shock level with each additional mistake. The other half were given a free choice of delivering or not delivering shocks each time the learner made a mistake. Pressed by the experimenter, almost 75% of the children from the first group continued to deliver shocks up to maximum voltage. Only 16% of the children who had a free choice went that far. The situational pressures were much more important than other factors, such as age or gender.

Shanab and Yahya (1977) rated the emotional responses of the subjects during the Milgram experiment, recording tense behavior (e.g., loud nervous laughter, lip biting, and trembling); if they exhibited 11 or more of these emotional behaviors, they were considered to display intense tension. Disturbingly, the number of children in the intense tension category significantly *decreased* with age. Of those who expressed intense tension, 44%, 25%, and 16% were in the age groups 6–8, 10–12, and 14–16, respectively. Although serious ethical doubts might be raised about the conduct of the highly intrusive experiment with adults, let alone with children, the virtual neglect of the findings from this stunning study (24 citations versus 984 citations of Milgram's 1963 paper; source: Web of Science, August 23, 2013) cannot be legitimized by such ethical concerns about the experiment itself.

Situational Donating

Examining the number of coins donated after the promotional UNICEF film discussed above, and then after the experimenter's probe, we analyzed the impact of situational pressure on donating. In two studies on seven-year-old children, a very small minority of children was inclined to donate any money spontaneously (see above for discussion of one of these studies). After being prompted by an experimenter to donate, the percentage of children who donated some or all of their money increased rather steeply from one-tenth to about two-thirds. The findings were remarkably similar across our two studies. The situational difference between watching a promotional video clip alone (including a call for donation) and being prompted by an experimenter afterward, explained around 40% of the variance in donating; only half as much was explained by background variables (age, maternal educational level). Dispositional (attachment) and constitutional (temperament, genetics) differences seemed irrelevant, at least as main effects.

The crucial question is whether situations can be created to channel participants' behavior into a prosocial direction. Fortunately, some experimental studies on adults suggest that this is possible, but research on children is scarce. Freeman et al. (2009) tested the influence of witnessing or reading about moral exemplars on donating to a charity. Students who watched a video clip that documented moral excellence or who read a story about an extraordinary moral act or person donated more money to a charity that promoted goals somewhat antithetical to their own political views. The experiments were based on Haidt's (2007) theory of moral elevation, leading to more intense moral emotions and moral acts. Witnessing an act of moral excellence would stimulate thoughts, emotions, and motivational states that encourage people to show more empathic concern and caring behavior.

Small situational changes, such as installing a security camera which implies the presence of an audience, have been shown to result in similar enhancement of prosocial behavior in a student sample (van Rompay et al. 2009). Students provided more help in collecting and sorting a pile of questionnaires accidentally fallen on the floor in the presence of a camera, although the camera did not affect the participants' reported donations to charitable organizations. The dispositional trait of need for social approval also explained some variance in helping behavior, on top of the situational characteristics.

A telling example of the power of modeling is provided by Kallgren et al. (2000), who tested the influence of the presence of a confederate picking up a crumpled fastfood bag from the floor of a parking garage. Participants were visitors to a public urban hospital who were returning to their cars. When participants reached their cars, they encountered handbills attached to their windshield. Throwing the handbills on the floor was the observed outcome. The simple witnessing of the confederate picking up a piece of litter decreased littering behavior from 43% to a mere 9.3%. A simple manipulation of the situation (setting an example, focusing on the prosocial norm) strongly stimulated prosocial behavior.

In behavioral economics, situational canalization of human behavior has become a central topic of research. In their book, *Nudge*, Thaler and Sunstein (2008) present a myriad of situational manipulations that effectively change human behavior in desirable directions without changing their moral reasoning, dispositions, or motivations. A nudge is defined as any aspect of the choice architecture that alters people's behavior in a predictable way without forbidding any alternative behavioral option. Some prime examples are the following: Putting healthy food on eye level and junk food on lower or higher levels in restaurants or shops increases significantly the choice for healthy food. Etching the image of a black housefly into the urinals of the men's rooms at airports reduces spillage by 80%. Emphasizing the majority of students who do not binge drink rather than stressing the problem of binge drinking with alarming percentages of those who do binge drink lowers the alcohol consumption significantly.

Promoting Prosociality

What kind of educational intervention is compatible with situational morality? To promote child prosocial development, a variety of answers have been posited (see Kagitcibasi and Britto as well as Nusseibeh, this volume). Here we focus on ways to use the concept of situational morality to reflect on potentially effective interventions (for a more extensive treatment, see van IJzendoorn et al. 2010; van IJzendoorn and Bakermans-Kranenburg 2011).

If the demand characteristics of the situation have the most impact on prosocial and antisocial behavior, the logical implication is to monitor and change the environment in which children are growing up and are being educated. We might need an ethics of situations; that is, of embodying high moral standards in environments that canalize individual prosocial behavior. In fact, if environments have both a physical and a social embodiment of high moral standards (e.g., in prosocial tutors and guidelines for proper behavior), they may be extremely powerful in canalizing prosocial behavior in children. This comes close to the Aristotelian concept of "habituation" through which virtuous affective dispositions are strengthened by conditioning behavior with reinforcing and punishing stimuli (Steutel and Spiecker 2004).

The just-community approach to moral education, originated by Kohlberg (1985; see also Power 1979; Oser et al. 2008), appears to come close to this, although its ethical inspiration is pertinently anti-Aristotelian. This project aimed to immerse students in an environment imbued with just and fair role models, rules, and interactions, and with concrete behavioral norms of an almost Aristotelian nature ("learning by doing" to be on time, to abstain from fighting). Most importantly, the peers in the just community embodied and sanctioned the socio-moral norms that canalized individual students' behavior. Kohlberg (1985:84) stressed that "the good as altruism is cultivated by a sense of community, by a feeling of group cohesion and solidarity." Essential ingredients were the community meeting for democratic decision making, the discipline committee for confronting individuals with their misbehavior and punishing and forgiving them, and moral dilemma discussions in the classroom to enhance the level of moral reasoning (Oser et al. 2008).

The just-community approach was a short-term success that elevated the moral judgment level of the students, but as Kohlberg (1985:80) stated: "While the intervention operation was a success, the patient died." One year after the conclusion of the experiment not a single teacher continued to have moral discussions. The successful failure of this just-community experiment may have at least two educational implications. First, implementation of a just community should be prolonged and sustained across several years to evoke effective change in the participants' moral behavior. In de Waal's (2008) intervention of mixing prosocial macaque and more aggressive rhesus monkeys, positive changes in the rhesus monkeys' interactions persisted within their own group after closure of the experiment, which lasted about two years on a human timescale (see also Maestripieri, this volume).

Second, part of moral education may consist of making individuals aware of the power of situations in determining their moral choices in experimental and natural settings. Teaching children and adolescents the experimental evidence of situational morality, such as the Stanford prison experiment (Zimbardo 2007) or the Milgram experiments (Milgram 1974), may lead to self-defeating prophecies and create opportunities to make moral choices that deviate from the situational pressures to act in a specific (immoral) way. Discussing with students some real examples of situational immorality, such as Auschwitz or Abu Ghraib, as well as examples of canalization of altruistic behavior, such as donating after the tsunami, may add to their understanding of the determinants of their own moral behavior. In fact, moral reasoning is also subjected to situational influences (Doris and the Moral Psychology Research Group 2010), and these influences might be used to enhance the level of reasoning as well as prosocial behavior. Whether enhanced moral reasoning and prosocial behavior contribute to a more peaceful society remains to be seen. Certainly it would help to level the social spirit (Wilkinson and Pickett 2010, see Steele et al., this volume) in the right direction and thus alleviate feelings of exclusion that leads to aggression.

Conclusion

There is not much evidence to support the popular notion that individual differences in prosocial behavior are determined by parenting and other childhood experiences. The role of attachment security and temperament seems disappointingly small. The same appears to hold for neurobiological influences. However, main effects of neurobiological and environmental factors might be hidden in their interactions, and research on interactions between neurobiology and environment is at an initial stage.

Moral *competence*—the ability to feel, reason and act prosocially—may be a universal human characteristic. However, the translation of this universal competence into prosocial *performance*—actual compassion and altruistic behavior—requires a *moral situation* with prosocial incentives and demand characteristics.

As research continues to address these issues, we suggest that attention be given to the following areas:

• Longitudinal studies across elementary and high school years tracking the development of observed prosocial behaviors, such as donating, are desperately needed.

• The influence of nudges to canalize prosocial behavior has been studied with students and adults, but only a few studies have examined similar processes in infants and young children.

• Can we support parents and other caregivers in creating a "moral" environment for the children in their care (e.g., by exposing them to moral exemplars)?

• The genetic component of prosocial behavior is elusive even in studies on gene-environment interaction. Gene-environment experiments are needed that include genetic pathways and epigenetic regulation of gene expression.

• Experimental studies with intranasal oxytocin administration must make clear for whom and under which conditions oxytocin might turn into a "peace hormone."

Acknowledgment

This chapter extends our earlier work (van IJzendoorn et al. 2010; van IJzendoorn and Bakermans-Kranenburg 2011) and builds on a presentation that we gave in 2011, "On situational and embodied morality," at the symposium on The Development of Character: The Aristotelian Tradition and Contemporary Developmental Psychology, Keble College, Oxford University, February 12–13, 2011. Our work is supported by awards from the Netherlands Organization for Scientific Research (MHvIJ: NWO SPINOZA prize; MJBK: VICI award no. 453-09-003), and by the Gravitation program of the Dutch Ministry of Education, Culture, and Science and the Netherlands Organization for Scientific Research (NWO grant number 024.001.003).

First column (top to bottom): Howard Steele, Marian Bakermans-Kranenburg,
Dario Maestripieri, Marian Bakermans-Kranenburg, Marinus van IJzendoorn,
Mary Dozier, Tom Boyce
Second column: Marinus van IJzendoorn, Nathan Fox, Heidi Keller, Howard Steele,
Dario Maestripieri, Heidi Keller, Hiltrud Otto
Third column: Tom Boyce, Hiltrud Otto, Paul Odhiambo Oburu, Mary Dozier,
Nathan Fox, Marian Bakermans-Kranenburg, Paul Odhiambo Oburu

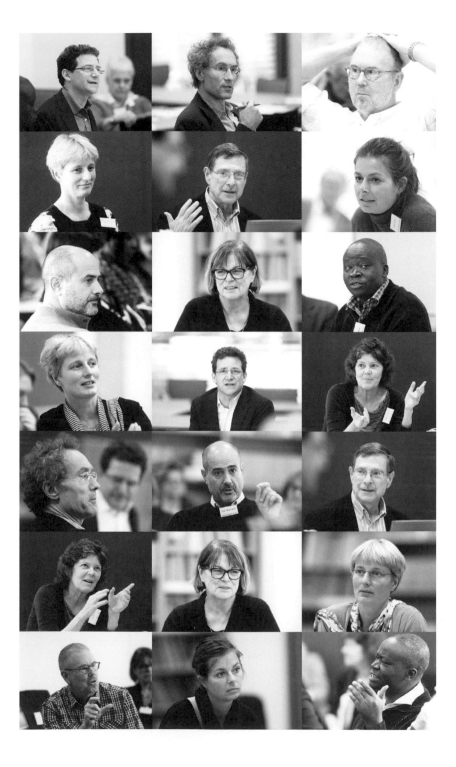

11

How Do Events and Relationships in Childhood Set the Stage for Peace at Personal and Social Levels?

Howard Steele, Marinus H. van IJzendoorn,
Marian J. Bakermans-Kranenburg, W. Thomas Boyce,
Mary Dozier, Nathan A. Fox, Heidi Keller,
Dario Maestripieri, Paul Odhiambo Oburu, and Hiltrud Otto

Abstract

This chapter focuses on early childhood experiences and how they may contribute to cooperative and peaceful behaviors and outcomes in the later childhood years and into adulthood. Five interrelated topics are explored: (a) universal tensions ever pushing us toward competition or cooperation; (b) socioeconomic inequities that powerfully constrain children's (and adult's) potential to contribute to and participate in a healthy and peaceful society; (c) the protective and enabling forces of the early caregiving environment when it is sensitive and responsive to children's needs; (d) the malevolent, if culturally understandable, influences of harsh parenting practices and child abuse; and (e) a summary of early psychological interventions that promote sensitive parenting and secure attachments well known to be associated with cooperative, nonviolent behaviors across childhood and beyond. Each section is punctuated by suggestions for further research and public policy developments (national and international) that could further advance the cause of peace.

Introduction

It is by no means novel to claim that early experiences with caregivers have an immediate, profound, and long-term influence on the developing child, contributing to whether the child as an older person will rely on cooperative (empathic) or competitive (aggressive) strategies when faced with frustration or distress. The power of early learning experiences is robustly evident in the tenets of ancient religions, just as it can be frequently heard in popular music, as in the 1971 Graham Nash song, "Teach your children well," first performed on the album *Déjà Vu*. "Already seen this/already been there" may be an apt description of the situation we find ourselves in vis-à-vis war and peace. For despite this music and its lyrics often being said to be among those influences that "shaped a generation," war and violence victimizing children remains a constant theme in human affairs, century upon century.

Graham Nash has commented that the immediate inspiration for the song came from a famous photograph by Diane Arbus, *Child with Toy Hand Grenade in Central Park*. The image, which depicts a child with an angry expression holding the toy weapon, prompted Nash to reflect on how children learn about and internalize war, and the (unfortunate) belief that acting aggressively appears at times the only way to defend our security, or the security of our family, community, or nation group referred to in social psychology as our "in-group" in contrast to an often feared and despised other "out-group." While we can celebrate attempts to encourage relinquishment of an "us versus them" mentality, and might adopt in its place an "us and them" perspective (Fry, this volume), it does appear that we live as individuals and groups situated between two poles, each having great motivational pull: (a) self- or status-preservative aggressive acts and (b) empathic or cooperative acts.

This chapter arises from an intensive group effort devoted to reviewing the current scientific evidence on just how early experiences in one's family, in the context of a wide range of moderating and mediating factors, may contribute to peace at the personal and social levels. Peace can be variously interpreted, and we do not attempt to define peace in any consistent or parallel way across various levels of discourse. Peace may be considered an outcome, as in a peace agreement between nations or as a peaceful reconciliation reached between sparring adversaries. Peace might also be used to label a state of mind, as in the sense of "inner peace." In addition, peace is a process, insofar as once achieved, it must be nurtured, protected, and maintained.

This chapter focuses on early childhood experiences and the diverse parenting and contextual factors that determine the likelihoods of children and families decreasing the use of violent force among individuals and groups, finding nonviolent ways to repair and reconcile relationships when conflict seems inevitable, and maintaining peace at the personal and societal levels. Five broad sections, focusing on different levels and domains of the problem, are addressed, and a summary of these interrelated topics follows:

1. Competition and cooperation: There are universal pressures, depending on the specific context and distribution of resources available, that may predict whether cooperation or competition between individuals will prevail at a given time. Robust data from human and animal studies show that cooperation enhances prosocial behavior toward others,

whereas competition often gives rise to aggression. This first section addresses aggressive and prosocial behavior from a functional perspective and describes their development in infants and children, with emphasis on the role of positive and negative emotions. We also discuss the role of children's social hierarchies— the visible, dominance-driven social orders that can be seen even in early childhood playgroups as well as the structures of preschool classrooms. Strategies for diminishing the severity of such hierarchies of dominance and subordination, with a consequent increase in cooperative, prosocial, and peaceful behavior, are presented, and we conclude with a discussion of the importance of training future leaders capable of creating social systems that are more egalitarian and peace-promotive, rather than despotic and violent.

2. Inequities in socioeconomic status: In developmental and epidemiologic research involving childhood experiences and health outcomes, socioeconomic status is by far the most powerful predictor for success. It is, in fact, such a powerful determinant that we question most associations not adjusted for confounding socioeconomic effects. Poverty, poor nutrition, and chronic stress are a breeding ground for marginalization and social exclusion, poor impulse control, disease, and violence.

3. Context of primary caregiving: The primary caregiving context into which each child is born, and which constitutes its main developmental niche over the first few years of life (including parents, siblings, grandparents, foster and adoptive parents) is fundamental to the child's early (and probably also later) possibilities for contributing to, and realizing, peaceable interactions with others. Context also provides the child, in optimal circumstances, with a safe haven to turn to when distressed and a secure base from which to safely explore and learn. As with competition and cooperation, attachment is a universal process, evolutionarily rooted, having emotional, cognitive and behavioral expressions, with links to neurobiology about which we are ever learning more. However, individual and cultural differences can be detected in how attachment is expressed, leading to patterns of attachment that may link up with steepness in dominance hierarchies, and correspondingly with more or less cooperation and competition (Troy and Sroufe 1987; Suess et al. 1992).

4. Treatment of children: Parents and teachers are challenged to set limits as they guide children toward peaceable behaviors regulated by inhibitory control. Parents and teachers differ in their capacity to set limits to violent interactions between siblings or pupils, and to promote cooperative empathic behaviors. Some err on the side of applying harsh practices to children, ranging from smacking to corporal punishment without leaving physical traces, and, at the extreme end, neglectful or abusive behaviors ("child maltreatment"), which is known to have highly adverse influences on children's behaviors, emotions,

cognitions, and brain circuitry (see Fox et al., this volume), creating fertile developmental ground for aggressive tendencies when conflicts arise. Top-down attempts to change harsh discipline practices of parents and teachers are reviewed in countries where legislation has been enacted to protect children, albeit with mixed results (Mweru 2010). Bottom-up strategies are encouraged for empowering parents and teachers to adopt a more flexible range of limit setting strategies, underpinned by warmth, understanding, and humor, so that children are more likely to learn peace-loving cooperative attitudes and nonviolent conflict resolution strategies and behaviors (see Hinde and Stevenson-Hinde, this volume).

5. Principles for interventions: When the well-being of children is endangered, and the prospects of peace for the child and his social environment are diminished, what principles should guide intervention efforts? The answer is robustly clear from many successful early intervention programs that are empowering parents to be more nurturing, more synchronous, and less frightening to (or frightened of) their infants. Recent scientific findings on genetic markers that support differential susceptibility theory are summarized. However, the weight of this discussion is on specific suggestions to those intervening with vulnerable parents so that they can maximize their chance to align themselves with parents' hopes and dreams for their children, providing them with a repertoire of nonviolent conflict management strategies.

Competition and Cooperation

A Functional Approach to Aggressive and Prosocial Behavior

Competition and cooperation are fundamental dimensions of life as social creatures. Competition occurs when individuals pursue their own interests, or the interests of their own group, at the expense of other individuals or other groups. Competition is driven by self-advancing motivation and can be expressed as aggressive behavior that directly or indirectly harms other individuals. Cooperation occurs when two or more individuals are more likely to achieve their goals by working together than by acting alone. Cooperation can be expressed as prosocial behavior that directly or indirectly benefits other individuals. Individuals are more or less likely to engage in competition or cooperation with others depending on the environment in which they find themselves (e.g., whether resources are scarce or abundant) and the identity of other individuals (e.g., whether they are family members or strangers). However, the tendency to engage in competition or cooperation can also depend on characteristics of the self, such as age, gender, temperament or personality, education, moral or religious beliefs, and financial resources. These individual characteristics can also influence how prosocial or aggressive behavior is expressed. For example, males at any age are more likely to engage in physical aggression, whereas females are more likely to engage in verbal or psychological aggression (Crick et al. 2006). From a functional perspective, everyone has the capacity for aggressive and prosocial behavior. Particular individual characteristics and contexts, however, can favor the expression of aggressive over prosocial behavior, or vice versa.

From a developmental perspective, the early emergence of empathic concern or feelings of compassion toward others is conducive to the later expression of prosocial behavior, whereas early selfish tendencies, coupled with negative emotions such as anxiety and anger, may result in later aggressiveness. Infants' initial emotional experience exists on a continuum from extreme distress (feeling unsafe or lacking containment) to extreme comfort (calm in the arms of a caregiver). Over time, comfort evolves into a smiling response and social laughter (by three to four months of age). Importantly, while congenitally blind children show a smiling response at the same time as typically developing babies, the smile never assumes the contours, range, and expressiveness of infants with sight. Just as the cry of the newborn functions to bring the outstretched arms of the caregiver, so too does the smile, a few months later, arise in the context of animated social exchanges. Emotions serve social functions and purposes. The infant needs the caregiver's contact, comfort, and protection; the infant's emotional life is influenced by interactions with the caregiver.

Prosocial and aggressive behavior can be seen clearly in the second year of life, with precursors evident in the first year. The function of prosocial behavior in young children is to invest in another individual who may be expected to show care or help in response (e.g., an adult caregiver or a friend). Aggression is typically shown toward others who are imagined to represent a threat to one's status. Already at this early age, prosocial and aggressive behavior occurs in very different contexts and may be affected by gender or socioeconomic status (see below). Moreover, two-year-old children may already evidence stronger prosocial or aggressive tendencies, depending on the experience acquired in their first year of life. Children exposed to sensitive parenting, who grow up in a predictable and supportive environment, are more likely to show empathic responses to others, inhibition of negative emotions, and prosocial behavior. In contrast, children exposed to insensitive or harsh parenting, or danger or trauma, may be less empathic, more prone to anxiety and anger, and more likely to be aggressive toward adults and other children.

Preschool children routinely cooperate with some children and compete with others, both in classroom settings and on the playground. Indeed, even preverbal human infants in the first year of life show mental representations of dominance relations, using relative size to predict the outcome of conflict between agents with opposing goals (Thomsen et al. 2011). Some children are more assertive than others or have better social skills which make them more popular and more effective at forming alliances with other children. These characteristics and skills influence the ranks that children occupy in their dominance hierarchies. Whether children have a high, middle, or low rank in these hierarchies may influence the probability of social marginalization and exclusion and of displaying or receiving aggressive or prosocial behavior from others. High-rank children may use bullying and other forms of intimidation toward lower-ranking children to maintain or reinforce their status. Such experiences of social marginality and bullying as well as their accompanying psychological pain have been shown to bear clear commonalities with physical pain, including the activation of the same cortical and limbic areas of the brain (Eisenberger and Lieberman 2004; Mee et al. 2006; cf. Cacioppo et al. 2013). Middle- and low-rank children may behave prosocially toward others to buffer themselves against aggression or intimidation, or to attempt to improve their status. In nonhuman primate societies, the steepness of the dominance hierarchy may influence the overall level of aggressive or prosocial behavior within a group. When the dominance hierarchy of a primate group has a steep slope, there is generally frequent and intense top-down aggression to maintain the status quo. The intense competition observed in these groups does not promote the expression of prosocial behavior. When the dominance hierarchy has a gentle slope, there is less top-down aggression and more cooperation and prosocial behavior being exchanged between individuals close or distant in ranks. In public kindergartens in Berkeley, California, where dominance hierarchies among five-year-old children have been observed and measured, the steepness of the social order may be markedly reduced by teachers who emphasize the unique strengths and assets of each child in the class (Boyce et al. 2012a). Concerns about status among children can also be minimized by teachers by introducing the value of fairness, resource sharing, turn-taking, and cognitive reframing. Teachers' interventions can thus reduce competition and aggression between children and promote cooperative and prosocial behavior.

Children may face power hierarchies not only at school but also in their families. In dysfunctional families, parents may insist on maintaining a steep hierarchy in their vertical relationships with their children and, correspondingly, are more likely to react to their children in ways that escalate quickly to the use of violence. In this way, parents assert their authority and show who is boss, modeling uncontrolled behavior which detracts from peaceful behavior. Such authoritarian parental behaviors make it more likely that children and adolescents will become rebellious and aggressive toward their parents or siblings. Thus we observe "chaotic" families where domestic violence and other adversities are prevalent, with family members moving in and out of the group. "Out" may mean prison. "In" may mean the return of a child who had been removed (for reasons of safety) to kinship or foster care. Well-adjusted families are those in which parents are authoritative (setting limits with humor, warmth, and control) instead of authoritarian and in which children learn to resolve conflicts through negotiation instead of aggression and violence.

Dominance hierarchies are ubiquitous in human societies, although there is great variation in the extent to which these societies are despotic or egalitarian (e.g., Fry 2006). It is important to emphasize that dominance hierarchies are not instrinsically "bad" or conducive to aggression and violence. It has been argued that the emergence of social dominance has adaptive advantages, in the form of divisions of labor, cooperative breeding, leadership provision, diminution of aggression, and constraints on the spread of infectious disease (Boyce et al. 2012a). Whether a social system with a hierarchical organization is characterized by cooperation and prosociality or competition and aggression may depend on how the power is handled by the leader of the group. In nonhuman primate societies, the personality of the alpha male can make a difference. A highly anxious and neurotic alpha male may attempt to control the behavior of other group members through aggression and intimidation, while a more relaxed and friendly alpha male will use his social skills to induce other group members to cooperate with him as well as with one another (e.g., Boehm 1999). The removal of domineering, aggressive individuals has been shown, in primate social groups, to alter the "culture" of a social group fundamentally toward a more pacific, egalitarian structure (Sapolsky and Share 2004). In human societies, it is possible to see the same processes at work insofar as some leaders appear bent on domination and control of their citizens and other nation groups such that outbreaks of violence are sudden and frequent, while other leaders appear to more easily achieve and maintain an egalitarian society where diverse competing groups share power with consequent reductions in violence. The task of leadership is complex and demanding.

Individuals who have the skills and opportunities to become leaders can be trained to understand that with power comes responsibilities and that leadership entails service to the community, not privilege. Training children to be good, effective leaders is vital for building peaceful societies; the length of childhood and adolescence offers multiple opportunities for such training. A moving example of a widely pursued strategy to train children to be leaders is reflected in an effort initiated by a Nigerian high school student in an urban slum that was related by the student's mother, Olayinka Omigbodun, a psychiatrist in Nigeria and coauthor of Britto, Salah et al. (this volume): With family support and sponsorship from a local university, the high school student applied fresh paint to a small hut and placed bookshelves inside and planks for children to sit on next to small tables. The neighborhood's children were then invited to learn to read. The guiding principle was "readers are leaders": an international and compelling concept with dedicated websites and Facebook pages that reflect similar efforts around the globe. In the Nigerian case, many hundreds of children (and their parents), Muslims and Christians, have been empowered by acquiring literacy skills in a place where despondency, under the weight of poverty, might otherwise prevail. The power of reading to lift underrepresented groups to positions of influence and inspired leadership has a celebrated history (Eagly and Carli 2007; Freire 1985). Civic programs at high schools and universities, public service (instead of mandatory military service), as well as sports teams (fertile ground for both cooperation and healthy competition) are all worthwhile efforts to build leadership capacities. The sports example highlights how leadership is a domain-specific skill, reflecting the variable character of natural talents. This creates opportunities for leaders of different strengths to meet and share insights on how best to motivate and serve one's constituency. There are socioemotional leaders as well as action-oriented leaders. All are needed to advance the cause of peace. Great leaders inhibit their selfishness and draw intrinsic rewards from helping others achieve their potential, motivated by a wish to live up to an ideal learned in childhood, or one acquired since.

Summary and Suggestions for Further Research and Policy

When young children express prosocial or aggressive behavior at home or with their peers, and when they occupy high-ranking or low-ranking positions in dominance hierarchies in the playground, they receive important feedback from the environment. This, in turn, influences their future behavior, psychological processes, and physiological reactions and canalizes their social development. Little is known about how this experience in the environment "gets under the skin" (see Carter and Porges, this volume). How is the brain of an eight-year-old boy affected by chronic social subordination (see Fox et al., this volume)? How are sex and stress hormones affected by social events that occur before and after puberty (e.g., being socially isolated or being at the center of a large network of family members and friends)?

There is an urgent need for research on the physiological consequences of dominance/subordination in children. At the same time, there is ongoing need for research that compares educational and social policy initiatives, so as to identify which approaches will best serve to level the playing field and create opportunities for all. (For a discussion on what has worked and why, see Kagitcibasi and Britto, this volume.)

Inequities in Socioeconomic Status

Social inequalities in health, development, and well-being are pervasive across the globe. Beginning early in life, impoverished children and families sustain higher rates of virtually every form of human malady: from low birth weight (Blumenshine et al. 2010) to traumatic injury (Brown and Davidson 1978); from infectious disease (Dowd et al. 2009) to dental caries (Boyce et al. 2010); from developmental disability (Msall et al. 1998) to poorer academic achievement (Kawachi et al. 2010). Both the perpetration of and victimization by violent acts also differ dramatically by socioeconomic conditions within families and neighborhoods (McCullough et al. 2013). Exposures to child abuse, aggression, and violence are associated, over the life course, with multiple comorbid outcomes, including school absenteeism and suspension (Ramirez et al. 2012), memory loss, substance use, and sexual dysfunction (Anda et al. 2006), disorders of mental health (Edward et al. 2003), and accelerated cellular aging (Shalev et al. 2013). Socioeconomic stratification of developmental psychopathology, which often emerges in preclinical form in the middle childhood years, exerts lasting influences on academic achievement, employment success, interpersonal relationships, and lifelong well-being (U.S. Dept of Health and Human Services 2011). These inequalities, moreover, have deep historical origins, and their consequences must be carefully documented, as they detract significantly from the possibility of health, economic security, and peace at personal and social levels.

Despite the universality and potency of societal disparities in health, it is only recently that socioeconomic status has become itself a focus of serious scientific study (Syme 2008). New studies of the socioeconomic status antecedents of population morbidities have recognized the extended influence of childhood social status on adult disease, even after controlling for socioeconomic status in adulthood (Cohen et al. 2010; Galobardes et al. 2004; Lawlor et al. 2006). Such evidence for lifelong effects of early disadvantage is rendered still more compelling by research that has documented the developmental origins of adult health and disease (Gluckman et al. 2005, 2009) and by epidemiologic work that has revealed systematic differences in nutrition (Khan and Bhutta 2010), access to medical care (Houweling and Kunst 2010), and physical environmental exposures (Gump et al. 2007) among children of differing social class.

Dramatic differences exist between countries and within countries going back through the centuries. From sixteenth-century English Poor Laws to contemporary concerns in the United States that "entitlements" must be cut back, there is consistent evidence that those at the top of the social hierarchy, often with justifications that suit them, work to undermine the possibilities of those at the bottom of the hierarchy. Socioeconomic differences are enacted and reinforced by those with political power. Children are differentially adversely influenced by this disparity between the wealthy and the poor.

There is research on how children reason about justice, equality, and fairness. Children from a very early age understand concepts of fairness. If you ask children to reason about fairness situations that they have experienced, they answer in ways that show their understanding of the need for equal distribution of resources. What's the relationship between their reasoning skills and their behavior? All of this depends on parents, teachers, and other caregivers. For example, when teachers emphasize and exacerbate the inequitable distribution, reasoning does not lead to just or fair behavior. However, when teachers set up the classroom on egalitarian principles, giving everyone access to all resources, then children's reasoning matches to this behavior. We learn about inequality from an early age, and we learn from parents and teachers.

At the same time, inequality in social stratification of groups is perhaps inevitable given the unequal distribution of natural talents that contribute to diversity, division of labor, and to the efficient production of socially valuable knowledge, goods, and services. Although unequal natural or inborn talents are basically undeserved, social inequality emerging from these natural inequalities may be defensible if the inequality works to the greatest advantage of the least privileged. This is the so-called "difference principle" in the theory of justice as fairness (Rawls 1971). Steep inequality gradients that have damaging effects on the lowest-ranking individuals are indefensible from the perspective of this difference principle.

Summary and Suggestions for Further Research and Policy

The sharp income gradient in the United States and other countries around the globe, as well as the stress that results, has immediate effects on health outcomes (Pickett and Wilkinson 2010). Lowering the gradient is vital to minimizing the toxic effects of poverty and stress on evolving brain circuitry, and improving health outcomes. Rank and resources are distinct aspects of socioeconomic status that may need to be separated out. Self-rank is different from objective income status, and lower self-ranking is a powerful predictor on its own of health and brain functioning (Fox et al., this volume). Opportunities for personal and social peace for children, parents, and society may be advanced if investments are made in teacher training programs as well as in the compensation (salaries) of teachers that reflect the vital influences they have on developing children.

The Primary Caregiving Context: Family

Moving from the socioeconomic level and questions about dominance hierarchies, let us focus on the first environmental context a child encounters; that is, his or her mother's body, biological systems, thoughts, feelings, and behaviors (see Keverne, this volume). Beginning with the newborn infant, and the infant's journey through conception and gestation, on through the first year of life, there is much to examine that may well set the stage for peace at the personal and social level across time. A report prepared for the World Health Organization some 65 years ago (Bowlby 1952) first signaled, to an international audience, the importance of early experiences with the mother or mother substitute. What was deemed vital for the child's immediate and long-term mental health was a relationship between child and mother, where each derived an enduring sense of joy. This report had been invited on account of the vast numbers of displaced and orphaned children in the years immediately following the Second World War. More than a half century later, and well into the 21st century, a wealth of data both confirms and qualifies Bowlby's 1952 hypothesis. Early experiences do matter greatly, but later experiences can either strengthen the effect of early experiences or, when prior experiences were adverse, diminish the effect of early experience and offer new more peaceful modes of relating to others.

The caregiver is the safe haven for the distressed child and the secure base from which the child ventures away to explore. A more or less continuous relationship to a caregiver is vital to every infant on account of the infant's biological and emotional needs for safety and protection. No child can survive and thrive on his or her own. Social bonds are essential, and the infant needs a primary caregiving relationship so that the infant knows where to turn for comfort and security. Around the globe, it is usually possible to identify a primary caregiver or caregivers responsible for each infant.

Cross-cultural research provides evidence that the number of primary caretakers and their acutal involvement in child rearing varies across cultures. Although the amount of alloparenting varies widely, alloparenting seems to be the rule in many societies, not the exception (Hrdy 2009). For example, Gottlieb (2004) reports that Beng newborns are greeted by the whole village on the first day of their life; Beng infants generally spend only few minutes on average with a caregiver before they are passed on to other caregivers in the community. For the Efe who live in the northern Congolese rain forest, alloparenting is completely normal, as it is with most hunter-gatherer groups (Hewlett and Lamb 2005). Until toddlerhood, an Efe infant rotates among multiple caregivers several times during a single hour, is comforted by multiple caretakers, and nursed by multiple women (Tronick et al. 1987). Similarly, Cameroonian infants are cared for by sibling caretakers as young as three years of age for most part of the day, who integrate the infants into their daily social life, work routines, and play (Lamm 2008). A transfer of responsibility to others (grandmothers, fathers, aunts, uncles, older siblings, or others) frequently occurs for short or long periods of time. Fostering peace in any one of these caregiving relationships—to the extent that they are more or less continuous, stable, and capable of providing an enduring sense of joy to caregiver and child— may be sufficient to insure that a child is capable of developing a healthy balance of cooperative and competitive behaviors so as to contribute to personal and social peace. When security prevails in primary caregiving relationships, children have a greater chance to be launched toward empathic relations and effective conflict resolution strategies with peers well into the school years and beyond (Troy and Sroufe 1987; Fearon et al. 2010; Steele and Steele 2005; Suess et al. 1992).

Security and trust are important ingredients for the development of empathy and prosocial behaviors, but we must be aware of cross-cultural differences. Research shows that parenting around the globe fosters two different aspects of security: psychological and physiological security. Both were originally addressed in the same way by Bowlby. Although both aspects of security are important for early child development, cultural contexts with their differential constraints and affordances obviously cause caregivers to emphasize these two forms differently: Highly educated middle-class families from Western cultures favor the development of psychological security from early on, as physiological security is taken for granted because medical care, hygiene, and food are provided for sufficiently. Studies show how the early communications of Western middle-class caregivers with infants instantiate the development of psychological security; that is, one caregiver directs undivided attention to the infant and responds immediately, adequately, and consistently to even subtle signals of the baby. Thereby, the baby learns that he/she is perceived as an independent agent with its own will and the right to express its own preferences and wishes. In contrast, caretakers in non-Western contexts that have high infant mortality rates, due to the existence of severe illnesses and the proneness of accidents, are more aware of the primary need for physical security. Here, parenting focuses on physical availability and closeness (e.g., through body contact and body stimulation), often without using verbal elaborations or mentalization skills (Keller 2007; Otto 2008). This attention to physical security by caregivers is found in most non-Western subsistence-based rural societies (e.g., the Efe, the Beng, the Nso).

Even in the best of circumstances, when caregivers aim to be sensitive and responsive, there are inevitably moments (for child and caregiver) of being misunderstood, neglected, or rejected, and over the lifespan there are inevitable separation and loss experiences. This is a feature of normal or typical development. When laboratory-based observations of mother-infant interactions are sorted into two groups, synchronous and asynchronous, only up to 50% of the interactions can be reliably judged as being synchronous or attuned (Tronick and Cohn 1989). For the other 50%, there are ruptures in synchrony. The vital question then becomes: How many of these ruptures are repaired or reconciled quickly? The answer leads into the subject of individual differences in infant-parent attachment security. Insecurity is typified by a history of interactions where ruptures were not quickly or not successfully repaired. Security is typified by reliably observed rupture-repair cycles, reconciling differences and expressing hope in continued connection and peaceable interactions.

This sensitive and responsive parenting style, which views synchronous turn-taking interactions as healthy, fosters the development of early agency in babies. Sensitive, responsive caretakers follow their children's signals; babies are encouraged to express their own will and to communicate their emotional states. Sensitive, responsive caretakers engage babies in conversations about their mental states, their preferences and their emotions, treating babies as individuals motivated by feelings, thoughts, and intentions. This discourse style has been labeled "mind-mindedness" by Meins and Fernyhough (1999), who suggested that mind-mindedness, in addition to sensitive parenting, leads to secure attachments. However, among non-Western rural subsistence-based societies, caregiver-infant discourse might occur somewhat differently: Some studies have found that it is characterized by rhythmic overlapping vocalizations/

verbalizations which may foster the experience of synchrony between the interaction partners (Keller et al. 2008). Nso mothers lead a highly normative hierarchical discourse, positioning the child to obey and to comply in a hierarchical set (Demuth 2008). This hierarchical normativity becomes particularly evident when the child performs socially undesirable behavior, just as may be the case in many Western contexts (see further discussion below on child maltreatment and limit setting). Some students of child development suggest that the use of a mind-minded style when interacting with infants may, however, be rare in some non-Western contexts (e.g., Cameroonian Nso mothers), as small babies are perceived as not yet capable of having intentions, preferences, or wishes (Otto and Keller 2014).

A central focus of successful intervention to promote positive parenting and secure child-parent relations must be to help parents accurately read the signals (nonverbal and verbal) given by their children and to respond sensitively to these signals. In addition to heeding signals to engage, sensitive caregivers must also heed signals to disengage. This is vital because none of us, and no infant for certain, can maintain a perpetual gaze into the face of the other. There is an ongoing need to look away that punctuates the wish to look. Homeostasis of emotion, attention, and physiological systems requires these "pauses" to one's social engagement. In adult conversation, identifiable speech turns are occasioned by switching pauses that signal to the listener that the speaker is ready to take a turn at listening. And so on. Switching pauses make possible rhythms of dialog (Jaffe et al. 2001). Infants need to pause as well. The extent of vocal synchrony in mother-infant interactions at four months is predictive of security of attachment to mother at 12 months (Jaffe et al. 2001). In addition, tighter synchrony at four months, suggesting a infant who habituates (processes information) quickly, is associated with higher cognitive development (Bayley scores) at 12 months. However, a caregiver who is unfamiliar with these universal rules of interaction (i.e., looking/speaking and looking away/silence) may interpret an infant who looks away as rejection and may react in kind: if the infant is angry, don't I have the right to be angry as well? This contagion of negative emotion is all the more marked when the caregiver has an internalized experience of rejection, loss, and trauma stemming from his/her past. Fraiberg first commented upon the phenomenon of unresolved loss/trauma from a parent's childhood having an intrusive and disruptive influence on the capacity to provide care to an infant. Fraiberg decribed this disruprive influence as something present in quieter (controlled) or louder (uncontrolled) forms in every nursery; namely, as "ghosts in the nursery" (Fraiberg et al. 1975). More recently, it has been acknowledged that in every nursery there are facilitative influences which empower the caregiver to respond appropriately to his or her infant based on appropriate lessons in caregiving in the caregiver's early history. These positive supportive influences have been termed "angels in the nursery" (Lieberman et al. 2005).

Autonomous exploration or play might be less valued in non-Western cultures, and socialization may focus more on the development of obedience, respect, and integration into the community. To develop intervention and prevention programs for non-Western populations, indigenous conceptions of relationship development, attachment, disorder, and risk need to be assessed and understood. In an intervention study on Turkish-Dutch immigrant families (Yagmur et al. 2014), adaptation of the Videofeedback Intervention to Promote Positive Parenting (VIPP-TM) in focus group discussions appeared to be minor, and the randomized control trial showed significant outcomes on sensitive parenting.

A fruitful approach to measuring "ghosts" (Fraiberg et al. 1975) versus "angels" (Lieberman 2007) in the nursery can be achieved with the Adult Attachment Interview, or AAI (Fonagy et al. 1993). AAI is a tool for assessing the caregiver's own childhood history and current state of mind about attachment, which is well established as the most powerful influence on whether the child will develop a secure attachment relationship by one year of age (Main et al. 1985) and has been confirmed by meta-analytic results (van IJzendoorn 1995). Paradoxically, perhaps, the central characteristic of a caregiver able to parent in a flexible, organized, and secure manner is the ability to describe and explain his or her own attachment history in a coherent, balanced manner that conveys a valuing of attachment (Main et al. 2008). The central feature of the parent's speech is adherence to the "cooperative principle" of conversation, deemed to be a universal characteristic of language (Grice 1975, 1989). Insofar as a healthy and robust capacity for cooperation is being advanced in this chapter (and others) as the behavior most relevant to achieving and maintaining peace at the personal and social level, the speech act comprising the "cooperative principle" merits attention. There are four maxims characterizing cooperative speech:

1. Truth, i.e., having evidence for what you claim.
2. Relation, i.e., staying on task and bringing information relevant to the topic.
3. Economy, i.e., saying neither too much, nor too little.
4. Manner, i.e., maintaining a level of politeness suitable to the context.

The maxim of truth has been posited as the vital core of attachment security in childhood and adulthood (Cassidy 2001). Truthfulness may also be vital to establishing and maintaining peace (e.g., truth and reconciliation commissions). Adherence to the cooperative principle in response to the AAI is linked to less aversive (amygdala) brain responses (fMRI) than speakers with low coherence (Riem et al. 2012).

What is the evidence that adherence to the "cooperative principle" is relevant to parenting and child outcomes? A parent's adherence to the "cooperative principle" predicts child-parent attachment security. This has been demonstrated with over 1,000 birth parents and their infants in multiple independent studies conducted in various cultural contexts and summarized in meta-analytic work (van IJzendoorn 1995), with caregivers who have no genetic link to their children including foster parents (Dozier et al. 2001) and adoptive parents (Steele et al. 2003, 2008), as well as with convergent evidence from cross-fostering work with primates (Maestripieri 2005a). This underscores the vital psychological and social (not genetic) influence that parents have on their children. Moreover, parents (including foster and adoptive parents) exert their influence upon their children in ways that impact brain development and functioning (Fox et al., this volume). This is compatible with the dialectical perspective advanced by Hinde and Stevenson-Hinde (this volume), where each context of development must be seen to be influencing, and to be influenced by, every other context. While further work needs to be done to consolidate the empirical evidence linking these contexts, which seem to be closely embedded in one another, with the parent-infant relationship having emergent properties for the contexts that follow (and contain) the first relationship, there is now robust intergenerational evidence from parent to child that is both social and biological. Indeed the very context of becoming a parent leads to hormonal changes (increases in oxytocin) that serve to promote affiliative bonding behaviors (Carter and Porges, this volume; Feldman et al. 2007). High levels of anxiety in pregnant women have long-term deleterious effects on an unborn child's ability to regulate emotions that are independent of maternal depression (O'Connor et al. 2002); this extends to cognitive abilities as well (Bergman et al. 2007). The mechanism of influence of these associations is an area of much current scientific inquiry. However the story unfolds, the take-home message is unlikely to change: Pregnant women should be helped to maintain a sense of peace (low anxiety) throughout the pregnancy, and to be able to provide a coherent account of their attachment history. Further work is needed to explore the extent to which adherence to the cooperative principle in conversations about one's attachment history is a universal phenomenon, as the theory predicts. Variations on the theme are to be expected, particularly with respect to the maxim of economy and the extent to which speakers speculate on the motivations guiding the behavior of one's parents, or one's children. The maxim of truth is likely to be the most universal maxim, since wherever one lives in the world, there is a story about one's experience that includes descriptions, memories, and evaluations that will resonate to the listener as more or less plausible/accurate/true.

With respect to peace at the personal and social level, attachment theory offers some potentially useful descriptive constructs that appear to have universal relevance to our human species and other animals (Maestripieri this volume, 2005a): These are the safe haven and secure base phenomena that appear to be readily observed across cultures, although other behaviors linked to attachment (e.g., stranger anxiety first typically observed at seven to nine months) are not observed across cultures (Keller 2003) or across primate groups (Maestripieri 2005a). It appears that in caregiving contexts where an infant is raised with a primary caregiver and many other kinfolk or neighbors nearby, stranger anxiety is less evident or absent (Gottlieb 2004; Otto 2008). Future research in diverse cultural contexts should investigate the prevalence of this phenomenon. Even if anxiety with strangers is absent, or there is a lack of visible distress on separation from the parent, the child may still show identifiable safe haven (proximity seeking/contact maintaining) behavior and secure base behavior (exploring away from primary caregiver but referencing back by the child).

In the world's most troubled, violent, and war-torn locations, transfer of care from the primary caregiver to others (typically kin, an older sibling, an aunt or uncle) is not uncommon (LeVine et al. 1996). In parts of Africa, where social ties are being broken and strained by the weight of the HIV epidemic, this is often the case. Poverty exacerbates the stress engendered by these circumstances. Nonetheless, in eastern and southern Africa, many children show remarkable resilience in the context of children raising other children, where young people are declaring: "I am my brother's keeper" (Bray 2003). This may be consistent with the developmental goal parents have for their children in African (and other) cultures; that is, be a socially responsible family member and fulfill your social role or duty. In Western industrialized locations, parents may place more emphasis upon a child becoming an autonomous and empathic individual (Keller 2003). In developmental research it is common within and between cultures to find evidence of equi-finality (children who show the same outcome via different developmental paths). From a child's perspective and that of the community in which the child lives, the chances of becoming an effective leader, and contributing to peace are increased when a secure base/safe haven is available over time (not necessarily from the same person).

Summary and Suggestions for Further Research and Policy

The early caregiving environment constitutes the fundamental influence over the course of a child's early, and to lesser or greater extents, long-term development. Separation and loss experiences are inevitable in an individual's life, and social support is vital to survival and thriving (see Britto, Salah et al., this volume). Parents and grandparents are the most typical caregivers to small children. However, siblings, other kin, foster and adoptive parents take on key caregiving roles vital to the well-being of children. Early trauma, loss, as well as domestic and political violence can exert long-term disruptive influences upon the ability to provide care, and may significantly diminish chances for personal and social peace. However, resilience is also widely observed. Further research is needed to chart the constituents of resilience and how this capacity can be promoted to rise above and beyond adversity (Cicchetti 2013; see Masten, this volume).

Child Maltreatment versus Limit Setting,
Spanking, and Harsh Parenting

Child maltreatment is a widespread, global phenomenon that affects the lives of millions of children all over the world (for a general description of the different types of maltreatment, see WHO 1999, Appendix A). WHO (1999) describes sexual abuse as the involvement of children in sexual activity that they do not fully understand, which they are unable to give informed consent to, for which they are not developmentally prepared, or that violates the standards of the society in which these children live. Physical abuse is defined as the infliction of potential or actual physical harm by a caregiver caused by interactions or lack of interactions that are reasonably in control of this caregiver. The description of emotional abuse includes the failure to provide a developmentally appropriate, supportive environment that allows the child to develop a stable and full range of emotional and social competencies, according to the child's personal potentials and in the context of the society in which the child grows up. Again, these acts should be reasonably within the control of the caregiver. Neglect, including physical, emotional, and educational neglect, is typified as the failure, within the limits of the caregivers' resources, to provide for the development of the child in all domains including health, education, emotional development, nutrition, shelter, and safe living conditions. Comorbidity between types of maltreatment seems to be more rule than exception (e.g., McGee et al. 1995; Menard et al. 2004).

In a series of meta-analyses, Stoltenborgh et al. (2012, 2013a, b) estimate the worldwide prevalence of child sexual, physical, and emotional abuse as well as of physical and emotional neglect, including 244 publications and 577 prevalence rates for the various types of maltreatment. The overall estimated prevalence rates for self-report studies were 76/1,000 for sexual abuse among boys and 180/1,000 for sexual abuse among girls, 226/1,000 for physical abuse, 363/1,000 for emotional abuse, 163/1,000 for physical neglect, 184/1,000 for emotional neglect. Although there is a dearth of studies on child maltreatment in low-income countries, the available evidence shows no differences between continents for prevalence of maltreatment modalities with the exception of the prevalence of sexual abuse. It should be noted that the prevalence rates for studies using informants other than the (potential) victims were considerably lower.

It is clear from a variety of studies that child maltreatment is one of the most important risk factors for the emergence of psychopathology (Felliti et al. 1998) and antisocial or externalizing behavior problems (Caspi et al. 2002). It is also clear that the boundaries between some types of child maltreatment and more typical parenting styles are somewhat vague and that these boundaries might also fluctuate according to cultural context. In the definitions provided by WHO (1999), this fluctuation seems to be addressed in their emphasis on the limits of caregivers' resources. It is important to note that there are many forms of child abuse, including sexual abuse, physical neglect, and emotional neglect; however, here we focus almost exclusively on physical abuse because it models violent behavioral interactions that seem inconsistent with peace. We will discuss the various ways in which parents might try to set limits to their children's non-obedient or aggressive behavior, using authoritative ways of explaining the reasons for the limits or more punitive styles such as spanking and other forms of harsh parenting. Whether these harsher forms of parental discipline should be considered as cultural specific and acceptable from the perspective of the child's development or whether they might foreshadow physical abuse in a more extreme sense is a central issue.

We argue that culture does not always mean difference, and that we may, and often do, find similarities across cultures, in particular in the perception, use, and consequences of harsh parenting practices. A report from five countries (China, Italy, Kenya, the Philippines, and Thailand) demonstrates that in every country more reliance on corporal punishment by parents was associated with greater anxiety and aggression in the children (Lansford et al. 2005). The severity and use of corporal punishment was greater when the parents believed it to be "normal." Frequent use of corporal punishment, and believed normalcy of the practice, appeared to be related to aggressive behavioral problems in childhood (Lansford et al. 2005). Beliefs, understanding, and practice are not always joined up against this ineffective and most certainly nonpeaceful punishing act, to which many parents and teachers still engage. Boys receive more corporal punishment than girls. Status considerations influence the use of corporal punishment: parents who want to exert their higher status may beat their children, and children with lower status have little choice but to accept it (and often believe it is deserved). Steep inequality gradients within the family might in the long run have similar detrimental effects on low-ranking family members as in other group contexts. Children who are abused may consider it normal, thus contributing to a future risk of becoming an abusing adult/parent later in life (Sroufe et al. 2005). Believing corporal punishment is useful contributes to intergenerational transfer, and such transfer may be more marked in those cultures or subcultures where parent-child relations are deeply hierarchical.

The world over, there have been efforts to eradicate this abusive form of limit setting traditionally imposed on children by parents and teachers. In 1947, Sweden began education and information campaigns to shift this parenting belief. It took some thirty years to enact the necessary legislations, but when corporal punishment was banned by law in 1979, the Swedish people were ready. By then, for the most part, Swedes no longer had a wish to apply corporal punishment and believed it to be ineffective. Research is plain on this latter point. Children only learn to try and avoid the punishment, and carry on with the behavior that elicited the punishment all the same, with a residue of anxiety and anger. In addition, children internalize the model of an abusive authority figure—something they may later act on when frustrated by another with similar or less power. Admittedly, some parents, especially among immigrant families, still apply smacking in their parenting practices. However, the situation in Sweden is better than in the United States, where no legislation exists to regulate corporal punishment, and none is expected due to prevailing perceptions against government interference in parenting practices. One can only hope that more sectors of the population become familiar with the literature showing the adverse nonpeaceful consequences of corporal punishment.

In Kenya, a law against physical punishment was enacted in 2001, but adherence to the law has been difficult to achieve. Why is it so difficult and time-consuming to halt physical violence against children? Even in areas where laws have been enacted and people understand that physical abuse is ineffective and wrong, physical punishment is still practiced (Mweru 2010). Clearly, more efforts are needed to equip parents and teachers with alternate limit-setting strategies. Top-down laws may be prescriptive but they are not necessarily influential. One exception to this can be found in Finland, where a top-down approach has proven useful: a law against spanking was introduced as a means of initiating a change in the beliefs so as to pave the way for changing practices. Perhaps a better approach would be to implement simultaneously a top-down and bottom-up process to alter beliefs and change in parenting practices (as in Sweden). Such an approach could be implemented locally: children could be educated about physical punishment and helped to realize that they do not deserve such treatment and that laws exist to protect them. In addition, educating and supporting teachers and parents are needed.

Given the widespread use of smacking and corporal punishment that does not leave a physical mark, it is tempting to think that such behavior is appropriate in some cultural contexts and that intervention is only warranted when punishment seriously harms a child beyond what is acceptable in a given culture. However, strong empirical evidence exists from many countries (including the culturally diverse United States, where 75–80% of parents spank their children) that spanking by parents is linked to aggressive outcomes in children. Children who experience corporal punishment are more likely to use such behavior with peers and, later, with their own children. Furthermore, when spanking is considered acceptable, it is just one step away from inadvertently or intentionally using forms of physical punishment that do leave marks on a child's body (i.e., physical abuse) and which violate the right of each child (Convention on Rights of the Child 1989).

Some 100 years ago it was common practice throughout the world for men to feel that it was their right, if not duty, to beat their wives. Today throughout the world we have strong laws against rape and sexual harassment, even though the incidence of this crime continues. No one would suggest that this means the act is anywhere acceptable. So, too, must the incidence of corporal punishment of children come to be seen as unacceptable. The use of corporal punishment by parents or teachers only serves to teach children that violence begets respect. Alternative modes of discipline, however, can equally teach that conversation, negotiation, and reconciliation deserve respect. Where laws forbidding corporal punishment of children do not exist, they should be enacted along with the necessary education, information, and support campaigns needed to provide a range of alternative limit-setting strategies and compliance to values that a child can internalize and embrace. In terms of the consequences of corporal punishment, gender is relevant: men most often mete out corporal punishment as teachers or fathers (just as it is men who typically rape), and boys are more likely to receive corporal punishment and more likely also to be diagnosed with externalizing or aggressive developmental disorders. Forms of disciplining children that include violence are accepted in some cultures (e.g., Afghanistan), but increasingly, as the goals of cooperation and equity in interpersonal exchanges advance, such violent practices will come to be regarded as unacceptable. Children's health and prospects for peace at personal and social levels depend on this.

From a well-known epidemiological study that included more than 10,000 respondents (Felitti et al. 1998), adverse childhood experiences over the first 18 years of life, including the experience of physical abuse that left a mark or a bruise, were measured and linked to a wide range of psychological and physical health problems, all of which detract significantly from a healthy peaceful life (Dube et al. 2001a). Children who have experienced harsh environments are prone to view neutral situations in hostile terms (Dodge et al. 1990), especially when they perceive a threat to the self (Dodge and Samberg 1987). Maltreated children are quick to judge anger on a neutral face long before it is typically judged to have morphed into an angry face (Pollak et al. 2000). Empathy is widely defined as feeling the distress of the other, and when empathy is really felt, empathic behavior is likely to follow. This was demonstrated in a recent study (Barhight et al. 2012) which showed that children who experienced an increase in heart rate (in response to a vignette of a child being bullied) were more likely to intervene in the classroom when a real child was being bullied.

Importantly, there is no evidence to suggest that children in any way deserve or attract (e.g., via a genetically based characteristic, gene-environment correlation) abusive parenting behavior. A large U.K. twin study showed that children's genetic characteristics may partly be linked up with being smacked by parents but not to being physically abused (Jaffee et al. 2004).

Summary and Suggestions for Further Research and Policy

More ecological and empirical work is needed to extend the findings on emerging natural experiments, where changes and continuity will exist in parenting practices and beliefs in relation to new legislation banning corporal punishment. In these contexts, hopefully many, important questions need to be asked about levels of child aggression before and after such changes, and the anticipated benefits to child, family and school life, if not also the wider community, that are expected to follow. For these benefits to be realized, "new" legislation needs to be joined up with a culture of peace; that is, new thoughts and feelings about the fair and peaceful manner in which children ought to be treated (see the Foreword, this volume).

Principles of Early Attachment-Based Interventions: Working with Parents to Help Them Raise Children with the Skills to Achieve Personal and Social Peace

It is vitally important for supportive parents to provide sensitive, responsive, and nurturing care of their children, and multiple well-informed intervention efforts are underway to achieve this (see Kagitcibasi and Britto, this volume). Here we review the shared principles of available interventions that are focused on promoting sensitive and responsive caregiving or secure infant-caregiver attachments, based on robust, published, empirical evidence. Rather than detail the specific components and results of various interventions, we will focus on global principles that have application whenever parents aim to do the right thing by their children.

Interventions with parents of infants share the aim of helping vulnerable parents to be more sensitive, responsive, and understanding toward their infants. Interventions with parents of toddlers and older children often include attention to limit setting as well as help in calming dysregulated children. Many of these interventions have empirical support as to their effectiveness in enhancing parental sensitivity and/or limit setting, on the one hand, and child behavioral and physiological regulations, on the other. Some have been tested and proven effective through randomized clinical trials, the gold standard for efficacy assessment (e.g., Bakermans-Kranenburg et al. 2008; Bernard et al. 2012; Toth et al. 2006; Van Zeijl et al. 2006).

Most interventions do not take a strong stand that parents must not physically punish their children; instead, interventions typically provide guidance toward a flexible range of sensitive limit-setting strategies. In addition, although the empirical evidence may not bear directly on these questions, these interventions seem likely to make children more peaceful in the following way: they aim to help children (and parents) make benign attributions toward others, develop or strengthen the capacity for inhibitory control, and negotiate interactions with others well.

Goals involve helping parents learn to recognize children's signals and respond in nurturing ways when children are distressed, to respond in contingent and engaged ways when children are not distressed, and to avoid frightening behaviors at all times. Among parents with children beyond infancy, interventions typically go beyond parental responsiveness to helping parents support children when they become frustrated or angry, and/or setting reliable contingencies.

Enhancing parental responsiveness and decreasing frightening behavior is expected to lead to changes in a child's ability to regulate attachment, behavior, emotions, and physiology. More specifically, effective interventions are expected to help children develop an organized attachment (not disorganized) and adequate regulatory abilities (behavior, emotion, attention, physiology), which enhance inhibitory control (i.e., the ability to "stop and think" before acting).

Effective interventions have several key components. First, emphasis is placed on building a strong working relationship between the parent coach (e.g., clinician, nurse) and the parent. Through a variety of means, parents are assisted to see themselves as efficacious. For example, some interventions emphasize the good intentions that parents have regarding their behavior toward their children (e.g., Lieberman and Van Horn 2011b). In others, parent coaches comment frequently on parents' behaviors that are in line with intervention targets, thus leading parents to have high success rates. In still other interventions (e.g., Olds 2006), nurses treat their relationship with the parent as a partnership.

Second, interventions need to specify process and outcomes. In addition, a methodology for monitoring fidelity must be utilized. Only recently have interventions for parents been "manualized"; this critical development has allowed for the specification of what occurs in each session. Nonetheless, a manualized intervention is not sufficient; both adherence to manual content and competence in implementation are key.

Interventions range in duration from brief periods (6–10 weeks) to much longer (weekly sessions for a year). A meta-analysis conducted by Bakermans-Kranenburg et al. (2003) found that shorter interventions were more powerful in effecting change in parental sensitivity. Nonetheless, some intervention developers make the case that intervening with vulnerable parents with multiple disadvantages (e.g., poverty, a history of adverse childhood experiences, domestic and neighborhood violence) may require more intensive, longer treatment, if only to create a setting in which parents are able to concentrate safely on improving the quality of interactions with their child.

Disseminating evidence-based interventions to community settings has proven difficult. Community settings present a range of challenges, including heterogeneous parent coaches, heterogeneous families, variability in agency commitment to the model, limited time for practice, and drift from the model. The "uptake" of models in the community (i.e., from the time when an evidence base is established until the model is used) is often quite long in mental health as it is in medicine. A relatively new area of study has developed—dissemination and implementation science—that focuses on moving interventions into communities successfully. Dissemination and implementation science is seen as a new frontier for training graduate students in psychology in the United States (Kazdin 2014). One of the key issues identified as critical for successful dissemination and implementation is identifying the mechanism of action of the intervention that has been proven effective. The mechanism of action refers to how and why an intervention has its effects. When a careful analysis has clearly identified the mechanism of action, the intervention can be modified for specific community needs without loss of effectiveness (Ronsaville et al. 2001). Fidelity monitoring methodology can be developed that carefully assesses and ensures that the essential features are implemented.

Notably, for many of these early interventions, efforts to demonstrate their effectiveness extend beyond questionnaires about parenting stress and observations of behavior (e.g., in the Ainsworth Strange Situation procedure) or interviews (e.g., the Adult Attachment Interview). Several interventions have been shown to enhance children's attachment quality (e.g., Bernard et al. 2012; Toth et al. 2006) and include neurophysiological and genetic measures to provide insights into the processes of change at these biological levels (see Fox et al., this volume).

One of the clear results from multiple studies is that an intervention may not be equally effective for every child (Bakermans-Kranenburg et al. 2008; Fox et al., this volume). In other words, children (and adults) show differential susceptibility to their developmental context for better *and* for worse, being more influenced by bad environments as well as by positive (interventions in) environments. This has led to a new model of development, and involves a switch from the diathesis-stress model to the differential susceptibility model. In the diathesis-stress model, the vulnerable and resilient child will develop similarly in positive environments; however, the vulnerable child encountering stress will suffer most; the resilient child who faces stress will not suffer. In the differential susceptibility model, the same child who is most strongly influenced by stress is predicted to respond best to positive changes in the environment (e.g., through intervention). Thus, in contrast to diathesis stress, more and less susceptible children will already follow different developmental pathways in positive environments (for a summary of this evidence, see van IJzendoorn and Bakermans-Kranenburg, this volume).

Ethical questions can arise. If we know who is suffering most or will profit most from the intervention, do we focus solely on this group? Given scarcity of resources, might we hope that the less susceptible will be left to their own? This would run counter to the UN's Convention on the Rights of the Child 1989, according to which an effective intervention should be universally available, just as education is available to all children. If levels of the behavioral disturbance (e.g., aggressive behavior) are similar across a whole group of children, we should apply the intervention and expect that some might profit more than others. Differential susceptibility might well be only one of the factors influencing the effectiveness of the intervention. David Olds (pers. comm.) saw differential effects of his home-visiting RN program across a wide range of domains and then made adjustment in the frequencies of contact. Who needs more got more, and who needs less received less. Allocation of scarce resources may thus be titrated to reach those who need it most. But can we always judge accurately who needs more and who needs less?

An intervention for parents of children who are behaviorally inhibited was developed and tested in a 15-year follow-up study by Rapee et al. (2005). The incidence of anxiety disorders is lowered at 15-year follow-up, but only for the group most at risk (i.e., the behaviorally inhibited). However, there may be other routes to anxiety disorders for which children need help. So, in ongoing work, best-fit psychosocial interventions must be sought.

Still, interventions must be more than psychosocial in nature. There are well-established beneficial effects that follow from changes in the physical environment and improvements to one's socioeconomic status, leading to healthier more peaceful behaviors and outcomes. Some toxins (e.g., lead, fluoride exposure) affect children more adversely than they do adults. The guiding principle must be: Protect all children so that everyone is protected. Advertising and the display of products or specific ways of sharing information have immediate effects on behavior. Epidemiologic data suggests that the decline in violent crime in the United States may be related to the decline in lead exposure—correlational data that is compatible with biological assumptions (Nevin 2000). Further work is clearly needed in this area as we gain new information about how best to structure "nudges" (Thaler and Sunstein 2008) in the physical contexts in which children are raised so that health and peace can be better fostered.

Summary and Suggestions for Further Research and Policy

Interventions with parents of infants typically help at-risk parents to be more sensitive and responsive toward their babies, whereas interventions with parents of preschool-aged children may incorporate a focus on limit setting and planful behavior. Interventions have been shown to be effective in enhancing children's attachment security as well as their ability to regulate behavior. As interventions are disseminated into the community, it is crucial for fidelity and adherence to the original model to be maintained.

With respect to the phenomenon of differential susceptibility (i.e., each of us is more or less sensitive to the caregiving environment), this has so far been studied primarily in children. Future research should explore the issue of differential susceptibility in adults, (parents), who often are the "receivers" of the intervention and mediators of the intervention effects on children?

Given that some intervention strategies for at-risk parents have established efficacy, moving interventions out into communities is an important next step. As interventions are moved into communities, it will be critical to monitor and ensure fidelity, and assess effectiveness, as well as to adapt the intervention as appropriate, and as allowable, to cultural norms.

Despite the existing evidence base of various interventions' effects on parent and child outcomes, the evidence that these interventions lead to more peaceful societies is speculative. Interventions lead to improved parent and child outcomes, including ones that should theoretically be linked with more peaceful members of the society and more peaceful societies. However, it is important to test this assumption empirically. There is a shared goal: that of creating a healthier, more peaceful society, where every child may live relatively free of fear, knowing well the experience of joy that emanates from positive interactions with family members, peers, teachers, and others.

Conclusion

In this chapter, we have explored five discrete but related topics relevant to the question: How do early childhood experiences contribute to personal and social peace? These topics should be seen as a presentation of the scientific evidence concerning the interacting influences of vital domains of social and emotional existence for humans and many other animals. This chapter should be read together with the figure and arguments presented by Hinde and Stevenson-Hinde (this volume), who chart bottom-up and top-down influences at work, among people and across the life span, that have a fundamental impact on prospects for realizing personal and social peace.

Here we have shown that the early caregiving environment and how a child's early attachments fare contribute directly to whether the child believes in empathic cooperative strategies, as opposed to aggressive competitite strategies, when conflict inevitably arises with others. By the second year of life, if not before, caregivers must enter into a form of confrontation with their children, by setting limits on the explorations of children (e.g., on crawling or walking) to protect the child from potential harm. Limit setting can become physical punishment or even maltreatment, when the caregiver exhibits poor impulse control, lives in social isolation, or has limited imagination. In this chapter, we have reviewed some of the well-known adverse consequences of child maltreatment, while pointing out discrepancies that ought to be resolved legislatively to protect children from physical discipline and parent/teacher beliefs and practices. The benefits of equitable interactions among children, as well as between children and teachers or parents have been discussed from a functional perspective of competition and cooperation—inevitable forces at work in human and other animal societies. In this context, the virtues of leveling dominance hierarchies were reviewed. Closely connected to this has been the focus on the powerful deleterious effects on health, which impact children in disproportionately large ways due to deep socioeconomic inequities. Such inequities are large, and are growing constantly within and between countries; this seriously detracts from the possibility of obtaining healthy, satisfying lives that may result in personal and social peace. Strategies for rectifying this have been suggested, including training and rewarding teachers to recognize the gifts of each student in their care, as a means of leveling the dominance hierarchy and training children in emotional and political literacy. Such training will help create responsible leaders committed to more equitable systems of access to resources. Finally, findings were presented of promising early interventions that help caregivers to provide sensitive and responsive care to their infants, and sensitive discipline to toddlers. How one fares in the early childhood years establishes, more often than not, how one continues in later life. However, the topic of intervention applies across the entire life span, because at no time in life is one impermeable to positive influences.

Challenges in Society

12

Mental Health and Development among Children Living in Violent Conditions

Underlying Processes for Promoting Peace

Raija-Leena Punamäki

Abstract

Peacebuilding is believed to be especially challenging among children who themselves fall victims to collective and interpersonal violence. An intriguing question is whether a focus on trauma, and on healing its negative impacts, is necessary for peacebuilding and societally harmonious human development. Some argue that suffering, pain, and injustice must be recognized and healed if peaceful and harmonious development is to be enabled; others emphasize the importance of positive outcomes despite violence. This chapter analyzes how forms of violence (military and domestic) influence the social, emotional, and cognitive development of children. Particular attention is given to the risks and negative impacts as well as the positive protective processes that promote meaningfulness. It also discusses how psychosocial interventions can enhance positive and peace-enhancing development in community and family domains. The core issue is to create political, societal, and cultural preconditions that will facilitate children's mental growth and generative resilience despite violence.

Introduction

Unfortunately, children often witness and are the targets of violence, both in their communities and homes. UNICEF (2009) estimates that over one billion children live in countries affected by wars, armed conflicts, and military violence, and experience human atrocities and material losses. Characteristic of modern wars is, indeed, the high level of civilian casualties. Violence in the home is a more invisible form of suffering. Childhood maltreatment (i.e., physical, emotional, and sexual abuse or neglect) is estimated globally to occur in 5–25% of families, based on retrospective self-reports (WHO 2007). Research shows linkages between collective and interpersonal violence: socioeconomic pressures and political insecurity increase the risk for domestic violence in war zones (Al-Krenawi et al. 2007; Panter-Brick et al. 2011).

Fortunately, research has also revealed a number of protective factors and healing processes that buffer children's well-being in violent conditions. Processes which foster resilience include creative narratives that provide cultural meaning to distressing experiences, supportive social relations, functional cognitive-emotional coping strategies, and biological plasticity (Masten 2011; Masten and Narayan 2012; Panter-Brick and Eggerman 2012). From a peacebuilding perspective, it is crucial to understand the mechanisms through which violence impacts child development, so that effective prevention and treatment can build on that knowledge to enhance positive outcomes. This chapter analyses the dynamics of children's social, emotional, and cognitive responses to military and domestic violence, both in terms of negative mental health and developmental outcomes as well as in terms of positive processes promoting meaningfulness and mental health. Thereafter, the effectiveness of available psychosocial interventions among war-affected children is evaluated and the core elements are analyzed that enhance developmentally salient generative and healing processes and potentiate peacebuilding capacities.

Nature of Violence and Child Development

Violence concerns any act that is likely to result in death, injury, psychological harm, developmental problems, or deprivation under civilian or war conditions (Evans et al. 2008). Interpersonal violence occurs in the context of close relationships (e.g., in families and schools), whereas large groups are the target of collective violence in political and military contexts, as in terrorism and war. Table 12.1 provides characteristics and examples of interpersonal (domestic) and collective (military) violence. As can be seen, violence differs in the way it impacts children's lives, its relationship to perpetrators, as well as the meanings ascribed to experiences.

Which form of violence is most salient? In the home, children experience direct physical violence from caregivers, or other familiar figures, in the forms of hitting, spanking, and burning, as well as psychological abuse, such as emotional neglect, ridicule, and isolation (Evans et al. 2008). In war zones, children are direct targets of explosions and bombardments, they witness atrocities and are subject to humiliation, and they experience loss of family and community members. In the face of both domestic and military violence, children try to make sense of their experiences; they actively attempt to mitigate harm and take responsibility for solving the problem. It is believed that violence experienced through intimate relations is more traumatic than war-related violence

Table 12.1 Characteristics and examples of interpersonal and collective violence.

Characteristics	Interpersonal (domestic) violence	Collective (military) violence
Ecological context	Home environment with own relatives	Political and military activity Stressful life events School and family environment
Role of parents	Presenting threat Neglect of children's need for protection	Protecting children Defending family safety Distracting attention from atrocities
Role of the child	Protecting siblings Isolation from parents	Collective responsibility Compensation for parental suffering
Nature of traumatic experiences	Protecting siblings Isolation from parents	Life danger and fear of being wounded Witnessing parents' humiliation or helplessness
Meanings of violence	Mistrust in human benevolence Fear for physical and psychological integrity	Loss of safety Threat to human dignity Seeking collective meaning
Emotions	Loss of safety Loss of human dignity Seeking personal meaning	Feelings of fear and anger Appraisal of hope for change

Examples	
Parental assault	*Military activity*
Hitting and slapping Head slamming Power and control behavior Verbal abuse and threats Humiliation and ridicule Witnessing violence Assaults on a parent Assaults on siblings	Witnessing shots, explosions, and shelling Being injured Losses and violence toward family Family evicted from home Injury of family members Witnessing violence Seeing people dying Killing or injuring of close relatives or friends

or natural disasters, despite exposure to life-threatening situations and the resulting insecurity that this brings. It is also possible that the nature of violence evokes specific responses, supportive actions, and coping strategies. For example, a study of Palestinian families found that exposure to childhood maltreatment was associated with decreased social support, whereas military violence

resulted in increased support; this was explained by the cultural values of heroism and collective appreciation of national sacrifice and by universal shame
related to family violence (Punamäki et al. 2005).

War itself can engender socioeconomic stressors that place families under
considerable strain and put children at prominent risk of depression or psychiatric distress (Catani et al. 2008; Eggerman and Panter-Brick 2010; Panter-
Brick et al. 2011). One longitudinal study analyzed the unique and cumulative
role of ethnic-political, intra-ethnic community, school, and family violence
on child mental health in a Middle Eastern context (Boxer et al. 2013; Dubow
et al. 2012). It found that family violence predicted increased peer aggression over time, beyond the effects of violence exposure in other contexts.
Universally, children seem to appraise violence toward their family members
as the most painful, and parents in turn feel guilty for their inability to protect their children in violent conditions (Punamäki 2006; Montgomery 2010).
Exposure to interpersonal violence shatters the core health-maintaining belief
that other humans are benevolent, fair, and predictable (Janoff-Bulman 2006).

These observations reveal the pivotal role of meaning in processing diverse experiences of violence. This has been emphasized in research on the
ideological expectations and attributions among war-affected youth (Barber
and Schluterman 2008), the cultural resources or dictates that promote hope
or suffering (Eggerman and Panter-Brick 2010, 2014), and ways to appraise
and cope with war experiences (Qouta et al. 2008a). Research based on interviews of both children and caregivers in Afghan families has revealed multiple
cultural-philosophical premises that exist to make sense of social suffering,
which include faith and religious world order, family unity and harmony, a disposition to individual effort and collective service to one's family and community, and moral codes of respect and honor (Eggerman and Panter-Brick 2010).
Children thus appraise and attribute their violent experiences in the context
of social and family rules, some of which are found throughout the world and
some of which are culturally bound.

Empirical evidence shows that both military and domestic violence pose
severe risks for the mental health of children and can compromise optimal
socioemotional development (Attanayake et al. 2009; Leeb et al. 2009). The
comprehensive impacts of violence on social development are commonly studied in terms of aggression, withdrawal, and marginalization. However, there is
well-argued criticism on the limitations of examining only pathological and
dysfunctional developmental processes, ignoring the generative and spiritual
aspects of children's capacity to grow up as resilient people and justice-mind-
ed, peacebuilding citizens (Panter-Brick and Eggerman 2012; Tol et al. 2014).
According to resilience-based approaches, the foci of research should be directed toward ways of enhancing hope and creating conditions under which
life can flourish, be strengthened, and be enhanced (Barber 2013; Eggerman
and Panter-Brick 2010; Masten 2011).

Some work on trauma maintains, however, that working through social suffering and family losses and repairing the rupture of children's cognitive-emotional development is necessary to the healing process (Brewin et al. 2010; Ehlers and Clarke 2000). For example, dismantling therapy studies maintain that traumatic memories should be vividly and experientially available for the survivors, so that they can alter both their meaning and content (Moser et al. 2010). This argument mirrors the belief in a kind of Jobian legacy: suffering creates conditions from which human virtues crystallize and flourish. This is articulated in the premises of posttraumatic growth, which encompass a new appreciation of life, strong affiliations to fellow humans, a realization of own and community's strength, and the experiencing of spirituality and faith (Tedeschi and Calhoun 2004). Evidence among adult trauma survivors confirms the possibility to change fragmented and distressing representations into new narratives that help in the acquisition of spiritual wisdom and a deep feeling of belonging to humanity (Salo et al. 2004; Zoellner et al. 2008). In addition, supportive parental relations, collective hope, and creative coping strategies have been reliably associated with positive developmental opportunities among both maltreated and war-affected children (Flores et al. 2005; Masten and Narayan 2012; Tol et al. 2013; Panter-Brick et al. 2014b). To understand how and why violence may result either in negative or positive developmental outcomes, it is urgent to learn about salient elements and processes that contribute to such a range of possible outcomes.

Underlying Mechanisms for Negative and Positive Outcomes

Human mind and behavior are not reflections of outside reality; they represent multiple, fundamental processes that may explain the possible link between exposure to violence and child development and mental health. Table 12.2 summarizes the risk and negative impacts that a host of psychosocial processes can have on development and suggests a variety of "counterforces" (left-hand column) to protect and promote children's healthy development. These counterforces make up the core elements applied to prevention and intervention with violence-affected children. Both negative and positive processes involve development in the social, emotional, cognitive, symbolic, and neurocognitive domains.

Peer and Sibling Relations

It has been suggested that life threats and war draw people together, as they attempt to survive, and bring out altruism and the willingness to share. Similarly, war violence has been viewed as leading to positive peer relationships that create feelings of safety and togetherness (Baker and Shalhoub-Kevorkian 1999). Empirical evidence is, however, less optimistic concerning children's

Table 12.2 Impacts of violence and trauma on developmental domains.

Developmental domains	Risks and negative impacts	Protective and positive processes
Social		
Peer and sibling relations	• Deterioration in intimate friendship • Sibling rivalry and conflicts • Difficulties to share traumatic experiences • Isolation and withdrawal	• Social sharing and listening to others' experiences • Disclosure of emotions • Enhancing empathy and prosocial behavior • Cohesive group processes • Conflict resolution (mediation, negotiation, dialog)
Parental relations	• Extensive clinging and need for safety • Compromised communication of trauma • Punitive and overcontrolling parenting • Rigid roles of strength and weakness	• Unique attachment-specific ways of trauma processing • Knowledge about a variety of trauma responses • Appreciating parents' motivation to protect their children • Sensitivity to children's specific attachment needs • Parent-child communication pointing to positive behavior • Attenuating aggression by storytelling and physical activity • Sharing family trauma narrative
Social support	• Intensive need for social support • Inadequate and disappointing support	• Learning repertoires of coping with violence • Proving and receiving help from each other • Cathartic feelings of being safe together
Emotional		
Emotion expression	• Lack of synchrony between feeling states, behavioral and physiology of emotions • Domination of behavioral urge to act at the expense of more reflecting emotions • Feelings of helplessness, shame, and guilt • Narrow repertoire of emotions	• Storytelling and communicating emotions • Sharing emotions in playful manners • Expressing multiple significant emotions verbally and bodily • Learning multisensory relaxation and mind-body integration

Developmental domains	Risks and negative impacts	Protective and positive processes
Emotion recognition	• Difficulty to name and differentiate strong emotional states • Dominance of negative persecution themes • Fragmented and nonnarrative reports • Difficulty to recognize complex emotions	• Empathy in cognitive (recognition) and affective domains • Recognition of own and others' bodily expressions • Integrative thinking and emotions • Joy of affective identification and modulation skills • Identify and enjoy a wide range of feelings
Emotion regulation	• Either underregulation (impulsiveness) or overregulation (numbing) • Dysfunctional regulation: distracting, suppression, repeating, and acting out	• Learning to frame (control) and ventilate (express) emotions in multimodal ways (bodily, verbally, symbolically) • Familiarity with various ways how emotions are helpful • Recognition of cues that evoke beneficial emotion • Training alternative regulation strategies in playful manner
Cognitive		
Appraisals attention	• Excessive vigilance for threat and danger • Automatic activation without cognitive feedback • Generalization of threat to neutral cues	• Recognition of own automatic processes • Learning about own threshold to endure threat • Replacing negative appraisals by positive
Memory	• Trauma image stays vivid and real; does not fade • Memory intensive as if happening here and now • Sensory, kinesthetic, and behavioral modalities dominate • Involuntary recall, evoked by arbitrary cues • No verbal access and difficult to share	• Processing memories on all senses (verbal, auditory, kinesthetic, touch, smell) • Inviting narrative stories (play, theater, songs, own biography) • Time-sequencing tools (diaries, praying, sleep hygiene) • Separating past from present
Attribution and explanation models	• Expecting people to be harmful and bad • Perceiving environment as globally unsafe • Self-blame and helplessness • Black and white world view	• Recognition of link between attributions and trauma symptoms • Replace negative attributions with hope and trust • Empowerment, self-efficacy, and agency
Problem solving	• Narrowing range of alternatives • Diminishing flexibility due to perceived danger • Problems of concentration	• Enrichment of thinking and creative tasks • Introducing multiple themes, solutions, and role change

Table 12.2 (continued)

Developmental domains	Risks and negative impacts	Protective and positive processes
Moral and ethical rules	• Dehumanization of enemy and perpetrator • Discourse of revenge	• Repertoires to explain human conduct • Forgiveness on affective, cognitive, and societal levels
Symbolic		
Play and games	• Lack of narrative and joy • Frightening and concrete themes • Ritualistic and repetitious	• Multiple themes and role changes • Anxiety transfers to excitement and relief • Imaginary themes and fantasy characters
Dreaming	• Lack of narrative contents • Realistic replication of reality • Narrow and negative themes • Bodily dream images without content	• Coherent narratives involving scene, participants, core event, and message • Symbolic stories, unseen shifts of events, fantasy figures, bizarre scenes, figures, and events • Repertoire of both positive and negative emotions
Fantasy	• Violent content • Unresolved aggression	• Multiple themes • Developmental and enriching themes
Neurocognitive		
Brain functioning	• Dysfunction in prefrontal cortex and executive functioning (shifting attention, filtering information, controlling)	• Extinguishing fear conditioning • Interpreting emotional cues • Strengthen executive functions
Brain architecture	• Hippocampal volume reduction (with high cortisol level and posttraumatic stress disorder)	• Emphasis in narrative quality of memories • Symptom reduction (intrusive, hyper arousal)
Psychophysiological processes	• Stress attenuation cortisol overdose • Functional abnormalities more among adults with childhood trauma → developmental plasticity	• Regulating physiological responses • Integrating bodily responses and thinking • Affect modulation and repertoire of coping strategies • Organizing fragmented trauma memories into integrated stories

age-bound social affiliation: war-related violence is likely to deteriorate rather than improve peer and friendship relations. For instance, in war zones of Uganda, children report insufficient support from their peers and friends (Paardekooper et al. 1999); in Palestine, children report loneliness and lack of intimate friendship when exposed to severe military violence (Peltonen et al. 2010). Similarly, maltreated children and those exposed to domestic violence report less social support and peer popularity in Western studies (Appleyard et al. 2010).

The reasons for deteriorated peer relations may lie in the changed behavior of children as well as in the fears and prejudices of their peers. Violence-affected children may withdraw from intimate contacts, because they feel that their experiences are too painful and shameful to be shared with peers (Hong et al. 2012). They may suffer from intrusive and uncontrollable memories and show vigilance for dangers, which seems odd to their peers. Children in war zones recount that the frightened or frightening behaviors of their friends upset them and they fear that intrusive and hypervigilant symptoms may be contagious (Diab et al. 2014).

Research shows both positive and negative impacts on sibling relations. Concerning domestic violence, a qualitative study revealed multiple outcomes, including distant and almost meaningless sibling relations with tendencies to reenact the family difficulties as well as positive and tight bonds between siblings that serve as a substitute for parental neglect (Leavitt et al. 1998). There is evidence that stressful civilian life events (e.g., divorce and unemployment) can improve sibling relations by increasing intimacy and decreasing rivalry (Jenkins Tucker et al. 2013), whereas war violence, atrocities, and losses can increase rivalry and conflicts in sibling relations (Diab 2011; Peltonen et al. 2010). There are observations that siblings show a "share of work" in their emotional responses in war-exposed families: one sibling can be "the symptom carrier" and suffer excessively, while another assumes a supporting and caring role, and still another shows greater endurance (Punamäki 2002).

Extensive evidence shows that social support and connectedness offer protection in terms of mental health in children exposed to military and domestic violence (Betancourt et al. 2013c; Cicchetti and Valentino 2006). For example, a study revealed that military violence did not increase depressive and anxiety symptoms among Palestinian children who enjoyed high intimacy and lacked rivalry with their siblings (Peltonen et al. 2010). Peer relations serve unique developmental functions, such as the learning of effective coping strategies, the shaping of world views, and the sharing of emotions and secrets. Making and maintaining friendships contribute to mental health. Thus estrangement from peers has, in general, devastating effects on children, especially in violent environments. The healing power of sufficient and adequate social support lies in (a) the creation of shared meanings and narratives, (b) a cathartic experience of expressing painful emotions, and (c) affiliating with others. In war violence, collective support contributes to the feeling of safety and, literally, to survival (Diab et al. 2014). Accordingly, the purpose of interventions that help violence-affected children is to encourage social sharing and the disclosure of emotions and to train cohesive group processes, including empathy and listening skills (Peltonen and Punamäki 2010; Tol et al. 2013).

Parenting and Family Support

Collective and interpersonal violence interferes dramatically with the core parental task of protecting children. In war, parents may face a dilemma of choosing between national aims of heroism and the safety needs of their family. In cases of maltreatment, parents are confusingly both the source of danger and protection. Assurance of safety is urgent for optimal development and health: in war, children must realize that parents are unable to protect them, whereas in maltreatment parents are unwilling. Violence, therefore, impacts the parent-child relationship, family communication, and attachment behaviors in multiple and complex ways.

There is evidence that everyday stressors, poverty, and the threat to life related to war strain family resources and result in harsh and punitive parenting (Quinlan 2007) as well as general negative family relations or even maltreatment (Boxer et al. 2013; Panter-Brick et al. 2011). Belsky (2008) argues that the increased punitive and harsh parenting serves a meaningful and life-protecting goal: parents attempt to prepare their children to adjust to the violent living conditions. Family-level studies show that war-related violence does not necessarily deteriorate parenting, but rather that parents attempt to compensate their children for the suffering through intensified loving and caring interactions (Punamäki 2006). Parents seem to share the work of monitoring and guiding their children in extreme violence. A Palestinian study found that a father's war-related trauma was transferred to his children's mental health and insecure attachment through his harsh and punitive fathering practices. In contrast, a mother's exposure to war trauma was associated with decreased punitive practices (Palosaari et al. 2013). Similarly, some studies among Holocaust survivors report that fathers exhibited more punishing and controlling parenting styles, while mothering styles remained intact (Kellerman 2001). However, maltreatment and domestic violence are consistently combined with poor parenting, characterized by insensitive interactions, punitive and unpredictable behaviors, and withdrawal or intrusive rearing practices (Sanders 2008).

Parents aim to safeguard their children from war trauma by hiding their own painful experiences. Children, for their part, protect parents from painful memories by pretending not to know about the family's traumatic past. The absence of generationally shared narratives, "the conspiracy of silence," has been documented among Holocaust and torture survivors (Bar-On 1999; Montgomery 2004). Children are highly sensitive to their parents' and siblings' security and well-being in violent conditions. They may constantly fear that something bad will happen to their family and adopt a responsible role in early age. These intensified feelings of burden, guilt, and helplessness have been described as a role-reversal pattern in the parent-child relationship (Wiseman et al. 2006). A study conducted after a major war in Palestine reported that 73.5% of children (ages 8–14 years) feared that they were going to die, 68% feared that shelling and bombardment would happen again, and 94% felt that adults were not able to protect them (Thabet et al. 2009). Political activity at an early age, typical of some contemporary conflicts, reflects a child's determination to save the nation, as their parents have failed.

A core finding of trauma research is the great individual and group differences when threatened by violence and danger (Janoff-Bulman 2006; Mikulincer et al. 2006). Attachment theory is informative for understanding how and why family members with secure, avoidant, or preoccupied attachment styles show unique ways to appraise threat, regulate and share overwhelming emotions, and make sense of violence (Bowlby 1982; Steele et al., this volume). Violence and trauma activate the attachment-specific behaviors of seeking safety and proximity; even older children cling to their parents (Mikulincer et al. 2006). Parental attachment style, in turn, predicts the degree and nature of emotional availability to the children: secure parents provide structured and sensitive care, whereas insecure parents show emotionally cautious or unpredictable care (Sroufe and Sampson 2000). Secure attachment is conceptualized as protective and insecure attachment as a risk in traumatic encounters; research has confirmed a link between insecure attachment patterns and heightened post-traumatic stress disorder among both adult (Ein-Dor et al. 2010) and younger (O'Connor and Elklit 2008) trauma survivors.

Family relations are obviously vulnerable in violent contexts, but they also possess immense protective powers. Under conditions of war, good and loving family relationships have been found to buffer children's mental health and to enhance creativity and skillful coping strategies. For instance, exposure to military violence in the Middle Eastern war context did not increase symptoms of aggression and depression in children if parents were not punitive and showed love, care, and wise guidance (Qouta et al. 2008b). Further, parental support and optimal monitoring protected adolescents from depression and aggression in war conditions in the former Yugoslavia (Durakovic-Belko et al. 2003) and Palestine (Barber 2001). A study in Afghan families has demonstrated that the maintenance of psychosocial family resources contributes to everyday resilience in children and that supportive networks offer the key protective factors for children's well-being (Eggerman and Panter-Brick 2014; Panter-Brick et al. 2011, 2014b).

Accordingly, the goal of psychosocial interventions is to support and improve parenting as a natural healing resource among war-affected children (e.g., van Ee et al. 2011). This typically involves creating a safe place and other attachment-inspired treatment elements, enriching parent-child communication, and encouraging family narratives to be shared, and increasing parental knowledge and competence. Parents are encouraged to serve as a secure base and to be emotionally available and responsive to their children's needs. Children, in turn, learn to expect and trust in adult protection and help. Family members are helped to mobilize their unique coping strategies and communication styles, thus allowing easier access to cultural resources and shared meanings (Shaver and Mikulincer 2002). Similarly, a meta-analysis on the treatment efficacy with maltreated and sexually abused children emphasized the beneficial role of improving everyday parent-child communication and emotional availability (Trask et al. 2011).

Emotion Expression, Regulation, and Recognition

Emotions organize human motivation and meaningful behavior and are pivotal for children's well-being. Their role in the regulation of overwhelming experiences is especially salient when exposure to violence and trauma is involved. Emotion regulation refers to the ways in which children modify, control, and maintain the valence, intensity, and duration of their emotional experiences (Sheppes et al. 2014). There is ample evidence that domestic violence and maltreatment constitute a risk for dysfunctional emotion regulation that involves both overregulation (suppression, numbing, and minimization of emotions) and underregulation (vigilance for treats, behavioral impulsiveness, and maximization of emotions) of feelings of anger, sadness, and fear (Cummings et al. 2009; Maughan and Cicchetti 2002). Both the minimization and maximization of emotions seems counterproductive in violent conditions. Denying emotions may defend children from painful experiences in these unpredictable and frightening environments, but it also blocks their access to wider developmental repertoires. Children with overwhelmed emotions face difficulties in attuning their excessive arousal and aggressive feelings, and this can result in social problems.

Research is scarce on emotion regulation in war conditions. Emotions have been implicitly conceptualized as distress, coping strategies, and temperamental characteristics, thus ignoring the more dynamic functions of emotion processing. A study found that high emotionality and poor self-regulation predicted severe posttraumatic stress disorder symptoms in U.S. children exposed to the 9/11 terrorist attacks. Emotion regulation was measured by irritability, impulsivity, inadequate attention regulation, and poor inhibitory control (Lengua et al. 2005). Emotion research posits that the basic emotions of joy, fear, sadness, anger, surprise, and disgust are universal, but that their expressions are culturally bound (Hutcherson and Gross 2011). A call for research has been made to situate analyses of the everyday lives of war-affected children in larger family and social contexts (Eggerman and Panter-Brick 2010; Tol et al. 2011). Emotion research could enrich these efforts because it has unique rules for emotion expression and shares fundamental principles for cultural scripts, social and moral order, and future hopes. This, in turn, can be used to guide children to recognize and screen dangerous cues versus protective shields in their everyday environments.

Functional emotion regulation requires the accurate identification of one's own emotional experiences as well as the recognition of feelings from significant others. Exposure to violence and trauma can impair emotion recognition, thus interfering with automated regulative processing. Children have been found to show narrow and biased recognition patterns of facial emotions which vary systematically according to the nature of the violence. Physically abused children are highly proficient in recognizing angry facial expressions but show deficiencies in recognizing emotions (e.g., sadness) in others, indicating a heightened alertness for danger (Pollak et al. 2000) as well as high vigilance for fear-evoking cues (Masten et al. 2008). Emotionally neglected children face difficulties in accurately differentiating between distinct emotions (e.g., fear and sadness); this suggests deprived learning experiences in early attachment relations (Pollak et al. 2000).

A similar pattern of biased negative emotion processing has been found in children exposed to war and military violence. Russian victims of a terrorist attack readily recognized threatening and angry emotions, and were generally sensitive to negative emotions, but they had difficulties in accurately recognizing sadness (Scrimin et al. 2009). Political prisoners exposed to severe torture showed negative feelings, narrow emotional repertoire, and unimodal reliance on behavioral emotion expression, whereas less-exposed prisoners were able to integrate feelings, thoughts and behavior into a coherent emotion repertoire (Näätänen et al. 2002).

Automatic or unconscious processes of emotion regulation and recognition provide dynamic information that can be used to tailor interventions for violence-affected children, as well as for peacebuilding programs. In a societal atmosphere of war propaganda, xenophobia, and ethnic hatred, "otherness" is emphasized. Children are primed to recognize negative qualities in other cultural groups and sensitized to attentional biases toward threat. The ability to recognize one's own as well as others' emotions underlies the potential for empathy and prosocial behavior (Michalik et al. 2007), both of which are the core elements in peace education and psychosocial interventions with violence-affected children.

Cognitive Processes of Appraisal, Memory, and Symbols

Children attempt to reconstruct, interpret, and understand their violent and traumatic experiences. Changes in thinking, world view, memory, attention, causal attributions, and appraisals reflect these processes. Again, it must be noted that cognitive changes can make children more vulnerable as well as help them rebuild their shattered lives by seeking creative resolutions. Posttraumatic cognition is an umbrella concept that refers to biased, narrowed, and negative ways of thinking after traumatic and violent experiences (Ehlers and Clark 2000;

multi-emotional, metaphoric, and happy-ending narrative. Among severely traumatized children, dreams often lack contents and stories, but involve frightening and distressing bodily feelings and themes of persecution (Punamäki 2007). Psychosocial interventions incorporate play therapeutic elements that counter these traumatic impacts and provide violence-affected children access to healing and recovery through symbolic expression and metaphoric activity.

The negative impacts of violence on representations and memories reflect a trap that violent environments place for healthy child development. Narrative and meaningful memories facilitate healthy child development and enable cultural sharing and future promises. However, violence interferes with vital functions. Trauma emerges in sensory and procedural memory systems, rather than in verbal and episodic memory domains (Rubin et al. 2008). Children thus face difficulties in narrating about upsetting and horrific scenes, because there are no words or coherent imageries available to describe them. Similarly, emotionally laden, symbolic dreams are associated with good mental health (Punamäki 2007), but traumatic events deprive children from these dream characteristics. This phenomenon reflects an interaction between the multiple domains of child development as a result of exposure to violence. Cultural values, histories of shared agony, and collective memories of endurance provide children with an anchor of resilience (Betancourt et al. 2013c; Eggerman and Panter-Brick 2010). Still, if children are not assisted, they can languish in social isolation and silence, partly due to trauma-related changes in cognitive-emotional processes (Bar-On 1999). To help violence-affected children endure, recover, and prosper, we must facilitate their natural healing processes; that is, their ability to create narrative memories and play, to share collective meanings, and to affiliate with others.

Neurocognitive Processes

Understanding the neurocognitive effects of collective and interpersonal violence is vital if we are to tailor treatments to improve children's learning, memory, emotion regulation, and mental health. Neurocognitive effects can serve as markers for vulnerability; they can indicate how violence negatively impacts crucial brain function and architecture; they also reveal the striking plasticity in brain development (Twardosz and Lutzker 2010). Identifying treatment-specific changes in neurobiological markers from involved brain regions provides information about what types of intervention elements work, for whom, and perhaps why (Carrion et al. 2013).

De Bellis and Thomas (2003) have suggested distinct and comprehensive impacts of childhood trauma on neurobiological development, and many problems (e.g., delayed cognitive development, disorganized attachment, hyperactivity, and attention deficits) have been attributed to abnormalities in the brain. It is agreed that violent experiences impact brain development through overburdening neurobiological stress responses (i.e., the sympathetic nervous system, the limbic-hypothalamic-pituitary-adrenal axis) and the serotonin systems) (De Bellis and Thomas 2003). Neuroimaging evidence (Hart and Rubia 2012) confirms that maltreatment is a risk for functional and anatomical changes in prefrontal cortex, which is active in planning, decision making, working memory, and inhibitory processes (conceptualized as executive functioning). The prefrontal cortex, in communication with amygdala in limbic system, is also crucial for fear conditioning, emotion regulation, impulse control, and in shifting attention. In adults who were subjected to maltreatment, smaller volume of hippocampus has been observed; results are inconclusive concerning maltreated children (Woon and Hedges 2008). Yet, elevated stress hormones and posttraumatic stress disorder symptoms can together predict a reduction of hippocampal volume (Carrion et al. 2013), which illuminates the neurobiological basis for intrusive memories, uncontrollable emotions, and disintegrated mental states among victims of violence.

Interventions and the Promotion of Peace among Children Affected by Violence

Optimal social, emotional, and cognitive processes are crucial in protecting healthy development in violent environments. If facilitated, they also provide healing elements for recovery, resilience, and posttraumatic growth. The available psychosocial interventions for children exposed to both collective and interpersonal violence aim to prevent problems and promote development in these domains. Consensus exists as to the evidence-based effectiveness of cognitive behavioral therapies in both war-affected and maltreated children (NICE 2014; Jordans et al. 2009). One of the core elements is narrating and sharing the traumatic experiences in a safe and supportive setting, which helps children organize their fragmented sensory and emotional memories. Moreover, cognitive behavioral therapy involves teaching emotion modulation, multiple coping strategies, and integrating cognitive and affective domains. An atmosphere of trust and safety is critical for disclosure, social sharing, and emotion expression, which, in turn, can contribute to recovery.

Concerning war-affected children, reduction of mood and anxiety disorders (especially posttraumatic stress disorder), and conduct problems are considered the main outcomes of effective interventions. A general call has been made to extend this to include access to optimal social and cultural resources (Jordans et al. 2009; Peltonen and Punamäki 2010). It is uncommon to assess explicitly the potential underlying mechanisms (mediators) that contribute to the outcomes, or preconditions for why and to whom the interventions work (moderators). It is also quite striking that protecting and healing elements on a community level are not the foci in interventions with war-affected children. In former Yugoslavia, only some psychosocial interventions focused on promoting peace, empathy, and prosocial behavior among children of former enemies

(Barath 2000; Woodside et al. 1999). With few exceptions (e.g., Meiser-Stedman et al. 2007), beneficial changes in social, emotional, cognitive, or neurobiological processes are not analyzed as contributors to growth, resilience, and recovery in intervention research. The same observations are also true for intervention studies involving children exposed to domestic violence and maltreatment (i.e., foci on symptom reduction as outcome and absence of underlying mediating and moderating mechanisms for change). Interestingly, enhancing family reconciliation and forgiveness are increasingly considered to be effective healing elements in these studies (Trask et al. 2011).

To understand how psychosocial interventions contribute to peacebuilding in violence-affected children, three alternative approaches should be considered. First, symptom-focused efforts aim to alleviate psychological distress, arguing that when children are free from depressive, intrusive and aggressive symptoms, they are able to prosper, show mental growth and accomplish their healthy development, including building peaceful societies. Second, a resilience-enhancing approach emphasizes the importance of positive and compensatory experiences, feelings of safety, agency and mastery, and effective coping and socioemotional skills that serve as a basis for good mental health that includes empathy, peacefulness, and prosocial attitudes and beneficial behaviors (Peltonen and Palosaari 2013). Third, by integrating mental health and peace promotion, elements of peacebuilding programs are included as an integral part in group and individual treatments among violence-affected children. The dynamic processes of forgiveness, reconciliation, cognitive and affective empathy, and dialogical interactions would serve well the aims of more comprehensive healing and growth (Abu-Nimer and Nasser, this volume). Empirical examples are available from the therapy literature, including adults with childhood sexual abuse (Hoyt et al. 2005), rather than from psychosocial interventions with war-affected children.

Sociopolitical Frames to Facilitate Peacebuilding

The current analysis of the underlying risk and protective processes was restricted to the levels of the individual, family, and school. From the perspective of promoting peace, it is important to understand the dynamics of societal, political, and cultural preconditions that facilitate the potential for endurance, resilience, and mental growth in violence-affected children. Obstacles to peace or nonviolence often relate to a cycle of revenge, heated by collective and individual memories of wrongdoing, injustice, and pain. It would be ignorant to argue that enhancing the mental health and optimal development of violence-affected children would guarantee world peace and family reconciliation. Still, research suggests that not working through, denying, or being obsessed with traumatic and violent experiences result in compromised developmental potential (Bar-On 1999; Ehlers and Clark 2000). Forgiveness, realistic views of the enemy, and a curiosity for universal and cultural virtues contribute to the ability to make peace-enhancing choices, but societal preconditions are necessary for such choices to be actualized.

There is a concern that violence can negatively affect the moral development of children, and that aggression begets aggression. On the positive side, struggling with real-life moral dilemmas contributes to a child's cognitive maturity, which is a precondition for high moral standards. Forgiveness serves an example of a complex process that (a) involves social, emotional, and spiritual elements and (b) results in the attenuation of angry emotions, resentful attitudes, and revengeful behavior. To enhance forgiveness and peacebuilding, both basic psychosocial and cultural processes must be combined. Forgiveness on a societal level, in turn, has multiple beneficial consequences for violence-affected families and children (Chapman 2007), including improved physical and mental health (Toussant and Webb 2005).

The bioecological model (Bronfenbrenner 2005; Cicchetti and Valentino 2006; Boxer et al. 2013; Britto et al., this volume) provides a framework in which multilevel influences on child development can be analyzed. It includes the positive and protective proximal and distal elements for healthy and generative developmental outcomes. The larger context (social, cultural, and political values, strategies and practices) is important to evaluate, as it provides the necessary, albeit insufficient, preconditions for peacebuilding. It is important to avoid an "either-or" mentality and focus on interactional dynamics between individual collective capacities. Empirical studies are, however, scarce: more studies are needed that articulate the multiple processes through which the distal frames (e.g., implicit and explicit cultural values, emotional scripts, political strategies, and attitudinal climate) interact with proximal phenomena (e.g., family's shared emotion expression, narratives, attribution strategies, and memories). The collective frames may facilitate, compensate, neutralize, or potentiate these more individual outcomes, whereas individual-level growth, accomplishment, and learning may, in turn, shape societal or even global developments. Combining these multilevel and dynamic influences will contribute to peacebuilding and help society make the vital changes toward a zero tolerance to both domestic and military violence.

13

Structural Violence and Early Childhood Development

Andrew Dawes and Amelia van der Merwe

Abstract

The first part of this chapter examines the influence of structural violence on early child development and the family environment. In contrast to direct violence, this form manifests as unequal exposure to protective and risk factors, inequitable access to the resources and services that could ameliorate risk and support positive development, and as unequal service quality. Similar to direct violence, the structural variant violates the rights of children and undermines the protective capacities of those who care for them. Insults to early development raise the probability of poor outcomes in the long term, including reduced capabilities for productive, prosocial, and peaceable citizenship.

The second part offers the example of an *essential package* of population-level, evidence-based services for young children and caregivers that has been developed in South Africa. These services aim to reduce exposure to risk factors that compromise developmental potential, and to increase protective and promotive influences in those most affected by poverty. It covers basic services designed to promote maternal and child health and nutrition, stimulation for early learning, social protection, child protection, and the well-being of primary caregivers. Provision of these services is seen as a social good (not just an investment in future productivity). They should be available to all, but particularly to those disadvantaged by poverty and other forms of deprivation occasioned by structural violence.

Introduction

Our contribution has two components: First, we examine the construct "structural violence" and its role in shaping the developmental environments and outcomes of young children. Second, we propose an *essential package* of evidence-based, population-level interventions for young children that reduces risk exposure and increases protective and promotive influences (see also Masten, this volume; Wachs and Rahman 2013). We see this package as a social good that must be available to all children. While relevant to child development in all countries, this part of the discussion focuses on a package appropriate for low- and middle-income countries using a South African example. These countries are particularly affected by structural violence, as a vast majority of children grow up facing significant risks to development in settings where resources for prevention and promotion are more limited than those in the Global North (Walker et al. 2007).

Definitions of early childhood commonly refer to the period zero to nine years (UNESCO 2007). Recognizing the crucial importance of development processes prior to birth, we include intrauterine development and focus our discussion on the period from then until five years of age (prior to school). Other contributors to this volume (particularly Chapters 4–10) explore the complex relationships between genes and environment, evolutionary processes, early relationship formation, and peace. We shall not go over this ground.

The Nature of Structural Violence

Distinctions between direct and structural violence are described in detail by Christie et al. (this volume). Essentially, direct violence is caused by persons, does harm to the body, is episodic (rather than chronic), and may kill rapidly. In contrast, structural violence is apparent in the nature of political, economic, and ideological systems. Galtung (1969) originally coined the term to describe any constraint, restriction, or limitation on human potential due to economic or political structures of power. Structural violence is ultimately an outcome of choices made. As Kent (2006:54–55) states: "Structural violence is harm imposed by some people on others indirectly, through the social system, as they pursue their own preferences" as in the case "when government leaders decide to purchase armaments rather than vaccines."

Above all, structural violence involves unequal access to resources, to political or economic power, to education or health care, to legal standing, and to inequitable quality in these services—all of which impact child development (Opotow 2001).

Structural violence is given *ideological* content when the ends and means of political action are justified (Eagleton 1991). Ideology also normalizes social relations, as when structural violence seems so commonplace as to be ordinary, which frequently makes it invisible (Winter and Leighton 2001). When unequal social conditions are *normalized* (i.e., rendered as natural, taken for granted as unquestionable conditions of the social order), those who are more fortunate are inclined to the belief—no, *the knowledge*—that the less fortunate have only themselves to blame for their condition.

The social psychological "just-world hypothesis" is relevant here. Individuals internalize principles of fairness and equity. However, when events occur to contradict this view, those who have access to resources tend to rationalize that those who do not simply get what they deserve (Lerner and Miller 1977), as in the case of the "undeserving poor." Just-world thinking also plays a role in sustaining an ideological position; that is, the need to believe that the world is fair and that people get what they deserve, particularly when they are perceived to be members of groups of lesser status.

A further ingredient of this process is *moral exclusion*. Group members develop a sense of the members of their moral community—those who share a network of relationships, ideological commonalities and notions of justice (e.g., family, friends, co-religionists, ethnic brothers and sisters). It is to them that we extend our sense of justice or fairness. Those outside this moral community are excluded on the basis of their real or imagined differences. They are seen as "expendable nonentities," and disadvantage, hardship, and exploitation that is inflicted upon them is perceived as "normal" and acceptable; as just "the way things are" (Opotow 2001:103). Poor treatment does not elicit remorse, outrage, or demand restitution.

The legitimacy or unacceptability of injustices is transmitted across generations through the socialization process. Everyday activities and discourse embedded in the practices (Miller and Goodnow 1995) of the home, community, and school expose young children to scripts for relating to others on the basis of similarity and difference (see also Christie et al., this volume). These may, for example, make race or class highly salient markers of difference. The ideological content of the scripts primes the child toward hostile, intolerant, or inclusive orientations toward others (Christie and Dawes 2001). The latter lays the foundation for potentially more peaceable orientations to others in later phases of development (for further elaboration, see Christie et al., this volume).

For all these reasons, social injustices may persist for generations.

Impact of Structural Violence on the Young Child

Inequality and Poverty

There is no simple or direct relationship between structural violence and early developmental outcomes. Its principle contribution is through the production of social injustice in the form of skewed exposure to developmental risk and opportunity, and inequitable access to the resources that can ameliorate risk and support positive development. As the social gradient steepens, the development of children at the bottom rung is compromised, while that of those at the top is enhanced (Wilkinson and Pickett 2010).

Evidence from around the world indicates that inequality is corrosive. Judt (2010:21) notes:

[Inequality] rots societies from within....(as) competition for status and goods
increases; people feel a growing sense of superiority (or inferiority) based on
their possessions; prejudice towards those on the lower ranks of the social ladder
hardens; crime spikes and the pathologies of social disadvantage become ever
more marked.

While poverty is not in itself structural violence, where income is highly
skewed, extensive poverty is one of its features. Galtung (1994:7) notes that
"the problem is not poverty as such, but the power of the affluent to tilt the use
of the world's resources to their favor."

Structural violence, through its production of inequity in resource distribution and service access, impacts on a wide range of developmental domains
in early childhood: for the good of the more fortunate, and to the detriment
of those at the other end of the social scale (Anastasi 1958; Huston 1994;
McLoyd 1998; Sen 1999). It affects the most vulnerable—women and children
in particular—who are exposed in great numbers across the world to a range of
social injustices (Schwebel and Christie 2001).

How are the impacts of structural violence on young children evident?
Access to the services and supports required for sound early development are
unevenly distributed both within and across nations (Schwebel and Christie
2001) and is correlated with indices of societal inequality (Sen 1999; Wilkinson
and Pickett 2010). Children living in poverty, particularly in low- and middle-income countries, have poor access to services such as potable water and
sanitation, food security, quality health care, and good education (Kent 2006;
Walker et al. 2007). This prevents millions of people from attaining their developmental potential (Engle et al. 2007; Jolly 2007; Nores and Barnett 2010).
UNICEF's statistical reports[1] provide useful country comparative data. Data
on child mortality (under five years of age) is more reliable than many other
indicators. An indicator of structural violence is the uneven distribution of
mortality across the world where it is concentrated in the poorest and often
very unequal societies. In 2011, about 80% of deaths that occurred in children under the age of five years took place in only 25 countries. About half of
these occurred in only five: India, Nigeria, China, Democratic Republic of the
Congo, and Pakistan (WHO 2013). Notably, the first three countries have also
experienced high rates of economic growth in recent times.

It is not only health- and education-related challenges that pose a risk to
the developmental potential of the young child. The well-being of the child's
caregiver plays a significant role in the level of stimulation and affectional
care that he or she is able to provide. Caregiver well-being and the capacity
to provide good care are comprised under conditions of poverty, particularly
when coupled with limited psychosocial support (Wachs and Rahman 2013;
Walker et al. 2007).

---

[1] http://www.unicef.org/statistics/ (accessed June 14, 2014).

Exposure to maltreatment and violence is a further risk factor that tends to correlate with social disadvantage in both rich and poor countries. Violence harms children leading to fear, psychic numbing, a sense of foreshortened future, and aggressive attitudes and behavior, all of which do not bode well for peace (Kostelny and Garbarino 2001). Chronic exposure in the early years of life is also associated with toxic stress reactions (McEwen 2012).

The South African Case

Among African countries colonized by the European powers (with the exception of Angola), South Africa has the longest history of structural violence and oppression of persons of color. Settlement by the Dutch in the seventeenth century was accompanied by the use of imported slave labor, a practice that was only terminated under British colonial rule in 1834. Violent suppression of hunter-gatherer indigenous peoples occurred from the beginning and continued until the early twentieth century. Khoikhoi (herder) and San (hunter-gatherer) populations were largely exterminated.

Forcible expropriation of the land of indigenous people was legislated in 1913 and 1936, leaving 87% of the land in the hands of whites. From 1948, the policy of apartheid ensured further dispossession and entrenched segregation in all areas of public and private life. Marriages across the color line were banned in 1949, and the Immorality Act of 1950 prohibited sexual relations between whites and other groups that formed part of the race classification system. These groups were administered separately. Vastly unequal state funding was allocated to the (segregated) health, education and welfare services, with whites receiving the most per capita. As recently as 1990, per capita education expenditure on black children was *one quarter* of that spent on white children (Dawes and Donald 1994). It is difficult to establish comparative health expenditure figures, but in 1984, for example, the per capita health expenditure in the four provinces of South Africa (mainly serving whites, people of mixed race, and Asian descent) was significantly higher than the expenditure in the areas in which blacks were required to reside. For example, public health expenditure in one of these provinces in 1984 was the equivalent of USD 68.00 per capita, while in Transkei (one of apartheid's so-called black homeland areas, now part of Eastern Cape Province), it was the equivalent of USD 14.00 (Benatar and Kirsch 1987). The impact of poverty and food insecurity in these years are evident in 1985 figures, when the physical growth of 41% of rural black children was stunted[2] compared to 4% of whites (Wilson and Ramphele 1989).

From the mid-1950s onward, oppression was increasingly met with resistance, and, of course, further repression followed, resulting in the banning of anti-apartheid political formations, detention without trial, and torture. The

---

[2] Stunting is an indicator of chronic malnutrition and is defined as height-for-age more than two standard deviations below the norm.

intensity and breadth of the South African struggle increased significantly in the period following the uprising of Soweto school pupils in 1976 (Pohlandt-McCormick 2000), when many thousands were plucked from their families and placed in detention without trial for extended periods (Reynolds and Dawes 1999).

South Africa, Post 1994: A Rights-Oriented Policy Regime

The legacy of exploitation, dispossession, and both direct and structural violence has marked South Africa's transition. Awareness of the need to address the legacy of the apartheid era informed many legislative and policy changes that were introduced, following the establishment of a democratic state in 1994 (Dawes et al. 2007).

South Africa is signatory to the United Nations Convention on the Rights of the Child (UNCRC 1989). Section 28 of the South African Constitution is aligned with this international instrument in providing children with the right to education, protection, basic nutrition, shelter, basic health and social services, and to nationality at birth. Legislation provides for early childhood services (e.g., the Children's Act 38 of 2005). Following the UNCRC, children's best interests are to be upheld in all matters. The fact that children's rights are entrenched in the Constitution of South Africa has been significant in advancing the services required to support child development, particularly among the poor (Dawes et al. 2007; Aber et al. 2013).

South Africa has pro-poor policies designed, as far as possible, to address the needs of those in poverty (the majority of the population); the highest shares of the 2013 budget went to social protection, education, and health. Schooling is free as are health services to pregnant women and children under six years of age who attend state services.

The constitutional right to social security for children has been used successfully to argue for the right of those eligible to access the Child Support Grant. Introduced in 1998, the Child Support Grant accounts for 3.5% of GDP; ZAR 300 (USD 28.00) per child is paid to beneficiaries who meet the means test.[3] Most recent figures indicate that 11 million children (60%) access the grant. There is substantial evidence that the grant is spent on food, education, and basic services, and has been shown to reduce malnutrition in beneficiaries under five years of age (Dept. of Social Development, SASSA and UNICEF 2012; Berry et al. 2013).

On one hand, these figures and outcomes are cause for celebration, as the social protection net is widely cast. However, the fact that such a high proportion of children are in need reflects a high level of structural violence.

---

[3]   Parents or guardians qualify if each earns less than ZAR 3,000 (USD 278) per month; conversion calculated on March 11, 2013: 1 US Dollar = 10.77 South African Rands (ZAR).

The right to health has ensured state provision of ante retroviral medication for the prevention of mother to child transmission of HIV. In addition, the right to shelter has made it the state's responsibility to provide housing for homeless indigent families with children.

In sum, there have been many gains since 1994; provision of health, social, and educational services for young children in poor communities has increased significantly. However, despite such gains, service delivery is constrained. There is little integration or coordination of services to ensure that the multidimensional needs of young children are met. There is insufficient quality to achieve good child outcomes, inadequate funding models, and ineffective targeting strategies (Richter et al. 2012).

South Africa remains a highly unequal society. The Gini coefficient, a measure of statistical dispersion intended to represent the income distribution of a nation's residents, is 0.68 (Finn and Leibrandt 2013). South Africa ranks as one of the most unequal countries in the world. Poverty levels are significant (Van den Berg 2010), and in the 2011 Census, 54% of all children were found to be living in households that expended less than USD 2.00 per day per capita. In consequence, the well-being of the majority of young children[4] in South Africa remains very unsatisfactory

Addressing the Consequences of Structural Inequalities for Young Children: A South African Example

Here we describe a package of services that have been deemed *essential* for the support of a strong early start to life. The Essential Package, as it is known, was designed by *Ilifa Labantwana*[5] (Ilifa) in 2013 and is currently being tested in pilot communities. Ilifa is a large-scale multifaceted donor-funded program that has been running since 2008 and will terminate in 2016/17. The focus is on children under the age of 6 and their families living below the poverty line (close to 60% of this age group) (Berry et al. 2013).

Ilifa is founded on the recognition of the structural inequities that face the majority of South African children and those who care for them. Its main goal is to provide the evidence to inform changes in government policy and provisioning for early childhood development, thus enabling a scale-up of essential services to ensure that children thrive, grow, and are ready to learn once they reach school. The main components of the program include:

- Interventions to improve systems of delivery of health, social, and early learning services.

---

[4] For current information on children in South Africa (e.g., their living conditions, care arrangements, health status, and access to schools and other services), see http://www.childrencount.ci.org.za/ (accessed June 14, 2014).

[5] For complete details, see http://www.ilifalabantwana.co.za/ (accessed June 14, 2014).

- A randomized trial to test the effectiveness of a parenting intervention to reduce harsh punishment and maltreatment.
- A trial to test the long-term impact (five years) of a short intervention delivered by paraprofessionals to promote maternal well-being and health, prevent malnutrition, and promote sensitive care.
- Interventions to test the effects of providing an essential package of services in target communities.
- Initiatives to strengthen human resource supply in the early childhood sector.
- Costing of home visits, playgroup and center-based interventions designed to promote the holistic development of children in poor rural communities.

The program operates in partnership with the government. All components are subject to evaluation using a range of methods (both quantitative and qualitative). Evaluations completed to date are available online.[6]

While not directly seeking to influence the production of future citizens with peaceful social orientations, evidence suggests that it is reasonable to propose that provision of a sound foundation for development will increase the number of future citizens with the capabilities required for constructive social engagement and productive lives. Likewise it will reduce the number who are unable to participate successfully in society, and who may be drawn into conduct that is contrary to peace.

It is essential, however, to recognize that many other risks to development are present in later years, and that these can both undo gains and compound earlier vulnerabilities. Early intervention does not offer a magic solution, but it has huge preventive and promotive potential to reduce the proportion of children who would otherwise have followed a negative developmental pathway. Longitudinal research on disadvantaged children who were provided with early interventions to improve health, nutrition, and early learning point to significant gains in adulthood capabilities that also promise a reduction in intergenerational poverty and inequality (e.g., Nores and Barnett 2010; Kagitcibasi et al. 2009; Hoddinott et al. 2008).

This Ilifa program does not address the need to eliminate structural violence. That is an issue of central *political* importance. Indeed, without political intervention to reduce, if not eliminate, both direct and structural violence, proposals such as that which follows may justifiably be viewed as long-term band-aids. While they may do important work to promote children's rights and enable a better future for the beneficiaries, they are certainly not sufficient in themselves to promote peaceful societal outcomes in the long term.

---

6   See 2012 Launch Publications at http://www.ilifalabantwana.co.za/ilifa-publications/publication-archive/ (accessed June 14, 2014).

The Ilifa Labantwana Essential Package of Early Childhood Services and Support

To improve the situation of young children, to reduce the loss of potential, and to contribute in the longer term to a more just society, it is necessary to develop comprehensive strategies to both reduce risks to early development and enhance protective factors at *population* level. To that end, *Ilifa Labantwana* developed an "essential package of services and support"[7] for children to be delivered from pregnancy to the end of the fifth year. It must be stressed that this package does *not* seek to cover every possible service that young children might need. It is designed to focus on the essentials, and to be aligned as closely as possible with current policies and programs mandated and supported by the South African State, and to be affordable for delivery at scale to those in the bottom two income quintiles.

Interventions in countries with limited resources and great demands on services need to take account of resource limitations and the need to reach the *majority* of affected children, often through paraprofessionals with limited education. That is the intent of the *Ilifa Labantwana Essential Package* (henceforth referred to as the Package).

The Package has been designed to be an attempt at promoting the delivery of evidence-based services that have potential to impact positively on significant numbers of children made vulnerable by poverty. The Package is aligned to policies and, where these are lacking, promotes transformation and service equity (these are aspirational goals that cannot be met under current conditions).

The Package must be viewed as complementing a broader set of provisions necessary to reduce inequality and promote survival and development. This includes poverty alleviation, food security, safe communities, and provision of basic household services (potable water, electricity, hygienic sanitation, and household infrastructure).

While it is recognized that all members of a family (whatever its form and structure) may play a role in the promotion of children's development, the focus of the Package is on the primary caregiver, and that usually refers to women.

The manner in which the Package addresses the consequences of structural violence is outlined in Table 13.1. It also recognizes that specific inputs are required at different stages of a child's early development and that it is necessary to build a developmentally appropriate continuum of services commencing with antenatal care, as illustrated with examples in Figure 13.1.

In the Package, five components are specified, each of which is considered essential for vulnerable children:

1. nutritional support (including to pregnant mothers),
2. primary level maternal and child health services,
3. social services,

---

[7] The Package may be accessed at www.Ilifalabantwana.co.za (accessed June 14, 2014).

Table 13.1 The Essential Package and structural violence.

Element of The Essential Package	Structural Violence Dimension Addressed
1. Nutritional support to pregnant women and children under 6 years.	Food insecurity and inadequate nutrition consequent on poverty. Provision of nutritional support is essential to prevent malnutrition and its consequences (poor school outcomes, drop out, risk of externalizing and antisocial behavior).
2. Primary level maternal and child health services	Inadequate supply of free public health services for pregnant women and young children living in poverty. Poverty presents a range of risks to maternal health during pregnancy, including heightened risk of maternal mortality and low birth weight. Prevalence of maternal illness (such as HIV and AIDS) poses significant risks to the child's development. Prevalence is elevated in poor communities and services are frequently inadequate. Poor early detection of developmental delay and disability results in these problems not receiving attention and impacting school performance in later years. Risk of morbidity and mortality is heightened in poverty environments; it is essential that children receive basic clinical services and that their health is regularly monitored.
3. Social services	Rights to protection from maltreatment, basic nutrition, shelter, basic health and social services and to nationality at birth are frequently violated. Birth registration enables access to a range of services. Income poverty impacts a very wide range of child outcomes. Provision of safety nets for children whose families do not have the financial means to provide adequate care and support for the child. Child abuse and neglect occur in all communities, but stresses on poor families elevate risk.
4. Support for primary caregivers (which recognizes the importance of caregiver health and well-being for early development and the prevention of risks during pregnancy)	Poverty impacts caregiving capacity, particularly the ability to provide nurturant and sensitive care. Programs to provide support to vulnerable caregivers are essential to improve their well-being and reduce the range of risks to child development that have been found to be associated with caregiver stress and poor coping.
5. Stimulation for early learning	Poor children have significantly more limited access to quality early learning opportunities than their better-off counterparts. Provision of early learning support in the preschool years (through cost-effective channels) has been shown to produce significant gains for children, including greater likelihood of good scholastic outcomes later in life and adult employment.

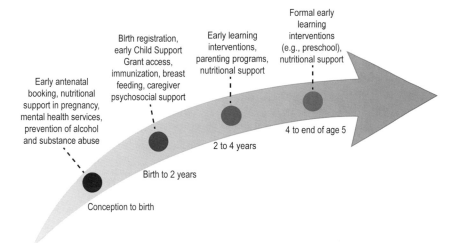

Early antenatal booking, nutritional support in pregnancy, mental health services, prevention of alcohol and substance abuse

Conception to birth

Birth registration, early Child Support Grant access, immunization, breast feeding, caregiver psychosocial support

Birth to 2 years

Early learning interventions, parenting programs, nutritional support

2 to 4 years

Formal early learning interventions (e.g., preschool), nutritional support

4 to end of age 5

Figure 13.1   Example of a developmental continuum of services and support.

4. support for primary caregivers (which recognizes the importance of caregiver health and well-being for early development and the prevention of risks during pregnancy), and
5. stimulation for early learning.

Some services target children with particular risk profiles (e.g., exposure to HIV via the mother during pregnancy). Others are necessary for all children.

Our experience is that in order to gain the buy in of government and other stakeholders, and to increase the chances of implementation, a Package of this sort should be aligned to services already provided in government policy and programs. It should also indicate those that must be provided where none are currently available (aspirational services).

Following Engle et al. (2011), the Package promotes intersectoral collaboration of early childhood services as far as possible. A number of channels of delivery that reach significant numbers of children are present in South Africa: public primary maternal and child health services, social welfare and social protection services, early learning services (including preschools and other channels for delivering early learning programs; Dawes et al. 2012) and programs that focus on early learning through a combination of home visits and group learning and support (e.g., the Turkish Early Enrichment Project and Mother Support Program; Kagitcibasi et al. 2009). Figure 13.2 illustrates the components of the Package, each of which will be briefly outlined below. The Package is primarily intended as a tool to assist service providers to monitor essential service delivery. Simple indicators of service delivery and for measuring success are provided.

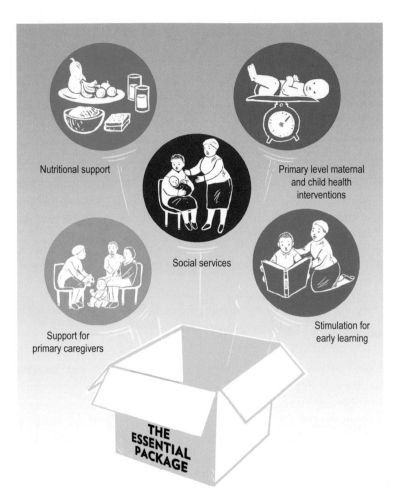

Figure 13.2   Components of the Ilifa Labantwana Essential Package.

Nutritional Support

Poor nutrition negatively impacts learning capacity and physical development and has serious consequences for adult productivity and economic development. Impact depends on the period during which it is experienced. Prenatal development and the first two years are particularly sensitive (Alderman et al. 2006; Dewey and Begum 2011). Poor fetal growth and stunting prior to age two leads to irreversible brain damage and, in the long term, to reduced human capital due to poor cognitive ability. Longitudinal study evidence suggests that malnutrition in year one plays a role in the development of violent conduct in adolescence (Galler et al. 2012). In the Mauritius longitudinal study, more severe malnutrition predicted higher rates of externalizing behavior (with other influences controlled) (Liu et al. 2004). Further work is required to examine the mechanisms involved.

The following are essential nutrition services to reduce the risk of low birth weight, postnatal malnutrition, and compromised neurological development:

1. During pregnancy, mothers are provided with education on breastfeeding and nutrition for children.
2. Pregnant women with micronutrient deficiencies are given nutritional support (iron, calcium and folate) and, up to 6 weeks postnatally, a high dose vitamin A capsule.
3. Children under 24 months who fail to thrive receive vitamin A and iron supplements.
4. Children aged one to five years are provided with deworming medication every six months.

Primary Level Maternal and Child Health Services

Chan (2013:1515) asserts that the health sector "has a unique responsibility, because it has the greatest reach to children and their families during pregnancy, birth, and early childhood. Universal health coverage provides the platform to achieve impact in a fair, integrated, and efficient way."

In South Africa, a key health-related threat to early development is poor antenatal care, which is associated with maternal mortality and low birth weight in surviving children (Saloojee 2007). Primary causes of death in children under the age of five years are preterm birth, asphyxia, infection, and AIDS-related illness and diarrheal disease (Saunders et al. 2010).

Maternal mental health receives scant attention, even though it is a key risk factor for poor child development outcomes (Wachs and Rahman 2013). Similarly, alcohol abuse and drug usage impacts fetal neurological development (Stratton et al. 1996). If we are to reduce their impact, screening and provision of primary level mental health support must be regarded as essential services (Honikman et al. 2012). Screening children for developmental delay and disabilities is an essential service if they are to be assisted.

It can be argued, however, that it is not ethical to screen if there is no accessible referral service, as is so often the case in low- and middle-income countries. There are, however, at least three counterarguments. First, from a right to health perspective, some form of basic service must be put in place, and this of course prompts us to seek low-cost interventions. Second, we argue that screening is essential as an advocacy tool, as it permits analysis of service needs. Third, in the case of developmental delay and/or disability, screening allows problems to be detected, some of which may be readily addressed (e.g., vision and hearing deficits; the need for an assistive device); others, if left unattended, constitute barriers to learning and result in preventable poor educational performance (Saloojee and Schneider 2007).

The services listed below reduce a range of risks to maternal and child health and promote survival and development:

1. Pregnant women are provided with basic antenatal care commencing in the first trimester.
2. Newborn health and exclusive breastfeeding is promoted through a home visit in the first six days after birth.
3. Pregnant women are screened for mental health conditions and alcohol and substance use, and referred for treatment where possible.
4. Prevention of mother-to-child-transmission (PMTCT) treatment is provided to HIV positive women.
5. HIV-exposed children receive PMTCT treatment.
6. Primary health care facilities are equipped to implement the WHO strategy of integrated management of childhood illness (WHO 2005).
7. Children are immunized.
8. Children are screened for developmental delay and disability and referred where possible.
9. Children who fail to thrive are screened for tuberculosis and, when positive, are treated.

Social Services

In South Africa, essential social services include birth registration social protection, Child Support Grant, and child protection (from maltreatment). Birth registration is a constitutional right that should be secured as early as possible, as it is required to access services including the Child Support Grant. This unconditional cash transfer lifts families in South Africa out of extreme poverty, increases food security, and reduces the risk of malnutrition (Aber et al. 2013).

While the right to protection from all forms of abuse and neglect is stated in the UNCRC as well as in the South African Constitution (Section 28, 1d), maltreatment poses a significant problem (Richter and Dawes 2008) that has major impacts on developing hormonal and neurological systems (McEwen 2012). Increased risk of dysregulation and later conduct problems are likely for large numbers of children.

Responsibility for the protection of children lies firstly with parents and caregivers; however, when a child is at risk or maltreated, the State becomes duty bearer. South Africa's Children's Act provides a range of provisions for child protection. Unfortunately, existing services are simply not sufficient to address present needs (Dawes and Ward 2008). Given what we know about the role of early maltreatment and exposure to violence in the evolution of aggressive conduct, early intervention is an essential ingredient in the prevention of population-level violence. The Package provides two services for child maltreatment that seek to track the responsiveness of the child protection system so that improvements can be made and the risk of secondary traumatization can be reduced. These must be complemented by preventive services such as parenting programs and caregiver support discussed in the next section.

Essential social services defined in the Package are as follows:

1. Children are registered within 30 days of birth.
2. Eligible children receive the Child Support Grant as soon as possible, but prior to their first birthday.
3. Children under six are provided with a child protection service that is responsive; that is, it processes reports efficiently and ensures prevention of secondary traumatization (trauma of the abuse is compounded by system inefficiencies and ineffectual service).
4. Children in the child protection system are provided with basic psychosocial support.

Support for Primary Caregivers

Support for primary caregivers includes parenting education and psychosocial support. Parent education may target specific populations, such as pregnant women, where the goal may be to prevent alcohol and drug use. Other programs may have a specific focus on caregiver/child relationships in the context of poverty, undernutrition, and mental health conditions (e.g., Rotherham-Borus et al. 2011), or on changing child behavior management through modeling and practice (e.g., Sanders 2003).

Nurturing and supportive parenting during the first years of a child's life has positive effects on social, emotional, and intellectual development. These capabilities are compromised in poverty and other stressful environments (Wachs and Rahmen 2013). Initiatives to support vulnerable caregivers and assist them to provide nurturant care must be regarded as an essential intervention, not only to promote the well-being of the caregiver but also to reduce the risk of neglect and undernutrition in the young child.

Low- and middle-income countries have few professional mental health services, particularly for children, and cannot afford long-term intensive programs (Tomlinson et al. 2012). Low-cost alternatives using paraprofessionals are needed and are indeed becoming available (Rotherham-Boris et al. 2011).

Essential support services for primary caregivers, who in the majority world are not necessarily parents, are listed below:

1. Caregivers have access to parenting education antenatally and thereafter. This includes (a) advice regarding smoking, alcohol and drug use, child neglect, and the dietary requirements of infants and (b) basic information on topics such as provision of affectional care and non-violent discipline, neonatal development, nutrition, health and safety (e.g., WHO Key Family Practices), injury prevention, developmental

milestones, stimulation of literacy, motor development and cognition, and social service access.

2. Caregivers identified as at high risk for mental health problems are provided with basic psychosocial support. South African examples include the Perinatal Mental Health Project[8] and the Philani Mother Mentor Project.[9]

3. Caregivers who work or for other reasons are unable to care for their children have access to childcare services that are monitored and subsidized.

Stimulation for Early Learning

Children whose early years are spent under impoverished conditions tend to be disadvantaged by inadequate preparation for the demands of schooling. This is a key contributor to poor scholastic outcomes and the negative consequences that follow. Evidence from across the world, including low-income countries, demonstrates that access to early learning stimulation in the preschool years significantly enhances the ability of children from impoverished backgrounds to benefit from schooling; it reduces the likelihood that they will drop out and increases the probability that they will be employed as adults (Nores and Barnett 2010). As in all other forms of intervention, the quality of early learning service provision is crucial. To make an impact, they need to be taken to scale in the most vulnerable populations. In low- and middle-income countries, preschools are not necessarily the answer, as they may be inaccessible to the majority of children. In South Africa, for example, only 20% of the poorest 40% of children attend. Thus other forms of early learning opportunity may be required (Richter et al. 2012).

Interventions to support early learning may be delivered through a number of channels. Examples include playgroups and home visiting programs (including group-based learning and support for parents) through which the abilities of caregivers to support early learning are enhanced (Grantham-McGregor et al. 1991a; Kagitcibasi et al. 2009).

In all cases, the use of evidence-based program and *quality assurance* is essential (but challenging). State subsidies (as is the case in South Africa) ensure greater participation and access to food provided as part of the daily program (Richter et al. 2012).

The Ilifa Package recommends that poor children have access to one of the following early learning programs:

---

[8] See www.pmhp.za.org (accessed June 14, 2014).

[9] See http://www.ilifalabantwana.co.za/2013/09/30/mentor-mothers-a-sustainable-paraprofessional-model/ (accessed June 14, 2014).

1. Children under three years: a free home visiting intervention in which stimulation for early learning is provided, preferably through inputs to both caregiver and child (Engel et al. 2007).
2. Children three to five years: a free or subsidized center-based program or a free weekly quality playgroup, with activities oriented toward readiness to learn in school (e.g., Dawes et al. 2012).
3. Toy and book libraries (including mobile services) that provide learning resources for children zero to five years in poor communities.

Conclusion

The status of early child development fundamentally reflects the social success of societies, both currently and in the future (Irwin et al. 2007). Irwin et al. argue that the extent to which a country is able to provide opportunities for optimal child development is the degree to which the well-being of its most susceptible and powerless members is upheld and supported.

The Essential Package of services and support to caregivers and children living in poverty described in this chapter draws on contemporary evidence and is designed to enhance South Africa's efforts to improve the well-being and development of its youngest children and their caregivers. While we await the results of evaluations, there is enough evidence to indicate that the delivery of a package that covers maternal and child health, nutrition, psychosocial support, social protection, and stimulation for early learning has the potential to mitigate the impact of poverty environments on children and their primary caregivers, and to promote sound developmental outcomes. This potential, however, will only be realized if the package components reach those for whom it is designed, are appropriately resourced, closely monitored, effectively delivered, and regularly reviewed.

The Essential Package of services presented here need not be specific to the South African context, but is offered as an approach that may be applicable in other countries affected by structural violence and poverty. By reducing risk and supporting sound development in all of its aspects, such a package has the potential to set the scene for *probabilistic* developmental trajectories that result in productive, peaceful citizens. However, access to a package of this nature will not guarantee the production of future generations of prosocial citizens committed to peace. This is because new risks and promotive opportunities impact children during other periods beyond the early years. These may build on or disrupt what has gone before.

In conclusion, in the absence of radical social change, structural violence will, to a greater or lesser degree, always be with us. While we work toward reducing inequality and convincing those in power as to its negative impact on societal well-being and its role in the generation of conflict, it is necessary to strive for effective interventions that protect the youngest and most vulnerable from its corrosive impact. This means that we must work to convince states to choose to allocate the necessary funds (or to seek the aid) required to provide the necessary services and support.

We suggest that one of our most important levers in this endeavor is the United Nations Convention on the Rights of the Child, which all the world with a few notable exceptions (e.g., the United States), has ratified. The Convention commits nations to act in the best interests of their children, and they can be held to account when they do not do so. It is critical, therefore, to incorporate a rights discourse in our arguments for formative childhoods as we endeavor to delineate a path toward building a more peaceful world.

We conclude with a summary of points that need to be addressed in future research:

1. Evaluate effectiveness and cost delivery of each component in the Essential Package when delivered at scale (reaching at least 90% children in the target community).
2. Develop culturally appropriate methods for screening the mental health of pregnant women (these are currently dominated by Western techniques).
3. Test and cost the effectiveness of culturally appropriate parenting programs delivered by community-based paraprofessionals to improve affectional caregiver care and reduce risk of harsh punishment particularly during the first 36 months of life.
4. Conduct follow-up studies to determine the extent to which children whose caregivers received a parenting program show reduced externalizing behavior at ages five and ten years, when compared to those from the same backgrounds who did not received the Package.
5. Develop effective models for changing dysfunctional systems of the Essential Package service delivery in state and nonprofit sectors.

14

Promoting the Capacity for Peace in Early Childhood

Perspectives from Research on Resilience in Children and Families

Ann S. Masten

Abstract

Lessons gleaned from five decades of research on resilience in children and youth exposed to trauma and adversity of many kinds, including war and family violence, may have important conceptual and practical implications for efforts to understand and promote pathways of peace in human adaptation and development. This chapter highlights concepts, approaches, findings, and controversies from studies of resilience that may prove informative for understanding and promoting pathways to peace in early childhood. These include a relational developmental systems perspective on peace; an emphasis on positive goals, processes, and pathways; issues in defining how well human systems at multiple levels are doing; delineation of adaptive systems that promote and protect peaceful function in interacting human systems; consideration of developmental timing and cascading influences among individual children and their nurturing environments; and the importance of intervention evidence for advancing a translational science agenda for peace. Resilience science also suggests that delineating processes of peace and peacebuilding in childhood requires attention to processes by which interacting systems shape the development and experiences of childhood pertinent to peace, particularly in the nurturing environments of childrearing and early education.

Resilience frameworks suggest three basic approaches to promoting capacity for peace in the lives of children: mitigating risk or preventing exposure to experiences that undermine capacity for peace; boosting resources and opportunities that nurture the capacity for peace; and mobilizing powerful adaptive systems that support and protect human capabilities for peace in hazardous circumstances. Theoretically, these strategies should contribute to building capacity among children for peace, as a foundation for learning peaceful means of social interactions, managing conflict, and responding to stress or trauma. Additionally, resilience frameworks emphasize the importance of strategic timing and targeting to interrupt negative and facilitate positive cascades in development and boost the return on investments in children. Findings from research on early onset pathways toward and away from violence are discussed, including preventive interventions that promote prosocial development while also reducing antisocial outcomes, including violence.

Key questions are raised for consideration by those aiming to promote peace through early childhood policies and practices. The first set of questions stems from the principle that "competence begets competence" in human development, asking whether building success in the developmental tasks of early childhood might also promote potential peace-related goals, attitudes, skills and processes in children and their ecologies, which could in turn contribute to peace at the level of families, communities, or societies. The second set considers whether reducing structural violence (i.e., inequalities in income, healthcare, education, and opportunities in early childhood) might promote peace along with better health and well-being at the level of individuals and societies. A third set raises provocative issues related to possibilities that capacities and skills intended to promote peace could also be applied to promote conflict and war and questions about whether violence can be adaptive or peace-promoting under some circumstances.

Introduction

Millions of children worldwide grow up in environments characterized by danger and scarcity of resources, often in combination (Masten 2013, 2014a; Lundberg and Wuermli 2012; Britto et al. 2013). Harsh or hazardous rearing circumstances and persistent poverty pose risks not only to child development, but also to the future economic, social, and political health of societies. Extreme deprivation, family violence, dangerous neighborhoods, and exposures to severe and persistent trauma or chaos of many kinds are associated with high risk for conduct problems and violence in childhood, adolescence, and beyond, as well as the risk for intergenerational transmission of vulnerabilities or problems related to conflict in relationships and communities (e.g., Dodge et al. 2008; Evans and Kim 2012; Loeber and Farrington 1998, 2012; Lösel and Farrington 2012; Masten and Narayan 2012). Conflict and violence show learning and "contagion effects" in children who experience violence, observe it in trusted adults, are coerced to perpetrate violence, or get involved in peer friendships and larger peer groups that encourage violence (Dishion and Tipscord 2011; Bushman and Newman 2013).

Yet many children who grow up under very challenging conditions or who experience appalling violence do not become violent, do not perpetuate it, or escape from a life of delinquency or interpersonal violence to become healthy adults contributing to their communities and raising children who are loving and getting along well in society (Cicchetti 2013a; Masten 2013, 2014a, b). Scientists and societies share an interest in such individuals (as well as their families and cultures) because they may offer clues to the processes that have the potential to promote peace-oriented human interactions and to prevent or mitigate risk for violence and its spreading effects over the life course or across groups and societies. In this chapter, I consider lessons for peacebuilding in early childhood that might be drawn from research on risk and resilience among children in contexts of extreme poverty, violence or war, and disaster.

Why would resilience theory and data be relevant to peacebuilding and the interrelated goal of reducing conflict and violent resolutions to conflict through interventions in childhood? There are multiple reasons. First, human resilience science is the study of processes involved in positive adaptation and development in the context of risks and threats to human function and development (Masten 2013, 2014a, b). Many of the situations studied in this literature are related to peace, directly or indirectly, including the study of individuals who experience violence in the family or in war zones yet become prosocial, loving adults and parents. Moreover, numerous studies in resilience science are focused on preventing or reducing violence and antisocial behaviors, with potential lessons for efforts to address violence in the context of promoting peace.

Second, focusing on peace or peacefulness as a goal in human interactions can be viewed as a specific subset of positive adaptation and development in human systems—one that is highly related to domains of competence at the individual and family[1] level that are targeted in many studies of resilience. These include, for example, caring relationships, learning, and prosocial behavior in individuals and families (Masten 2007; Masten and Monn 2014). In other words, there is conceptual overlap in the criteria by which "resilience" and "peacefulness" of a given person or group may be judged.

Third, and relatedly, peace and positive adaptation at multiple levels may be influenced by overlapping promotive and protective processes. Additionally, common foundational processes may be involved in meeting the developmental tasks shared by many families and communities around the world, and in achieving peaceful relationships and nonviolent conflict resolution in interpersonal and societal relationships. Individual or collective self-regulation and problem-solving skills in a child, family, or community may contribute to harmonious relationships and conflict resolution that serve "good outcomes," as defined by seekers of peace and social justice, as well as interventions or policies to promote healthy child and family development.

There are convergent findings in research on early risk factors for later violence and conduct problems and research on interventions which promote developmental competence in children or reduce the risk for later antisocial behavior. Theory and empirical findings on antecedents and prevention of violence in children and youth, along with research on building resilience in children at risk for violence and related problems, suggest key strategies for laying a foundation in early childhood for peace (or at least the tools to learn peaceful ways of living):

---

[1]   Note: the term "family" is used to describe a group of people bound together by kinship, roles in caring for each other, cultural traditions, or close affiliation.

1. Protect brain development.
2. Prevent exposure to cumulative trauma and violence in the family, community, and media.
3. Support positive attachment bonds with caregivers.
4. Protect family function.
5. Promote self-regulation capabilities.
6. Foster prosocial skills.

At the same time, it seems clear that foundational tools in early childhood are insufficient to yield a lifetime of peaceful behavior or prevent violent conflict resolution, because they could potentially be utilized at a later period of development in ways counterproductive to peace in peer groups, classrooms, neighborhoods, or larger macrosystem contexts.

Fourth, there are common issues faced by scientists and policy makers who aim to promote resilience or peace. These include issues of defining "peace" and "resilience" in dynamic interacting systems and the problem of adaptive human skills and tools being directed at goals at odds with peace or healthy development.

In this chapter, I consider how the literature on resilience in children may be helpful to scientists, practitioners, and policy makers who seek to understand and promote peace in human development. I begin with a discussion of the conceptual parallels between "peace" and "resilience" in developmental science before considering lessons from resilience science focused on mass trauma. Research on pathways and prevention of violence are discussed, followed by a description of a resilience framework for peacebuilding. A set of provocative issues from the resilience literature are raised that may likely confront those aiming to promote peace, and directions for the future will be highlighted.

Conceptual Parallels in Defining Peace and Resilience

Peace, like resilience, is a complex concept with multiple meanings, ranging from a state-of-mind to nonviolent conflict resolution between individuals or nations, or to social justice. It can be construed as a disposition, process, outcome, or a culture (Leckman et al., this volume). It can be defined in negative terms (e.g., "not at war" or "nonviolent conflict resolution") or in positive terms ("harmonious interactions" or "calm"). The concept of resilience in human development also has multiple meanings, although all of them are related to adaptation in the context of adversity; human resilience has been defined as a trait, a process, or an outcome (Masten 2011, 2014a, b).

Over the decades, definitions of resilience have become more dynamic, reflecting a broad transformation of developmental science toward systems theory. In relational developmental systems theory, development and adaptation emerge from the interaction of many systems within and between individuals, social groups, and the physical environment. From this perspective, "resilience" refers to the capacity for adapting successfully to disturbances that threaten the viability, function, or development of a system (Masten 2011, 2014a, b). Living human systems are continually interacting with many other systems, including other living systems, the physical world, and technological systems, such as computers and software systems. Good adaptation in individual human lives can be defined by achieving success in expected domains of behavior for a given period of development, culture, and time in history (called developmental task domains). However, resilience can also be defined by negative criteria, such as avoiding mental health problems despite exposure to severe neglect or maltreatment.

Resilience is manifested in the presence of a disturbance; if the system has not experienced a significant threat, then the capacity to adapt may be assumed but is not clearly established. The capacity for resilience in an individual arises from the interaction of many adaptive systems within a person and in their environment, including the family. Moreover, because all these systems are constantly changing, resilience is dynamic. The capacity to adapt can be depleted by overloading of stress, exhaustion, or aging. Individual resilience can also be promoted by development, learning, better nutrition, sleep, better parenting, school, or social support, and many other changes at multiple levels. These changes can arise from any level, with cascading consequences across levels.

Because resilience reflects dynamic processes that link many systems, it is not a "trait" of an individual system at any level. Individuals have the capacity for adaptation to disturbances impinging on them because of the resources and capabilities available to them at any given time; however, the manifestation of resilience emerges through many interactions and processes. The resilience of children often depends on the resilience of families, which in turn depends on the resilience of their communities. The capacity for adapting to challenges at a given time, potentially drawing on any available human or social capital, economic resources, or other forms of help, comprises resilience; however, this capacity is distributed among interdependent systems and is not an attribute of a single system. Thus individual resilience is better viewed as a set of changing capabilities and resources that arise from the interplay of many systems available to the individual and not as a single trait. Debates about the meaning of peace also likely reflect the dynamic reality of interacting systems involving many processes over time.

Defining resilience always involves two components: some kind of risk or threat and indicators of positive adaptation (Luthar et al. 2000; Masten 2001). These "two judgments" reflect evaluations of how well a system is functioning during or following a significant disturbance or threat to system function or viability. In human developmental science focused on individuals, good adaptation is often defined in relation to *developmental tasks,* which refer to the expected achievements of individuals at different periods of development, defined in the context of culture and history as well as developmental perspectives (McCormick et al. 2011).

Similarly, family resilience can be defined in terms of threats to family function and the expected functions of families in a particular culture or period of history (Masten and Monn 2014). Families have life cycles with changing roles as they form and develop (Goldenberg and Goldenberg 2013). In most cultures, families with young children are expected, for example, to care for and protect their children, support them economically, and socialize them for appropriate roles in their society. Families may be judged by how well children in the family are doing as well as according to their fulfillment of other expected functions. Family function can be challenged by adversity, and stress on a family system can disrupt the quality of parenting in many different ways (Walsh 2006).

The criteria by which good adaptation in individuals is judged in resilience science are typically multidimensional, varying with development and culture. In the Project Competence Longitudinal Study, for example, criteria for competence in childhood include the developmental tasks of academic achievement, getting along with other children, and rule-abiding conduct (Masten and Tellegen 2012). As children grow older, criteria change to reflect later developmental tasks, such as work or parenting success. In some studies, negative criteria have been utilized to define adaptation, such as whether or not war survivors have posttraumatic symptoms or mental health problems (Masten et al. 2014). A purely negative definition of doing well in life, however, has serious limitations, including the observation that parents, young people, communities, and other stakeholders rarely define their goals for children or self in life in terms of avoiding negative outcomes.

Peace, similarly, can be defined in multidimensional ways, by negative as well as positive criteria, as is evident in this volume. Leckman et al. (this volume) delineate four elements for peace, each with negative and positive meanings. Moreover, it seems unlikely that a definition of peace signified by the avoidance of violence or war alone, at any level (from the individual to national or international system levels), would be satisfactory to those hoping for harmonious relations and social justice among people and political entities.

Resilience involves more than simply doing well in life. At the individual (or family) level, resilience implies the potential or demonstrated capability for responding effectively to significant challenges. Some investigators require resilience to be manifested in the presence or aftermath of such challenges, whereas others acknowledge that humans often assume the capacity for adaptation from observing the presence of well-functioning adaptive systems known on the basis of evidence to facilitate resilience in the presence of disturbances. In either case, it is conceivable that a child who is developing well in low-risk conditions may not have the capacity to adapt under extremely hazardous conditions. Moreover, it is widely assumed that some exposure to stress (system disturbance) is important for developing the capacities for good adaptation in the presence of adversity, sometimes called "steeling effects" or "stress inoculation" (Masten 2014b; Rutter 2012). In other words, some adaptive systems may require a degree of challenge in order to calibrate appropriately to the expected environment (Ellis and Del Guidice 2014).

In the context of "peacebuilding," I would argue that peace implies more than simply harmonious relationships or a tranquil state of mind. Concepts of peace, peaceful relationships, or states of mind suggest the capacity or demonstrated capabilities for effectively resolving conflicts (disturbances to peace or peacefulness) without resorting to violence and war. As with resilience, it might be argued that the adaptive skills and capabilities for peace develop in children (or communities or nations) and similarly may require some exposure to challenges (e.g., conflicts) that train the individual (or community or nation) to manage conflicts.

One of the primary goals of resilience studies in children has been to identify the promotive and protective processes or experiences that foster resilience. Initially, in the first wave of resilience science, these factors were identified as predictors of good adaptation (by specified criteria) among children who experienced adversity (Masten 2007). Subsequently, in the second wave, research has focused on understanding protective processes (i.e., how these factors worked to promote resilience). The third wave focused on testing these processes using experiments that promote good adaptation among children at risk for problems related to adverse childhood experiences. Currently, there is growing interest in delineating how adaptive systems work across multiple levels of analysis, from molecular to social and ecological levels, as interdependent systems. Integrated multiple-systems approaches characterize the fourth wave of resilience science (Masten 2007, 2014b).

Over the years, investigators have noted a striking consistency across diverse studies in the factors associated with resilience, suggesting that there are fundamental adaptive systems that play a substantial role in resilience (see Masten 2001, 2007, 2014b). These include internal adaptive systems, the processes underlying cognitive skills, motivation, and self-regulation capabilities as well as relational adaptive systems, such as close relationships with competent and caring adults and well-functioning families. Effective school systems and community support systems have also been implicated in resilience science, and in recent work, the roles of cultural adaptive systems, long neglected, have been given much more attention (see Ungar et al. 2013).

Resilience scientists have noted that the tools we encourage children to develop for learning (e.g., social success, prosocial behavior, and other aspects of success in life) could be co-opted or "hijacked" later in development by various combinations of unmet needs, negative role models, lack of opportunities, recruitment into antisocial causes that are highly rewarding, and other incentives (Masten 2014b). In other words, the skills that contribute to positive adaptation or development could potentially be applied toward other goals that parents or a society might not approve. For example, gang leaders can be persuasive in recruiting able young people in a context of injustice and limited mainstream opportunities. Children can also be forced into violence, for example, when they are kidnapped to be a child soldier or threatened with death unless they join a gang. Having the capabilities for positive adaptation does not mean that the skills will be applied for goals that various stakeholders would approve.

In addition, resilience investigators recognize that there are multiple pathways to positive adaptation and development, reflecting the myriad influences that shape and threaten development and the importance of context and timing (Masten 2014b; Masten and Narayan 2012). There is no single pathway to resilience. Similarly, there are likely to be many pathways to peace and ways of peacebuilding. Concomitantly, there are multiple pathways to violence and engagement in conflict, and some of the key influences on these pathways may emerge after early childhood.

Mass Trauma and Resilience

The systematic study of resilience emerged in the aftermath of World War II, when global attention was directed toward the plight of and cost to children as a result of the war (Masten 2013, 2014a; Masten et al. 2014; Werner 2000). Millions of children died, but many survived great peril. Huge numbers of children around the world were orphaned, displaced, raped, starved, and forced to suffer the consequences of horrific injuries or trauma. In this setting, the United Nations Children's Emergency Fund (UNICEF) was founded, as was CARE in the United States, now international and renamed the "Cooperative for Assistance and Relief Everywhere." These organizations and many others mobilized to aid war-affected children, especially in Europe. Clinicians were called on during and after the war to help child survivors who were exposed to unspeakable atrocities and loss. Some research was conducted on the effects of trauma on children during and after the war, but strong designs were not usually feasible. Nonetheless, observers noted that children fared much better when they experienced danger and war in close proximity to their caregivers. They also noticed individual differences and recovery patterns.

The consequences of exposure to mass trauma experiences, in war or disaster, held great interest and importance for the early resilience researchers (e.g., Garmezy 1983) because these events exposed large numbers of children to adversity and clearly called for efforts to mitigate risk and promote recovery. War and disaster exact a toll of mass destruction on the lives of children and highlight the interdependence of children, families, and other systems (Masten and Narayan 2012; Masten et al. 2014). Children did not fare well when families were gravely affected or when they were separated from family. Families did not fare well when community and national systems collapsed.

Violence enters the family system in regions experiencing prolonged conflict. In Belfast, Ireland, political violence in the community appeared to affect children indirectly through effects on family function, such as increased marital conflict (Cummings et al. 2012). Research by Boxer et al. (2013) in the Middle East, discussed further below, suggests that political violence at the macro level cascades across system levels to affect youth microsystems, such as families and schools, which in turn contribute to increasing aggression in young people. These findings in conflicted regions are congruent with other research on macro-level effects of stress on families that alters family function to effect children in the family (Masten and Monn 2014). Family stress theory was proposed to explain the processes by which economic stress alters family and child function (e.g., Conger et al. 2010; Elder 1974/1999). Similar processes may unfold in situations of inequality (structural violence), although in a more insidious and less acute form (see Dawes and van der Merwe, this volume).

Over time it also became clear that a given exposure to traumatic violence in the context of war, political conflict, or disaster had worse effects on children when they were experienced in a context where adversity already had occurred or was ongoing before and after the acute exposure. For example, Israeli adolescents exposed to political conflict had more posttraumatic stress disorder symptoms, substance use, and violence perpetration if they had been maltreated in childhood (Schiff et al. 2012). In Sri Lanka, the 2004 tsunami was associated with worse outcomes for children who had been living in the war zones of Sri Lanka (Catani et al. 2010). The combination of war-related violence and exposure to family violence appears to be particularly problematic for children and youth (Masten et al. 2014; Panter-Brick and Leckman 2013). Cumulative risk matters, there may be sensitization effects, and the quality of the recovery context is important (Masten and Narayan 2012; Masten et al. 2014).

Research on risk and resilience in extreme political violence, both war and prolonged conflicts, has highlighted issues related to the *engagement* of children and youth in warfare (Barber 2009a, 2013). Some young people participate voluntarily whereas others are kidnapped to be child soldiers and forced to kill or maim others. Research on these young people has underscored the complexity of these situations and the importance of understanding the historical and sociocultural context in relation to individual youth, the meaning of conflict, and their engagement.

There is a distinctive literature on young people engaged in ethnopolitical conflicts, such as the Palestinian-Israeli conflict (Barber 2009a, 2013; Cummings et al. 2012; Dimitry 2012). Some of the findings are provocative. For example, youth in these conflicts sometimes gain a sense of identity and agency through their engagement, despite the dangers of participation (Barber 2009b, 2013). One study found that the functioning of young Palestinians was better at extremely high levels of exposure to political violence (compared to lower levels of exposure), which led to the suggestion that in extreme situations, youth may be inspired to greater involvement and heroism (Qouta et al. 2008a). During recovery in child soldiers of Mozambique, Boothby et al. (2006) found differences that were dependent on time in captivity. Boys who had spent six months or less in captivity viewed themselves as victims, whereas boys who spent a year or longer as child soldiers viewed themselves as *members* of the army. The latter made comments like the following (Boothby et al. 2006:244): "I could have escaped but I didn't because I had a good position." "I first served as his personal servant. Then he made me chief of a group of other boys. I had power."

Evidence is limited on the cross-level effects of violence, moving upward or downward in level, from the neurobiological levels to behavioral to social to family or intergroup function to community or cultural or societal. A recent and rare longitudinal study of cascading effects across ecological levels tested a model grounded in Bronfenbrenner's ecological theory (Bronfenbrenner and Morris 2006), employing a cohort sequential design. Boxer et al. (2013) demonstrated a top-down cascade of violence from the macro (political) to the micro (family, school, community) to the individual level. Based on structural equation modeling of data from three waves for three ages of Palestinian and Israeli youth (initially ages 8, 11, and 14), violence at the political level predicted violence at the community, school, and family levels, which predicted increases in individual violence. This study serves as a reminder that violence may cascade or spread across human systems from the "top down," the "bottom up," or both. Thus, it may be crucial to identify the best level or levels of intervention for impacting change.

For some time, there has been concern about the possibility of long-term and spreading effects of mass trauma experiences on development, over the life span as well as across generations (La Greca et al. 2010; Masten and Narayan 2012; Masten et al. 2014). Longitudinal data have hinted at long-term sequelae of early trauma experiences, and recent research on epigenetic transmission of trauma effects has opened a new dialog on the processes by which such transmission might occur. Yehuda and colleagues, for example, have studied prenatal exposure to war and terrorism, and suggest that long-term alterations in stress-regulation systems (congruent with recent models of gene expression for glucocorticoid and related genes) may be associated with lifelong health issues and intergenerational vulnerability or risk for posttraumatic stress disorder (e.g., Yehuda and Bierer 2009; Yehuda et al. 2005). There is growing interest in the possibility that long-term effects of early exposure to trauma or violence could be interrupted, for example, by *reprogramming* adaptive systems that have gone awry through various means, including therapy or reopening windows of plasticity in brain development in a context of positive opportunities or directly intervening to promote specific epigenetic changes (Karatoreos and McEwen 2013; Masten 2014a, b; Panter-Brick and Leckman 2013).

Research on rehabilitation of child soldiers and interventions for children affected by war is limited in quantity and quality, although it is improving (Betancourt et al. 2013a, b; Boothby et al. 2006; Masten and Narayan 2012;

Masten et al. 2014; Peltonen and **Punamäki 2010**). Little is known about the potential of media and social networking for prevention and intervention in the context of mass violence. However, promising strategies have focused on social support, cultural practices, and opportunities for education and work. Restoring family or sociocultural routines and practices appears to be fruitful. Betancourt et al. (2013b) are now following former child soldiers from Sierra Leone as they form their own families, to learn more about the long-term patterns of their lives, especially as they parent the next generation.

Early Pathways to Violence and Prevention Research

Research on the antecedents to antisocial behavior and violence has implicated early experiences of poor parenting and family violence as risk factors for later conduct problems (Farrington et al. 2012; Loeber and Farrington 1998; Lösel and Farrington 2012; Van Horn and Lieberman 2012). Early child behaviors associated with these family problems include poor self-regulation skills and noncompliant behavior, which appear to set the stage for early problems in the school context with learning and social relationships. Early problems of aggression and self-control emerging in the family and early school contexts appear to spread over time or to result in problems in other contexts and domains, with elevated risks for antisocial behavior and violence (Dodge et al. 2008; Masten and Cicchetti 2010; Moffitt et al. 2011; Shaw and Gross 2008). Basic research on child maltreatment indicates an elevated risk for difficulties in attachment relationships, self-regulation, and later externalizing behaviors (Cicchetti 2010, 2013). Generally, the evidence on early onset "pathways" toward antisocial behavior and various conduct problems has led numerous prevention scientists toward early intervention, with the expectation that early development is a window of opportunity for high return on investment (Heckman 2006; Masten et al. 2009; Reynolds et al. 2010).

International data on 24 countries drawn from UNICEF's Multiple Indicator Cluster Survey of developing nations provides interesting findings. Results suggest associations between physical violence (and nonviolence), as used in parenting practices and discipline for two- to four-year-old children, and country-level indicators of life expectancy, educational attainment, and economic well-being (Lansford and Deater-Deckard 2012). As observed in numerous other studies, harsh discipline carried out by caregivers was related to lower level of education. Causes for these observed linkages are undoubtedly complex, potentially reflecting interactions of parent, child, and country parameters at multiple levels in the context of developmental, cultural, and historical changes. Processes may involve cultural norms and attitudes toward parenting and physical punishment, socialization practices, and the role of verbal capabilities in self-control. Lansford and Deater-Deckard (2012) suggest that parental values and knowledge about effective discipline and parenting may shift as they acquire more education, perhaps leading to reductions in violence along with improvements in child competence and later achievements, although these causal pathways remain speculative. Growing evidence also suggests that cumulative exposure to poverty and violence may take a toll on multiple domains of health and well-being in development, including the capacities that support learning and later parenting (Shonkoff et al. 2012).

Prevention research aimed specifically at reducing risk for later misconduct or violence has increasingly turned toward early intervention strategies focused on improving parenting or parent-child bonds to prevent maltreatment, improve child compliance, and boost child self-regulation skills (Cicchetti 2013; Piquero et al. 2009; Sandler et al. 2011). Among the better-validated interventions with effects on later antisocial behavior are the Nurse-Family Partnership pioneered by David Olds and colleagues (Olds 2006), parent training methods developed by the Oregon Social Learning Center (Patterson et al. 2010), and the Family Check-up (Dishion et al. 2008; Shaw et al. 2006). In early interventions specifically developed to reduce child maltreatment, the focus has been on improving the quality of attachment relationships and caregiving as well as specifically on fostering sensitivity in the caregiver (Chaffin et al. 2004; Lieberman and Van Horn 2011a; Thomas and Zimmer-Gembeck 2011; Toth and Gravener 2012). Findings from this body of work corroborate, through intervention experiments, the basic research findings that implicate a causal role of parenting quality in early pathways toward conduct problems and violence.

Recent studies also suggest that early exposure to what is now often referred to as "toxic stress" (prenatal or postnatal) may create vulnerabilities in children that compound the problems of later exposure to family, peer, or community violence (Shonkoff et al. 2012). Stress-regulation systems may be altered by maternal exposure to trauma during pregnancy or early postnatal experiences of children to maltreatment or neglect (Cicchetti 2013; Gunnar and Herrera 2013). Repeated exposure to stress hormones can be harmful to the developing brain, damaging the neural systems that support the development of self-control and learning. Some children may be more genetically sensitive to these exposure effects while others may develop greater "sensitivity to context" as a result of adversity experiences (Belsky et al. 2007; Boyce 2007; Ellis and Del Guidice 2014; Obradović and Boyce 2012). In some children, stress systems may downregulate in response to sustained adversity, resulting in insensitivity to stress, which can protect the brain from excessive exposure to stress hormones and related damage but interferes with efficient stress regulation (Gunnar and Herrera 2013).

Interventions that focus on quality early child care or education, particularly those with effective parent engagement, appear to reduce the risk for later antisocial behavior (e.g., Reynolds et al. 2011; O'Connell et al. 2009). These interventions may work in multiple ways to reduce risk for antisocial behavior and/or promote prosocial conduct. In addition, they may simultaneously support better parenting, reduce family stress, provide positive adult and peer role models, and foster the development of self-regulation and other learning skills in children.

Conclusions from the prevention literature suggest that the prevention of problems and the promotion of healthy child development depend largely on the improvement in the quality of *nurturing environments* (Biglan et al. 2012). Based on prevention science, Biglan et al. (2012) summarized the characteristics of nurturing environments as follows: Nurturing environments minimize toxic experiences; they promote prosocial behavior and other aspects of competence needed for a productive adulthood in society; they monitor and limit opportunities for negative or problematic behavior and foster mindful psychological flexibility. They argue further that families and schools are the highest priority targets for fostering nurturing environments.

A Resilience Framework for Promoting Peace

A resilience framework may be useful when conceptualizing methods and issues related to the question: What kinds of early childhood interventions and investments may have the potential for promoting peace? This question can be addressed from several different perspectives.

First, it is important to note that this question is posed in a positive way. Promoting peace may not be the same task as reducing violence or conflict, although risk reduction is an important element of translational resilience science. Lowering the risk of violent conflicts at individual, family, community, cultural, or national levels may well play a role in promoting peace. Similarly, reducing exposure to stressors that have damaging effects on development of tools for self-regulation or problem solving may also have indirect benefits for peaceful conflict resolution and problem solving that averts violent conflict. However, peacebuilding may also involve processes orthogonal to or somewhat independent of violence-focused risk reduction. A recovering child soldier, for example, may be "prevented" or diverted from engaging in violence in various ways when he or she returns to the community; however, this differs from efforts that would help the same youth meet developmental task expectations of the community to form a family, rear respectful children, work, or contribute in other ways to the good of the family or community.

Resilience frameworks focus on pathways *toward* the desired outcomes (e.g., children who are equipped to learn peaceful ways or are "peace prone") in addition to pathways *away* from the undesired outcomes (e.g., children who are vulnerable to violence or are "conflict prone"). At the same time, resilience perspectives recognize that there will be many pathways away from the same starting point to different outcomes (multifinality) and to the same outcomes from different starting points (equifinality) (Cicchetti and Rogosch 1996). Multiple pathways result from the many interacting influences across levels of function (e.g., molecular, neural, behavioral, contextual) that shape the life course (Overton 2013). There are many paths toward peace-oriented children and many paths toward and away from violence and conflict. Experimentally induced pathways toward desired goals hold particular value in resilience research because such examples inform theory as well as practice (Panter-Brick and Leckman 2013).

A resilience-based approach suggests three primary strategies for promoting desirable (to a community or society) outcomes in children at risk for developing problems (of health, behavior, or well-being) due to extremely adverse childhood experiences (Masten 2011):

1. Prevent or reduce risk exposure.
2. Boost resources (increase assets or promotive factors) that facilitate desired outcomes (these work at any level of risk).
3. Mobilize or nurture protective systems, such as relationships with caring adults or mentors and cultural practices, that foster the desired outcomes or reduce the impacts of hazardous experiences (i.e., play a special role in the context of high adversity or risk exposure).

This framework could prove useful in delineating strategies to promote peace in the context of direct or structural violence (Dawes and van der Merwe, this volume; Christie et al., this volume). This approach requires a delineation of goals (the nature of the "desired outcome") at multiple levels (e.g., individual, family, school, community, cultural, national). In addition, it is important to build a knowledge base on how the desired outcomes at one or more levels are linked to risks, resources, or protective systems that are preventable, promotable, and/or malleable. In situations where children are exposed to direct violence, this framework suggests intervention approaches would be implemented to (a) reduce violence or exposure to violence; (b) increase resources or access to resources that promote peace or peaceful outcomes (or the capacities that support these outcomes); and (c) mobilize or nurture adaptive systems that protect child development or foster the capacity for peaceful behavior in the context of violence exposure.

In the context of structural violence, this framework suggests that interventions aim:

1. to reduce inequality and exposure to developmental risks and adversities related to inequality,
2. to build resources and access to essential assets for healthy child development, and
3. to nurture and support systems that protect positive development in the context of structural violence (until inequality can be addressed).

This perspective is congruent with recommendations by Dawes and van der Merwe (this volume). In either context of violence (direct or structural), examples of strategies to promote the capacity for peace in children might include the following: protect healthy brain development and self-regulation skills through a reduction of toxic stress exposure; increase food security and access to medical care; and foster effective parenting and child learning through supports to families and access to quality early childhood education.

A resilience approach to intervention also emphasizes windows of opportunity for change and multiple levels of consideration for intervention (Cicchetti 2013; Masten 2011; Panter-Brick and Leckman 2013; Wachs and Rahman 2013). To leverage the desired change most effectively, interventions can be strategically planned and targeted to (a) the right time in development, (b) individual differences, (c) contextual differences, or (d) system level. Well-timed, targeted interventions have the potential to interrupt negative impacts, thereby instigating positive effects that will cascade over time to yield high ratios of benefit to cost. Evidence on risk and resilience pertinent to violence suggests several early windows of opportunity: a prenatal window (e.g., the mitigation of prenatal exposures to stress), an early childhood window (e.g., for early promotion of secure attachment bonds with parents and prevention of child abuse), and an early childhood education window (e.g., promoting self-regulation and socialized conduct).

Resilience models encourage consideration of multiple levels of intervention and target processes that link levels, such as intergenerational programs aimed at child and parent or family. Sometimes the potential for change may be optimized at the level of schools or peer interaction (e.g., to prevent bullying or reduce intergroup conflict), whereas at other times this may occur in the family (e.g., to promote early attachment bonds or compliance). Some situations (e.g., major disasters) require intervention across multiple levels simultaneously to address emergency needs for food, water, shelter, and rescue or medical care as well as subsequent needs for restoring electricity, reuniting families, and restoring normal community routines or school.

As fundamentally observed in resilience science, the capacity for resilience is distributed across interacting systems (Masten 2014a, b). Similarly, the capacity for peace is distributed across individuals, families, classroom, communities, and many other levels of culture, media, and society. Concepts of *peace* or *peacefulness*, like the concept of resilience, can be applied to many systems and levels. To achieve peace at the level of regions or nations, we must understand how these levels are interrelated.

In the case of achieving peace (or building a capacity for peace) through early childhood policies and programs, considerable work lies ahead to build a conceptual framework, methods, and knowledge base. The contributions from this Forum reflect a broad consideration of the processes, disciplines, sectors, and levels of analysis that might be involved in this effort, ranging from research on brain development and the promotion of empathy to peace education.

In resilience science, more is often known about defining and measuring the processes that lead to an undesired outcome (e.g., violence or conflict) than the desired outcome itself (e.g., peace or peaceful conflict resolution). It is important to build the positive case but nonetheless valuable to consider options built on a good understanding of the processes leading to war, political conflict, or interpersonal violence. Considerable literature exists on the pathways to violence at various levels of analysis (neurobiological, behavioral, social, intergroup, ethnic, or political) regarding children at risk for violence due to maltreatment or exposure to family or community violence.

Competence Begets Competence but Does It Promote Peace?

Evidence on the predictive significance of success in early developmental task accomplishments for later competence in academic achievement, peer relations, and adult work provides a substantial data base of basic and intervention findings to support the idea that competence begets competence while also lowering risk for future problems, including antisocial behavior (Heckman 2006; Masten 2013). The positive, forward cascade of competence observed in childhood, when early achievements in key developmental areas (e.g., positive attachment relationships, compliance, and self-regulation skills) lead to later successes in development (e.g., learning, good conduct, social skills, and work skills), aligns with the high return on investment in early childhood interventions, particularly for high-risk children.

When considering the goal of peacebuilding through early childhood policy and programming, we must ask whether the building of tools required for competency can also provide the foundation needed for peacebuilding. Clearly, skills like problem solving and self-control would be helpful to any type of learning or social interaction, and perhaps especially helpful in a context of threat or challenge. But is this enough?

Later influences in life, such as, youth violence in the school or community context (e.g., intergroup conflict, gang activity, and bullying) involve group and political dynamics in antagonistic or rival groups as well as other processes beyond the individual (see Morrill 2013; Morrill and Musheno 2013; Motti-Stefanidi et al. 2012). Most successful interventions with children and youth involved in intergroup conflict have focused on group-level dynamics, using strategies that mobilize children to achieve superordinate goals or increase positive intergroup interactions. Some of these strategies date back to classic studies in intergroup relations, such as the Robber's Cave experiment by Sherif et al. (1954/1961), in which intergroup conflict was experimentally fostered through competition and then reduced through cooperative activities to achieve superordinate goals. Interventions to reduce intergroup conflicts in schools based on race or ethnicity or nationality have shown some success (e.g., Spiel and Strohmeier 2012).

Does Reducing Inequalities in Health, Education, and Opportunities Promote Peace?

Ongoing war and political conflicts that affect millions of children globally often occur in low- and middle-income countries (Engle et al. 2011; Reed et al. 2012). Huge numbers of children in high-conflict, low-income regions are traumatized, displaced, orphaned, unable to go to school, exploited, and exposed to many other known risks to human development, including extreme violence. As noted above and discussed by Dawes and van der Merwe (this volume) as well as Christie et al. (this volume), inequality of this kind is often described as structural violence. Among humanitarian and economic development agencies and advocates, including UNICEF and the World Bank, there is growing consensus that early intervention (particularly in low- and middle-income countries) is essential to address global inequalities in health, education, and economic opportunities related to poverty and ongoing conflicts (e.g., Engle et al. 2011; Lundberg and Wuermli 2012; Britto et al. 2013). Early interventions focus on clean water, medical care, adequate nutrition, parent education about nutrition and child development, and high-quality early childhood programs. Interventions for older children and youth focus primarily on education and occupational training, except in cases of rehabilitation of child soldiers or severely traumatized children. In the latter situations, a range of mental health services, often based in schools, provides young people the help needed to recover (Masten et al. 2014).

Recovery for children depends on the function of families, schools, and other interdependent systems (Masten and Narayan 2012; Masten et al. 2014). For younger children, it is particularly important for family routines to be restored as soon as possible. In addition, the resumption of school (and childcare programs) appears to symbolize recovery for adults as well as children.

A key question that arose from this Forum is whether addressing the well-being of children in extremely poor and conflict-affected areas will contribute to peace as well as health, education, and improved economic prosperity. Are children more inclined to live in peace and support peaceful solutions at the community and government level when they are healthy, have strong attachments to adults and peers, normal learning and self-regulation capabilities, educational opportunities, and belief systems that hold that life has meaning and the future holds promise? If we invest in the capabilities and successes of young children for early developmental task attainment—a strategy that appears to yield wide-ranging benefits for later success at the individual and societal level—will we also be building a solid foundation for peace?

Christie et al. as well as Dawes and van der Merwe (both this volume) argue persuasively that promoting healthy development and equality of opportunity also promotes a solid foundation for peace. However, would this foundation be sufficient? That seems unlikely and begs for a developmental set of related questions: How do we build a strong foundation for peace through investments in early childhood? What needs to be done at later stages of development (through different contexts, policies, or practices, at local, national, and international levels) to reinforce the foundation for peace that has been laid in early childhood?

Three Provocative Questions

It has been noted in the resilience literature that the capabilities and skills required for competence and success in many developmental tasks across the life span can also be directed at goals at odds with those of the family or society (Masten 2014b). Moreover, what is viewed as maladaptive in one time frame or context may be viewed as adaptive from another perspective. Those who aim to promote peace through programs and interventions to influence child development would be wise to consider the issues posed by three provocative questions:

1. Can skills intended for peace contribute to violence?
2. Can violence lead to peace?
3. When is conflict or violence adaptive?

These questions address in different ways the judgments that are always involved in defining desirable outcomes and processes, including "peace" and "good development." The same behavior, such as skilled leadership, can function to promote success in war or peace. Gang leaders recruit talented young members by providing opportunities for agency and leadership directed at illegal activities. Moreover, leading a gang effectively requires social skills and knowledge of intergroup relations. Nations sometimes wage war with the explicit goal of achieving peace or halting violence, such as the efforts by a multinational coalition to stop Hitler in World War II. Violence enacted in self-defense or in the defense of others is often viewed as heroic or justified.

The literature on young people engaged in ongoing political conflicts highlights the complexities of promoting peace in situations where young people may be inspired or motivated to engage in violence to resist oppression actively, express identity, or gain a sense of control over their destinies (Barber 2009a, b, 2013; Boothby et al. 2006). Indoctrination of child soldiers, in a context where violence is the only option for survival, can result in a sense of pride, power, and belonging that may protect the individual from hopelessness and despair (Masten et al. 2014). Thoughtful attention to the adaptive function of violence in these situations may be crucial when designing interventions to promote peace.

Peace and peacebuilding (like resilience and interventions to promote resilience) always have a context. Training children in skills that promote peaceful interactions among children at school could conceivably endanger children who return home to a very different context, perhaps fraught with dangers not imagined by the teachers at school. Fostering "adaptation" to structural violence rather than intervening to address inequalities could serve to perpetuate pernicious forms of societal-level maltreatment of children.

Conclusions

Peace and peacebuilding are complex concepts that have much in common with the concepts and goals of developmental resilience science. Peace can refer to goals, states of being, or processes and pathways leading to harmonious or calm interactions within a single individual, in small and large groups of individuals, or among nation-states. The capacity for peace likely involves the interplay of many systems within children, as well as between children and other systems, which together shape development of skills and capabilities that make it possible to respond effectively to challenges that could otherwise produce violence as well as to act on behalf of peace. Such capacity and associated skills are likely to require learning about conflict and experiences engaging in and resolving conflicts with tools other than violence, just as some experience with adversity and stress appears to facilitate adaptive capabilities for handling challenges in human development. Defining, understanding, and promoting peace requires a dynamic perspective on human interaction and development across multiple systems, including individuals, families, communities, cultures, and societies.

Evidence from research on risk and resilience pertinent to direct and structural violence suggests that pathways of peace may overlap with pathways of resilience more broadly defined. Literature on preventing violence in youth and evidence on promoting resilience in young people who have experienced violence earlier in life align in suggesting that efforts to promote competence and positive development and build or support nurturing environments in early childhood have capacity-building implications for peace as well as competence in human development. Important capabilities and protective influences implicated by the literature on peace and violence, as well as effective adaptation to adversity more broadly defined in the resilience literature, include warm relationships with competent and caring adults who provide emotional security along with child-appropriate limit-setting and monitoring, prosocial values and behavior, self-regulation skills and flexible thinking, empathy and social understanding, and opportunities for intergroup learning and experience handling conflicts and manageable challenges.

Research explicitly focused on linking the conceptual and empirical work on risk and resilience to peace is limited to date, although this volume provides many ideas for future research across multiple levels of analysis, from molecular genetics to cultural processes. Prevention and intervention experiments designed to promote the processes or outcomes defined as peacebuilding, peace, or tools for peace offer the most powerful evidence that investments in early childhood can contribute to the goals of peace. However, there appears to be considerable work to do in delineating the meaning of peace at multiple levels and identifying important processes along the potential pathways to peace.

Peace can be viewed as a domain of competence in human systems (at multiple levels) which must be nurtured and can be threatened by adversities. Risks, promotive factors, and protective factors for peace-oriented children described in this volume show striking similarities to influences widely implicated as important for human development in diverse studies of risk and resilience (Masten 2014b; Panter-Brick and Leckman 2013; Wachs and Rahman 2013). The lessons gleaned from nearly five decades of conceptual and empirical work in resilience science in young people offer potentially helpful ideas, methods, findings, intervention strategies, and issues to inform the emerging science and practice of peace and peacebuilding in child development.

Summary Points and Questions for Future Research

1. Five decades of research on resilience in children offer helpful concepts, findings, and issues that can inform efforts to promote the capacity for peace in child development.

    - How are pathways to peace related to pathways of positive development more broadly defined in the research on risk and resilience?
    - Are there promotive or protective influences in early development for peace and how do these overlap with widely reported predictors of positive child development or adaptation in adversity?

2. Investments in children and families that promote normal brain development and function, self-regulation skills, learning, and prosocial behavior may also reduce risk for antisocial behavior and violence.

    - When and how do adaptive skills such as self-regulation, learning, and prosocial behavior contribute to peace or violence in different cultural and sociopolitical contexts?

3. Family context, early child care, and educational settings are promising targets for interventions to build nurturing environments for healthy child development that also hold promise for promoting the capacity for peace in human development.

    - What are the best combinations of family-focused and educationally focused interventions to enhance nurturing environments for children in ways that promote peace?
    - How do families promote skills for harmonious social interactions and effective conflict resolution in young children at home before and after their children begin formal schooling?

- What are effective classroom- and school-based strategies during the primary education period for promoting peace in early and later human development?

4. Building the skills and capacity for harmonious and equitable human relationships at the individual or group level involves engaging effectively in conflict resolution.

- What are the most effective strategies in early child development for fostering later intergroup harmony and conflict resolution skills?

5. Given that the capacity for peace involves interactions across levels of human function and organization, research is needed on strategic timing and targeting of interventions to promote peace.

- What are the features of multisystem, integrated programs in early childhood that show promise for promoting the capacity for peace in children, families, and their communities?
- What are the cost-effective and promising targets as well as windows of opportunity for leveraging peace-relevant developmental changes in children or families?

Acknowledgments

Preparation of this chapter was supported in part by grants to the University of Minnesota from the Institute of Education Sciences (IES #R305A110528; Masten, Carlson, and Zelazo, Co-PIs) and from the National Institute of Mental Health (NIMH #P20 MH085987; August PI). The opinions expressed are those of the author and do not necessarily represent the views of IES, NIMH, or her collaborators.

First column (top to bottom): Daniel Christie, Jere Behrman, Mark Tomlinson, Catherine Panter-Brick, Raija-Leena Punamäki, Mark Tomlinson, Raija-Leena Punamäki
Second column: Catherine Panter-Brick, Jacqueline Hayden, Jim Cochrane, Kirstin Goth, Jacqueline Hayden, Ann Masten, Jere Behrman
Third column: Andrew Dawes, Jim Cochrane, Kirstin Goth, Daniel Christie, Ann Masten, Ilham Nasser, Andrew Dawes

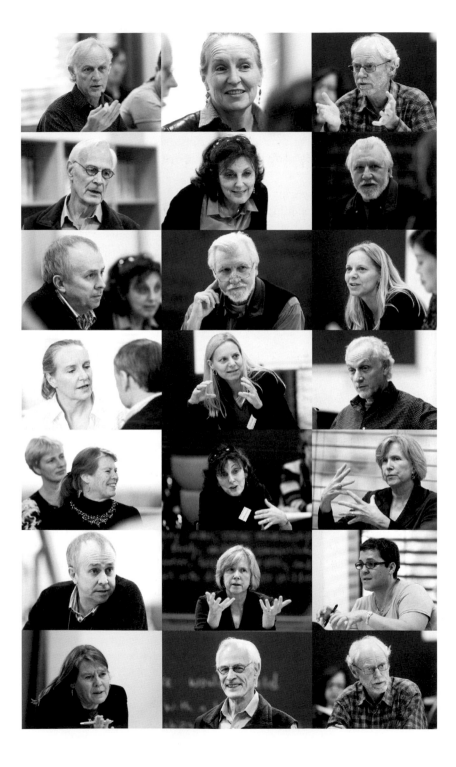

15

Healthy Human Development as a Path to Peace

Daniel J. Christie, Catherine Panter-Brick, Jere R. Behrman,
James R. Cochrane, Andrew Dawes, Kirstin Goth,
Jacqueline Hayden, Ann S. Masten, Ilham Nasser,
Raija-Leena Punamäki, and Mark Tomlinson

Abstract

What is the potential role of early childhood interventions for promoting peace? From
our perspective, healthy human development during early childhood can lay the foundation for the child's acquisition of complex and specific capacities required to engage
in peace-promoting behavior. This chapter focuses on children's capacity to create,
maintain, and restore harmonious and equitable relationships with others. Obstacles
and catalysts for healthy human development are identified, as are the competencies
required for children to engage in harmonious and equitable relationships. Sustainable
peace in a society requires a "systems approach" that reduces both direct and structural
violence and promotes peaceful means and socially just ends. A model is proposed
based on four sequential foundations: healthy human development, healthy primary relationships, prosocial interpersonal relations, and the adoption of a peace and social justice orientation toward out-group members. Three case studies are presented to clarify
the key concepts and propositions we advance. Drawing on an agentic perspective, in
which the child is a producer as well as the product of social environments, our concept
of *peaceful* children implies not only healthy human development and the acquisition
of specific developmental capacities for peace, but also the child's internalization of
a set of values that support a commitment to relational harmony and social justice. In
conclusion, suggestions for future research are offered.

Introduction

In this chapter, we offer evidence for the proposition that healthy human development lays the foundation for the development of peaceful children. When
we refer to *peaceful* children, we are not implying docility in any form. To
the contrary, our use of the term "peaceful" comports with the way in which

scholars from the transdisciplinary field of peace and conflict studies use the term; namely, as the nonviolent pursuit of socially just arrangements between individuals and groups (Galtung 1996). We also share with peace scholars the view that peace is not sustainable without an approach that integrates non-violence with justice; moving seamlessly from justice to peace is what has been referred to as "justpeace" (Lederach 1999). Accordingly, we begin by discussing the meaning of peace and violence. Because we view healthy human development as one of the foundations for the development of peaceful children, we then examine what we know about barriers and catalysts for healthy development.

Our group, with representatives from anthropology, economics, psychology, and peace studies, began with wide-ranging discussions. We agreed that there is a sequence of developmental tasks and corresponding foundations that favor the development of a prosocial orientation in children. Prosocial children tend to be healthy, form secure attachments, engage in self-regulation, have a stable social identity, exercise agency, have well-honed social skills, and the capacity to reason and communicate (van IJzendoorn and Bakermans-Kranenburg, this volume). *Peaceful* children, in addition to having a general propensity toward prosocial behavior, appear to have specific capabilities that are particularly well-suited for engaging in peaceful behavior: the capacity for empathy, respect for others, and a commitment to fairness and trust in relationships with other individuals and groups. These capabilities, combined with peace-promoting social ecologies, leave the prosocial child well positioned to pursue peace and social justice in relation to others who are outside the child's reference or identity group.

Throughout this chapter, we emphasize the importance of a strong developmental approach that will accommodate notions of sequential development, optimal timing for interventions, and multiple trajectories. Most importantly, we contend that pathways to peace vary with geohistorical contexts. In contexts where unfair conditions persist and pose risks to child development, the primary task is the mitigation of structural violence: a more equitable structural arrangement in access to resources is needed for healthy human development. In contexts of direct violence, the immediate goal of interventions is the creation of social ecologies (environments) that restore peace in and around the child. In contexts characterized by deep divisions between groups and conflictual relationships, the primary goal is to maximize the child's engagement with harmonious relationships. When social injustices are the dominant feature of the geohistorical landscape, nurturing the child's awakening sense of social injustice, agency, and nonviolent social activism is the most relevant intervention and pathway to peace.

In summary, from our perspective, *peaceful* children have the capacity to create, maintain, and restore harmonious and equitable relationships. Because these peace-promoting capacities are complex, we view healthy human development as potentially contributing to their development. We recognize that children's commitment to relational harmony and social equity suggests an internalized set of values, in addition to being healthy and developing peace-promoting capabilities. Moreover, we recognize that there are gaps in our knowledge about paths favoring the development of peaceful children.

Peace and Violence

World War II made it abundantly clear that the field of international relations and its central organizing principle, *political realism,* could not deliver on the promise of preventing war. Shortly thereafter, the term "peace" entered the lexicon of social scientists and two academic cultures emerged: (a) *peace science*, which emphasized objective, quantitative, and analytical approaches to the generation of knowledge within the positivist tradition (Isaard and Smith 1982), and (b) *peace and conflict studies*, a transdisciplinary and value-explicit approach dedicated not only to an analysis of the causes and consequences of violence but also to the reduction and elimination of violence combined with the promotion of human well-being (Clemens 2012).

When "peace" entered the social science lexicon, scholars in the United States tended to focus on the causes and consequences of conflict, rather than on peace itself, in part because "peace" was associated with normative concepts and was politically suspect, especially during the McCarthy era (Kelman 1981). Our perspective here is more closely aligned with peace scholars in Europe (Galtung 1969, 1996) and the academic space occupied by peace and conflict studies, which examines not only the mitigation of direct interpersonal and collective violence but also structural violence. The latter is a pernicious form of violence that kills people just as surely as direct violence, but does so insiduously by depriving them of basic human need satisfaction. Worldwide, it has been estimated that about 1.5 million people per year die from direct violence (WHO 2009), while annually 14–18 million deaths are due to the structural violence of hunger, unsanitary water, and a lack of access to medical care (Gilligan 1997).

Direct and Structural Violence

Structural violence is reflected in vast disparities in income, wealth, health, and access to services, both within and between societies (Galtung 1969). It occurs where people are socially dominated, politically oppressed, or economically exploited. One way to think about structural violence is the number of deaths that could be avoided if human needs were satisfied equitably. For instance, structural violence occurs where relevant health care facilities exist in one area, but some people are persistently marginalized in terms of their access to quality care.

Direct and structural violence can be distinguished in a number of ways (Christie 2006): Direct violence kills directly and quickly through bodily harm, whereas structural violence kills people indirectly and slowly though the deprivation of human need satisfaction. Direct violence is intermittent, dramatic, and often personal, whereas structural violence is chronic, normalized, and impersonal. On a global scale, structural violence can occur through (Kabeer 2010):

1. social inequalities that marginalize, devalue, and discriminate against people on the basis of their identity;
2. economic inequalities that distribute assets and opportunities unequally.
3. political inequalities that deprive people of voice and representation in matters that affect their well-being; and
4. spatial inequality in which geographic location can make it less likely that people will have access to goods and services.

In the context of early childhood, structural violence can be evidenced in the unequal exposure to risk and protective factors (Dawes and van der Merwe, this volume). As a form of structural violence, global poverty and inequality creates difficult life conditions for caregivers and puts children at risk for malnourishment, infectious diseases, and a host of other debilitating problems that adversely affect human development (Leon and Walt 2001). While the global poverty landscape has been changing rapidly, due largely to the dynamic emerging economies in Asia, there are hundreds of millions of people that are still trying to eke out survival near or below international poverty lines (Chandy and Gertz 2011). As Harper et al. (2012:48) notes:

> Whichever way one frames the problem of chronic poverty—as human suffering, as vulnerability, as a basic needs failure, as the abrogation of human rights, as degraded citizenship—widespread chronic poverty occurs in a world that has the knowledge and resources to eradicate it. Tackling chronic poverty is therefore the global priority for our generation and is vital if our world is to achieve an acceptable level of justice and fairness.

The issue of social justice also looms large even in high-income countries. In their examination of 23 high-income countries, Wilkinson and Pickett (2009) found a strong positive correlation between income inequality and a wide range of health and well-being variables, including life expectancy, infant mortality, mental illness, educational achievement, teen birth rates, homicides, rates of imprisonment, levels of social trust, and social mobility.

Healthy Human Development: Barriers and Catalysts

In this section, we examine well-documented barriers to the reduction of structural violence in children's social ecologies and their untoward impact on the child's development. Thereafter, we identify some catalysts of healthy human development. Our view is that healthy human development is promoted when the social ecologies in which children are embedded are relatively peaceful (i.e., when structural and direct violence are low). Accordingly, we examine the barriers and catalysts that can reduce structural violence and promote healthy human development.

Barriers to Healthy Human Development

Physical and social settings that are relevant to human development encompass household composition, physical infrastructures and spaces used for play or recreation, essential services or resources such as water or electricity, as well as geographical location. In addition, political and socioeconomic forces shape social and economic equity in terms of rights and opportunities to enhance well-being. The force of these arrangements may impact directly on the young child in several ways: (a) when potable water is not available, risk of infection is heightened; (b) when financial resources are limited, the range of stimulation opportunities may be limited; (c) when nutrition is limited by food insecurity, growth status may be compromised.

Physical and social settings also influence parenting and child outcomes (Gehlert et al. 2008). Crucial factors are the quality of the child's nutrition, health care, caregiving relationships, and stimulation for early learning (Steele et al., this volume). Caregiver mental health is a key concern throughout the parenting experience. Most research on the impact of caregiver health has been conducted on mothers, rather than fathers or other primary caregivers (Panter-Brick et al. 2014a). For mothers, rates of depression during the perinatal period are particularly high in low- and middle-income countries, where rates range from 18–33% (Fisher et al. 2012). Numerous studies have shown the negative effects of maternal depression on early interaction, child care, and parenting practices (Wachs et al. 2009). Maternal depression has been associated with infant growth and stunting (Stewart et al. 2008; Wachs and Rahman 2013). The relationship between maternal depression and compromised child development is, however, complex, in that the risk factors of poverty, stress, poor support, and low levels of education are implicated in both (Tomlinson et al. 2014a).

Threats to sound cognitive, language, and socioemotional development in the years prior to school include poor self-regulation abilities, which may be the result of neglect and harsh parenting in the first years, and limited stimulation of developmental capacities required for children to be ready to learn. Children from low-income settings, who have not benefitted from some form of early stimulation programs, are commonly exposed to forms of early stimulation that are not aligned with the skill requirements of the schooling system. Early language development provides an example. The richness of the language environment in the home varies along a socioeconomic gradient. As a result, as the classic U.S. study by Hart and Risley (1995) showed, differences in language ability between children of wealthy and poor backgrounds become apparent prior to age three. The gap widens through the school years, resulting in very different educational outcomes and life chances that are a function of class background.

Reduction of poverty and inequality are central priorities if we are to promote the development of healthy and peaceful children. Foundational skills important for prosocial behavior depend on brain development, and many other aspects of healthy development, which can be compromised, for example, by inadequate nutrition, poor caregiving, exposure to toxic substances, and lack of learning opportunities. Prenatally, exposure to neurotoxins, maternal malnutrition, and maternal stress or trauma have been linked to alterations in a child's developing neurological systems important for later self-regulation and other neurobiological functions related to prosocial and antisocial behavior (Mendes et al. 2009; Masten and Narayan 2012; Shonkoff et al. 2012; Gunnar and Herrera 2013).

The first thousand days (pregnancy through the first two years) are particularly sensitive: the outcomes of early prolonged malnutrition may be difficult to reverse (Victora et al. 2008; Yousafzai et al. 2013), although recent studies indicate that substantial growth faltering and growth recovery, associated with child cognitive development, occurs after early childhood (Crookston et al. 2013; Schott et al. 2013). Postnatally, malnutrition remains one of the most common preventable threats to normal neurological development and intellectual functioning. Impact depends on the period of life during which it is experienced and the duration of exposure (Fox et al., this volume). Links between stunting and externalizing behavior in childhood have been established in recent cohort studies (Liu et al. 2004; Liu 2011; Galler et al. 2012). These studies posit an indirect relationship between malnutrition and violent conduct in which stunting affects executive functioning, which in turn impacts school performance: children are more likely to drop out of school and, in the teenage years, are more likely to become involved in antisocial activity, including interpersonal violence.

The majority of the world's young children live in environments in which the necessary affordances for a sound foundation in health, nutrition, and cognitive and language development are inadequate. Under these circumstances, a chain of developmental consequences (known as "development cascades") ensues (Masten and Cicchetti 2010): individual potential is compromised, and children are less likely to develop the capabilities required to benefit from schooling and ultimately to become productive adult members of society. Developmental outcomes such as violent conduct become more probable (Walker et al. 2007).

Referring to children in challenging environments, Richter (2013:7) explains that "as time goes by, difficulties grow because they build on each other. A small, sickly child may make fewer friends and learn less, they may get shouted at because they're slow, and their self-esteem may suffer. All these conditions worsen if the child goes to school later, is held back in class, is teased by others and has few supportive adults to turn to. Such accumulating problems get harder to overcome, more needs to be done to address them, at greater cost, and with diminishing possibilities for success."

In regard to interventions, Shah and Beinecke (2009) describe three barriers to the implementation of comprehensive family-based strategies that have particular relevance in low-income countries, but which also pertain to resource-rich countries: scarcity, inequity, and inefficiency. There is a lack of funding; available resources are concentrated in urban areas rather than in rural areas. There is a lack of adequately trained and supervised workers as well as leadership and public health skills across sectors (Saraceno et al. 2007). Models of intervention are urgently needed that focus on early parenting, familial cohesion, illness detection, appropriate health-seeking behavior, cognitive-behavioral strategies of behavior change, the linking of people to poverty alleviation programs, and comprehensive strategies that begin early in life and continue over time (Tomlinson et al. 2011).

Catalysts for Healthy Human Development

It is important to remember that competence and adaptive success also cascade: "competence begets competence" in human development (Heckman 2006; Masten 2011; Masten, this volume). Strategic interventions can be designed to initiate positive cascades, and when such interventions are well-timed and targeted, there can be lasting and spreading effects across multiple domains, associated with a high return on investment. This is the basis for the argument of resilience-focused interventions in child development to promote well-being (Panter-Brick and Leckman 2013).

Figure 15.1 illustrates an integrated and aspirational framework for understanding key developmental opportunities for intervention. The X axis describes what we know about child development; caregiver roles are depicted on the Y axis, with dispositional and context factors on the Z axis. The dotted line along the X axis depicts the fluidity of caregiving roles across childhood; while parental sensitivity and mutual regulation, for instance, are separated in the diagram for heuristic purposes, they are necessarily part of the same caregiving function. No one intervention can cover all these bases. However, all areas should optimally be addressed in interventions that seek to prevent violence and enhance the probability of child outcomes oriented toward pro-social behavior.

There is clear evidence that interventions to promote maternal health and nutrition and reduce intake of substances (e.g., alcohol) during pregnancy reduces the risk of neurological insult to the developing fetus. Promotion of maternal health is therefore a priority. We also know that perinatal depression is highly prevalent in poor communities, in both high- and low-income countries. While not directly associated with the development of externalizing behavior and adult violence, perinatal depression compromises the capacity to provide

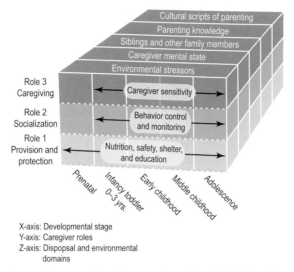

Role 3
Caregiving

Role 2
Socialization

Role 1
Provision and
protection

Cultural scripts of parenting
Parenting knowledge
Siblings and other family members
Caregiver mental state
Environmental stressors

Caregiver sensitivity

Behavior control
and monitoring

Nutrition, safety, shelter,
and education

Prenatal   Infancy toddler   Early childhood   Middle childhood   Adolescence
0–3 yrs.

X-axis: Developmental stage
Y-axis: Caregiver roles
Z-axis: Dispopsal and environmental
domains

Figure 15.1 A matrix approach to interventions through childhood and adolescence (provided by Tomlinson et al. 2012, after Rosenberg and Knox 2005).

responsive affectionate care and is predictive of a broad range of risks to young children (Wachs and Rahman 2013). Thus, the provisions of primary mental health interventions for vulnerable mothers and other primary caregivers have the potential to reduce risks substantially to a large number of young children while promoting caregiver well-being. For example, evidence indicates that home visits by professionals or paraprofessionals, who provide support for vulnerable pregnant mothers from low-income households, can have a positive impact on maternal and child health. The first case study (presented below) describes one such program in Khayelitsha, South Africa (Rotheram-Borus et al. 2011; LeRoux et al. 2013; Tomlinson et al. 2014b).

There is limited evidence of a direct link between exposure to early stimulation programs in the preschool years and externalizing behavior. However, an evaluation of Early Head Start[1] in the United States (which provides intensive support to low-income vulnerable caregivers from birth), reports reduced aggressive behavior in beneficiaries five years of age. There is also evidence that children from economically disadvantaged homes, who do not have formal early learning opportunities, are at greater risk for a cascade of increasingly negative outcomes (e.g., school failure, early drop out, and involvement in crime). A range of studies from both low- and high-income countries show the benefits of either formal preschool education or home- and community-based initiatives for at-risk children, in promoting long-term positive outcomes

---

[1] See http://www.acf.hhs.gov/sites/default/files/opre/prekindergarten_followup.pdf (accessed June 14, 2014).

through to adulthood and on to the next generation (Engle et al. 2007, 2011; Heckman 2008; Heckman et al. 2009; Hoddinott et al. 2008; Behrman et al. 2009; Kagitcibasi et al. 2009; Maluccio et al. 2009; Nores and Barnett 2010; Walker et al. 2007).

Program intervention may be designed to support internalized cultural scripts for child rearing and serve as a catalyst for healthy human development. Cultural scripts[2] can provide the caregiver with direction in terms of what forms of care are appropriate, at a particular point in development, and what intellectual, moral, and behavioral orientations are to be valued in the child (LeVine 1990; Rogoff 2003; Harkness and Super 2012). These may include orientations toward respect for social hierarchy, empathic concern for the less fortunate, cooperative rather than competitive behavior with peers, and inclusion or exclusion of those defined as "other," such as cultural minorities or people with disabilities (Hoffman 2000).

Taken together, we suggest that the effectiveness of a program designed to promote healthy human development depends on the alignment of actions vertically and simultaneously through multiple levels of social systems (individual to policy level), building on deep values, goals, assets, and institutions already present in a community (Britto, Gordon et al., this volume). Measurable costs and outcomes are also essential for evidence-based approaches. To assess the feasibility of programs and to justify continued streams of funding, benefit-cost analyses are useful. As Panter-Brick and Leckman (2013) have shown, emphasis is placed on being strategic in the targeting of interventions for developmental timing and program effectiveness. The scale-up and sustainability of programs seems most likely when interventions are deeply relevant to cultural practices and existing institutions. Successful programs are often those that employ a participatory approach, in which program design and implementation is carried out in partnership with local stakeholders and is built on local wisdom. Broadly speaking, context sensitivity and local input seem important for "buy-in" (i.e., the commitment of interested or affected parties to a decision) and sustainability, along with the aligning of strategies, agendas, and institutions. An example of a program in which buy-in was particularly noteworthy is described in the second case study (Skoufias 2001; Levy 2006; Behrman 2010).

Case Study 1: The Philani Project in Khayelitsha, South Africa

Context: The Philani project is being conducted in Khayelitsha, South Africa, to address a matrix of extremely serious social problems, including widespread

---

[2] The term "cultural scripts" refers to the articulation of cultural norms, values, and practices in terms that are clear, precise, and accessible to cultural insiders as well as to cultural outsiders. They are not intended to provide an account of real life social interactions but rather descriptions of commonly held assumptions about how "people think" about social interaction.

poverty, poor nutrition, HIV and TB infection, substance abuse, sexual abuse, and violence in the home.

Program features: The Philani paraprofessional "mentor mothers" project aims to improve the health and well-being of vulnerable pregnant mothers, infants, and children from low-income households, through a strategy of home visits by specially trained "mentor mothers." Mentor mothers deliver a home-based intervention that assists mothers to ensure that they (a) gain access to the most appropriate health services for themselves and their babies, (b) reduce or eliminate alcohol consumption during pregnancy, (c) improve nutrition for both themselves and their babies, and (d) prepare more effectively for the baby's arrival. The mothers also learn about breast-feeding options and a range of effective parenting techniques. Related topics include caring for their own physical and mental health. The Philani approach builds on the cultural values of the beneficiaries. Mentor mothers are drawn from the neighborhoods where the program is implemented and go through a comprehensive training program. They engage in conversation with these women and other household members in an informal, interactive, and nonthreatening way, providing the necessary advice and support in the process.

Outcomes: The outcomes of the study have been very positive. Mothers who have received the intervention are less likely to engage in hazardous drinking during pregnancy and less likely to have a low birth weight infant. They are more likely to breast-feed longer and to breast-feed exclusively for six months. In the case of HIV infection, they are more likely to adhere to the complete protocol for prevention of mother to child transmission of HIV, including adherence to antiretroviral medication. Their infants are likely to experience fewer episodes of diarrhea and require fewer clinic visits. At 18 months, children whose mothers received the intervention were less likely to be malnourished than those whose mothers were not involved in the program. The children of antenatally depressed mothers receiving the intervention were also more likely to have better growth and cognitive development at 6 and 18 months of age, respectively.

Lessons from the field: In contexts of high adversity with severe resource constraints, local women can be recruited from the community, trained and supervised to deliver successfully a cost-effective homebased intervention that improves maternal and child health across a range of domains.

Case Study 2: The PROGRESA/Oportunidades Conditional
Cash Transfer (CCT) Program in Mexico

Context: Mexico has a long history of considerable inequality and poverty (Gasparini and Lustig 2011). As in most countries, poverty is particularly concentrated in small poor rural communities. Before PROGRESA was introduced, substantial resources were utilized to subsidize urban tortilla consumption, providing subsidies across the board because everyone eats tortillas.

Program features: Established in 1997, PROGRESA provides cash transfers to mothers in households that are designated as eligible on the basis of a proxy poverty index, conditional on fulfillment of "co-responsibilities," such as attending regular information and check-up sessions at health clinics and an 85% school attendance rate for their children. PROGRESA initially focused on small communities with populations less than 2,500 in which many of the poorest Mexicans live (but was implemented with primary schools, which excluded the smallest and most remote communities). The program was "top-down," as part of an effort to reorder governmental expenses after the 1996 "peso crisis," and had two important features:

1. Monitoring and evaluation was a central component: The first sample consisted of 508 poor eligible communities with ~125,000 individuals, using random assignment for those receiving program benefits and others phased in two years later (note: the latter were not informed of that initially so as to avoid program anticipation effects). Baseline and periodic follow-up longitudinal data were collected (initially every six months), and an initial evaluation was conducted by an international institution (selected to increase credibility of quality and "arms-length" evaluation). A number of evaluation reports are in the public domain, data are available for public use by other researchers, and over 100 academic articles have been published in international peer-reviewed journals.

2. "Buy-in" was critical at various levels:

    •   Co-responsibilities rather than "handouts" were used for both poor and nonpoor households.

    •   Poor communities met to determine who would be eligible and assigned to the program.

    •   The Mexican Congress played a critical role in maintaining and expanding the program, due to evidence of program effectiveness.

    •   Despite a historical change in leadership in 2000, Mexican presidents accepted and extended the program with minor modifications rather than abandon the program for new ones of their own making. For example, they changed its name to Oportunidades and increased coverage to urban areas. This was because of the credible evidence of program effectiveness.

    •   PROGRESA began under the Zedillo government in 1997 and was entirely financed through Mexican funds; this made it possible for the people of Mexico to view the program as "home grown," as it operated independently of international agencies. Later, however, the World Bank and Inter-American Development Bank became strong advocates of the program and provided support at critical junctures, as a result of positive evaluations.

Outcomes: Evaluation results suggest significant positive effects that are well-targeted on children's schooling and health, as well as positive effects on adults, with benefit-cost ratios significantly greater than one for real resource costs (not including transfers per se but including public and private costs). The program was rapidly expanded to cover over 30 million poor Mexicans and has been emulated broadly, with adaptations at various levels, in over 30 countries.

Lessons from the field: Important aspects of success, including scaling-up, were Mexican ownership, alignment of "buy-in" at many levels, and serious efforts to monitor and evaluate.

From Healthy to *Peaceful* Human Development

In the previous sections we identified barriers and catalysts in relation to healthy human development. Here, we offer evidence for the proposition that healthy human development during childhood lays the foundation for the child's acquisition of the complex and specific capabilities required to engage in peace-promoting behavior. We begin by situating the child within a level of analysis framework and then discuss social ecologies that foster the development of *peaceful* children.

Levels of Analysis

A requisite question for scholarly inquiry into any behavioral or social phenomena, including "peaceful children," is the question of what unit or level of analysis will be chosen for systematic inquiry. As Lewin (1951:157) stated, "the first prerequisite of a successful observation in any science is a definite understanding about what size of unit one is going to observe at a given time."

Our unit of analysis is the individual child, though we recognize that the child is continuously interacting with other systems (Overton 2013). The individual child is embedded in multiple ecologies (Bronfenbrenner 1979) and networks of influence, some of which are proximal and others more distal. At the most distal level, "peace" engenders international- and societal-level structures along with associated norms and collective narratives that reduce direct and structural violence, while promoting relational harmony and equitable well-being. More proximal to the child, prevention and promotion processes take place in the child's community and, most importantly, family. At the individual level, "peace" involves subjective states and actions aimed at the prevention of direct and structural violence and the promotion of nonviolence and social justice. These levels are interdependent and interactive; that is, individuals and groups are influenced by distal processes and, conversely, the functioning of the macro system depends on the behavior of individuals and groups (Suedfeld et al. 2012). In relation to violence and peace, prevention and promotion processes operate within levels but also across levels. As Cacioppo and Berntson (1992) have noted, a target event at one level of analysis may have multiple determinants both within and across levels of analysis.

Research on cascades, positive or negative, across levels of analysis over time, are extremely rare. One recent example of these multilevel dynamics is provided by Boxer et al. (2013), who studied the effects of societal level violence on the more proximal systems of youth life and the cascading effects on youth aggression. Data from their longitudinal study of Palestinian and Israeli youth indicate that ethnopolitical violence at the macro levels spills over to violence in proximal systems in the community, family, and school, and is associated with increases in the aggression of individual youth. The same arguments have been made in Afghanistan and Sri Lanka for linking collective violence with interpersonal violence in humanitarian settings (Panter-Brick et al. 2011). Research demonstrating the impact of macro-level systems of violence on micro systems, such as the family, underscore the importance of reducing violence and promoting peace at multiple levels of analysis: from structural levels to the level of the individual child.

Social Ecologies and the Peaceful Child

While structural violence within and between societies is a problem in and of itself, structural violence also undergirds direct forms of violence. This is not necessarily because those at the bottom of society are likely to get agitated and violent, although this does happen (see Smith et al. 2012), but because those on the top are invested in the status quo and will take action to maintain their status, using a variety of narratives to justify system-based inequalities (Jost et al. 2002).

Conversely, direct violence contributes to structural violence. For example, pervasive armed conflict has a direct impact on economic development and the equitable satisfaction of human needs. The percentage of global poverty concentrated in fragile states has grown considerably in recent years and is expected to exceed 50% by 2014 according to some recent estimates (Chandy and Gertz 2011). Clearly, because direct and structural violence form interlocking systems of violence, sustainable peace requires a systems approach that reduces both direct and structural violence and promotes peaceful means and socially just ends (Christie and Montiel 2013).

Notwithstanding the systemic quality of violence, it may seem unwieldy to frame the concept of peace broadly, to include both the amelioration of direct and structural violence. However, an exclusive focus on the reduction of direct violence between individuals and collectivities leaves open the possibility of maintaining "peace" through coercive means. Examples include authoritarian parenting at the family level and a doctrine of deterrence at the international level. Similarly, an exclusive focus on the reduction of structural violence, without attending to direct violence, leaves open the possibility of pursuing socially just ends through violent means.

Because sustainable peace requires the reduction of structural as well as direct violence, we adopt a broad view of peace—one that includes the prevention and mitigation of both direct and structural violence. From our perspective, the development of *peaceful* children is most likely under conditions in which (a) healthy human development is fostered and (b) social ecologies are relatively free of both structural and direct forms of violence.

So How Do We Conceptualize *Peaceful* Children?

While the reduction and elimination of direct and structural violence in the child's social ecologies make an important contribution to the development of *peaceful* children, the child, in turn, brings certain peace-promoting competencies to bear on social ecologies. Accordingly, when conceptualizing *peaceful* children, we adopted an approach that emphasizes children's promotion of peace and arrived at a consensus on the capacities of peaceful children:

> Peaceful children are healthy, self-regulated children who have a sense of identity, agency, social skills, the capacity to reason and communicate, as well as the capacity to form trusting relationships with other individuals and groups.

To be clear, we do not mean to imply that *peaceful* children are passive. To the contrary, we view children from an agentic perspective, in which children are both the product and the producer of the social ecologies in which they are embedded (Bandura 2000).

Our assumption is that the child's peacebuilding capacities allow the child to engage in harmonious relations and internalize the pursuit of equitable well-being within and across social systems. The peace-promoting constructs of harmonious relations and equitable well-being may be orthogonal. However, they are indivisible for sustainable peace, as we have suggested, and compatible when social justice is pursued through nonviolent means; that is, when (structural) peace is pursued through peaceful means (Galtung 1996). Although "speaking truth to power" creates tension in relationships (Montiel 2001), the importance of reconciling differences and restoring harmony in relationships remains a hallmark of peaceful approaches to social transformation. The prototypical manifestation of such an approach is Gandhi's experiments with truth (Gandhi 1948), which underscore "peace" as both a process and an outcome.

Our discussion now turns to the child's capacities in relation to the development of competence and skills in the resolution of conflict, which is essential for the creation, maintenance, and restoration of harmonious relationships. Thereafter we examine some of the psychosocial mechanisms involved in the child's internalization of a social justice orientation and pursuit of equitable relations with others.

Harmonious Relations and the Role of Conflict Resolution

Even under ideal conditions, children experience conflict in their lives. Peace scholars have defined conflict in various ways: as opposing preferences (Carnevale and Pruitt 1992), antagonistic feelings (Fisher 1990), perceptions of divergent interests whether real or imagined (Rubin and Levinger 1995), or differences in views, interests, or goals (Deutsch 1977). Taken together, these definitions of conflict contrast sharply with the meaning of direct violence. Conflict is primarily a cognitive and affective experience, whereas direct violence has behavioral referents that are manifest, for example, in interpersonal aggression at the micro level or organized efforts to inflict casualties on other groups at the macro level of analysis. In addition, in contrast to direct violence, conflict is ubiquitous and inevitable in human relations.

The distinction between conflict and direct violence opens the possibility of managing the former to prevent the latter. As Deutsch (1977) pointed out, conflicts are inevitable—the key question is whether conflicts will be managed in constructive ways that strengthen relationships or destructive ways that harm relationships. Among the most widely used constructive methods to manage conflict is a principled approach that encourages opposite parties to understand their interests and work toward a mutually beneficial outcome (Fisher and Ury 1983). Not surprisingly, empathy is a key mechanism involved in this principled approach, as well as in many other approaches that seek to resolve conflicts, promote interpersonal and intergroup understanding, and improve relationships (Wagner 2012).

In the developmental psychology literature, there is a distinction between cognitive and affective empathy (Decety and Jackson 2004; Preston and de Waal 2002). Cognitive empathy occurs when children can effectively comprehend a distressing situation experienced by someone else, recognize another's emotional state, and assume another person's perspective. Affective empathy occurs when children actually experience a vicarious emotional response to someone else's expressed emotion. Both types of empathy are typically encouraged in programs designed to enhance social and emotional learning in children, though arguably greater emphasis is placed on cognitive empathy (i.e., perspective taking) in programs that are specifically designed to induce cooperation and learning (Johnson and Johnson 1990).

A growing number of studies demonstrate that when groups in conflict are brought together, cognitive and affective empathy can play a role in the improvement of intergroup relations and reduction of prejudice. This research indicates that intergroup contact is positively associated with empathy and, in turn, empathy is negatively associated with prejudice (Pettigrew and Tropp 2006; Pagotto et al. 2010).

In addition to intergroup empathy, children's perceptions of social norms also influence whether increased contact is associated with more positive attitudes. A longitudinal study of German and Turkish children in Germany offers hints regarding the causal direction between increases in direct intergroup contact and positive attitudinal changes (Feddes et al. 2009). The relationship between contact and attitudinal change was partially mediated by social norms: How do you think other German children or other Turkish children would feel about your playing with members of the other group? This suggests that increased contact led to changes in perceived norms, which in turn led to more positive attitudes. These findings were obtained with majority status Germans but not minority status Turkish children, a generalization problem that is common in studies which employ the contact hypothesis. Interestingly, Killen and Rutland (2011) speculate that the lack of contact effects among minority group members may be due to their awareness of their group's lower status.

Just as conflicts in relationships are inevitable, the sense of being treated unfairly, aggrieved, or hurt is, at times, also part of the human condition. Under these conditions, the restoration of harmony in relationships may require forgiveness, defined as the process of releasing negative thoughts, feelings, and behaviors toward a transgressor and transforming these negative reactions into more positive thoughts, feelings, and behaviors (Thompson et al. 2005). At the societal level, collective forgiveness can serve as a mechanism to restore harmony and peace. For example, in countries such as Jordan and Egypt, the collective rituals of reconciliation (known as Sulha) draw on local cultural constructs as a basis for individual forgiveness and to diminish negative feelings toward one's self and others (Nasser et al. 2014).

Not only is there a strong correlation between the degree to which forgiveness occurs and the victim's experience of empathy for the transgressor, the likelihood of victims accepting an apology and forgiving a transgressor is almost totally mediated by the victim's empathy for the transgressor (McCullough et al. 1998). Similar findings have been obtained in field-based programs. In Northern Ireland, for example, Tam et al. (2008) found that empathy mediated forgiveness and reduced discriminatory behavior toward out-group members.

At present, there is no consensus on the relative effectiveness of cognitive and affective forms of empathy in the forgiveness process. Hodgson and Wertheim (2007) provide evidence that perspective taking is most consistently associated with the tendency to forgive, although other investigators place affective empathy and compassion at the center of the forgiveness process (Enright 2001). In a review of research on intergroup contact and forgiveness, Swart and Hewstone (2012) invoke both forms of empathy and complicate the picture by noting that forgiveness is mediated by a number of emotional and cognitive factors, including increases in perspective taking, affective empathy, intergroup empathy, and the reduction of anger-related emotions.

Emotion regulation also plays a role in forgiveness. Research indicates that those who are able to manage their emotions (i.e., attend to and repair their emotions) and refrain from being overwhelmed by their emotions, are more likely to forgive others; the relationship between emotion regulation and forgiveness is mediated by the tendency to view situations from the perspectives of others (Hodgson and Wertheim 2007). Similarly, in a content analysis of 14 forgiveness-promoting programs, Wade and Worthington (2005) found that all programs had an empathy component and that most programs explicitly encouraged participants to view the transgressor within the context of the situation in which the transgression took place, thereby inducing perspective taking and situational rather than dispositional attributions.

We offer, however, a cautionary note. While a great deal of research has underscored the importance of empathy for maintaining and restoring harmony in interpersonal and intergroup relationships, nearly all of this research has originated in the West. In East Asian and other collectivistic cultures, for example, harmony in relationships is highly valued, and a robust finding is that conflicts are avoided between individuals and groups (Leung et al. 2002). In the Middle East and other contexts where religious teachings are central cultural assets, religious beliefs and family-based narratives are used to teach forgiveness (Abu-Nimer and Nasser 2013). Taken together, these cultural variations demonstrate that what matters most for the child is the acquisition of culture-specific competence to guide actions that create, maintain, and restore relationships. The importance of taking cultural considerations into account is illustrated in the third case study, based in Afghanistan (Eggerman and Panter-Brick 2010; Panter-Brick et al. 2011; Omidian and Lawrence 2007).

Case Study 3: Focusing Interventions and Promoting Family "Unity and Harmony" in Afghanistan

Context: For the past thirty years, Afghans have endured pervasive violence, rising inequality, and noxious poverty. Layers of war-related, structural, and interpersonal violence intersect: in the wake of war and displacement, the everyday reality of social and economic stressors, which permeate life slowly but steadily, unhinge men and women to commit acts of violence within and outside the home.

Critical ingredients for intervention: Focusing is a technique used to teach a culturally grounded technique of "mindfulness." It has been taught to over 400,000 women in small workshops throughout Afghanistan. As a technique it is aligned with Sufism and allows perpetrators and victims of violence to reach an inner state of safety and calm. Using specific focusing techniques, individuals distance themselves from threats and anxiety to rebuild their emotional and social lives. A sense of safety, calmness, and peace are precursors for interrupting the practices of domestic violence.

In the absence of job security and effective governance, strong families and strong cultural values remain the main anchor of hope and resilience. "Family unity and harmony" is a salient value in the Afghan culture, the bedrock of resilience in the face of life adversity. Seeking to address the culture of violence in domestic settings, one intervention sought to give voice to Afghan children on the radio: the children clearly distinguished between acceptable

both laboratory- and field-based research indicate that appeals to empathy are more likely to be associated with helping in-group than out-group members (Stürmer et al. 2005). A related phenomenon has been observed in resource allocation games: children between 4.5 and 6 years of age prefer equitable division of resources with friends, but treat nonfriends less well (Moore 2009).

The power of social categorization to undermine more positive peace-promoting behaviors is most apparent at the intergroup level of analysis, where social categorization processes are foundational in identity-based conflicts between groups. Kelman (1999) notes, for instance, that some of the most intractable conflicts in the world are characterized by social identities that are negatively interdependent, such that the assertion of one group's identity negates the other group's identity. Social categorization can also be seen in intergroup conflicts that occur when groups have overlapping territorial self-images, with each side claiming a sovereign right to the territory in dispute (Liu and Paez 2012).

Viewed within a developmental framework, the categorization of "us and them" is a fundamental and universal process in humans. In his classic work on prejudice, Allport (1954:20) notes:

> The human mind must think with the aid of categories....Once formed, categories are the basis for normal prejudgment. We cannot possibly avoid this process. Orderly living depends on it.

Infants become aware of social categories and exhibit visual preferences for members who belong to their own social category (own-race) by three months of age (Kelly et al. 2005). Importantly, these preferences are not observable at birth. Moreover, infants who have considerable cross-race exposure during the first few months after birth do not show same-race bias (Bar-Haim et al. 2006). These findings indicate that own-race preference is learned and likely due to differential exposure to one's own race versus others.

As children begin to engage in self-categorization, the potential for excluding others on the basis of social category membership becomes an important consideration for interpersonal peace and a sense of social justice. Self-categorization produces an in-group bias in which there is a preference favoring one's own group over out-group members (Brewer 1999). In-group bias has been demonstrated in numerous "minimal cue experiments" designed so that individuals are classified and groups are formed on the basis of some minor, artificial, distinguishing feature, such as the color of one's hat (e.g., randomly chosen red hats versus blue hats). Under certain conditions, the in-group bias can lay the foundation for prejudice toward others.

The early development of an in-group bias combined with the development of prejudice underscores the importance of the early childhood period. Research findings indicate that racial out-group attitudes either remain stable through middle childhood and adulthood or become even more negative (Nesdale 2008). Clearly, children's sense of morality is shaped in large part by social category awareness, combined with attachment and identification with peer group norms of inclusion or exclusion—all of which takes place by the time children are eight years old. When considering equity in human relations, children must somehow navigate between the force of moral principles and group identity.

Children sometimes exclude others when their skill set does not match the task at hand, not because of antipathy. However, when social exclusion is accompanied by prejudice, the situation is ripe for conflict and violence. Prejudice is typically defined as negative evaluations of others, because of the social groups to which they belong (Brown 2011); this contrasts with in-group bias, which refers to bias in favor of one's own group over out-groups (Brewer 1999).

Importantly, while in-group bias is consistently activated whenever social identities are constructed, in-group favoritism does not have to be accompanied by out-group derogation (Brewer 1999). A rather dramatic example of the independence of in-group favoritism and out-group derogation was demonstrated in factor analytic research with college students, where "patriotism" and "nationalism" were shown to be independent constructs (Kosterman and Feshbach 1989): love of country (patriotism) does not require enmity toward others (nationalism). For children, negative attitudes toward out-group members can be activated by a host of variables, including the strength of their ethnic identification, the degree to which the in-group norms denigrate or exclude out-group members, and whether or not the out-group is perceived as a threat to social identity (Killen and Rutland 2011).

The malleability of social exclusion and out-group prejudice has been demonstrated in numerous studies designed to encourage children to develop a common in-group identity (e.g., shared school, community, or national identity) that effectively reduces bias against members of other ethnic groups (Cameron et al. 2006). In addition to reducing bias and increasing positive evaluations of out-group members, a common in-group identity has been shown to increase trust, forgiveness, and helpfulness (Dovidio et al. 2009). In a demonstration of the common in-group identity model, Jewish students were more willing to forgive Germans for the Holocaust and decreased their expectation that Germans should feel collective guilt when category membership was increased from intergroup (us and them) to the level of common humanity (Wohl and Branscombe 2005).

In a carefully designed meta-analytic study, Pettigrew and Tropp (2006) found that higher levels of intergroup contact are associated with lower levels of intergroup prejudice. This effect can be enhanced when Allport's (1954) four primary conditions are met; that is, when contact is cooperative, between equal status groups, supported by institutional authorities, and based on common goals. In addition, because intergroup friendships have been found to have a powerful influence on the reduction of prejudice, Pettigrew (1998:76) added a fifth condition to the contact hypothesis, noting that the "contact situation must provide the participants with the opportunity to become friends."

Cross-group friendships are characterized by close personal relationships in which individuals are free to share intimate information (e.g., points of view, feelings, and desires). Research evidence indicates that both implicit and explicit forms of prejudice can be reduced through cross-group friendships, and some mechanisms involved include empathy, trust, self-disclosure, and the reduction of intergroup anxiety (Turner et al. 2007). Knowing that other in-group members have experienced positive contacts with out-group members can motivate in-group members to have more positive attitudes toward out-group members (Wright et al. 1997). In light of the "extended contact" effects of knowing someone who has a friend in the out-group, it is perhaps not surprising that children who experience extended contact vicariously, through stories, report an increase in positive attitudes toward out-group members (Cameron et al. 2006).

Taken together, research findings on the development of inclusion and a social justice orientation indicate that children's understanding of morality changes from concrete moral principles that emphasize sharing, turn-taking, and not inflicting physical harm, to more abstract moral principles that emerge in adolescence and take into account contextual considerations such as the individual's intention, the group's power and status, as well as the traditions, customs, and rituals of a society (Killen and Rutland 2011). As children develop, their foundation for a life in pursuit of social justice would seem most likely if they are raised with an inductive approach, develop an accurate theory of mind, are exposed to conversations within the family that discourage exclusion and encourage inclusion as a principle of morality, have peers who similarly value inclusion, live in a society with norms of inclusion, develop an inclusive group identity, have direct contact with out-group members under conditions that enhance the intergroup contact effect, know of friends who have befriended out-group members, and are exposed to media that encourage an inclusive social justice orientation.

A Developmental Path to a Peace and Social Justice Orientation

Although we agree that there are multiple pathways to peace, in Figure 15.2 we propose a model developmental pathway that could lead to children capable of adopting a peace and social justice orientation toward out-group members. The model is based on our group's consensus and relevant research findings. In Figure 15.2, a cumulative process is proposed in which each foundation builds on the next over time. Beginning on the left, foundation 1 (maternal health, adequate nutrition, and other factors) results in healthy human development during the prenatal period. When foundation 1 is combined with responsive care, stimulation, and other factors depicted in foundation 2 during the infant and toddler period, the second developmental task is met: healthy primary relationships are constructed. Given healthy primary relationships, the next task

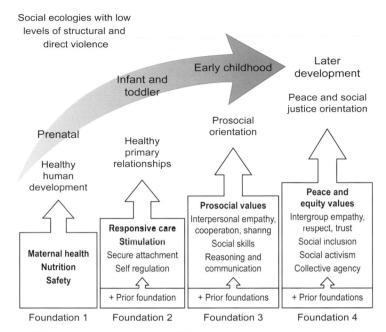

Figure 15.2   Model pathway for a child to develop an orientation toward peace and social justice as a function of targeted foundations and social ecologies. Boldfaced text denotes contributions of caregivers; normal typeface depicts contributions of the child.

to emerge during early childhood is a prosocial orientation toward others who comprise the children's in-group. Foundation 3 provides the requisite experience and skills for the child to engage in prosocial actions. Having realized a prosocial orientation toward in-group members in early childhood, the child is prepared to develop a peace and social justice orientation toward out-group members and will engage in the pursuit of relational harmony and equitable well-being if the requisite foundation is put in place (foundation 4).

In short, given a healthy start, children proceed to establish harmonious relations in primary relationships followed by prosocial interpersonal relationships in early childhood. A peace and social justice orientation lies beyond early childhood and requires the extension of harmonious relations and equity to out-group members. The model underscores the central importance of developmental timing in which interventions target the foundations that support specific developmental tasks. Each foundation is a window of opportunity for certain kinds of interventions. For example, prenatal interventions focus on nutrition as well as the mother's safety and well-being; interventions during infancy and toddlerhood promote secure attachments, self-regulation, and responsive and affectionate care; during early childhood, interventions are tailored to the child's development of interpersonal competencies and skills; thereafter, emphasis is on competencies, skills, and values that support the creation, maintenance, and restoration of harmonious intergroup relations combined with an orientation toward equitable well-being.

Any path toward a peace and social justice orientation is necessarily embedded within a larger geohistorical context, depicted as social ecologies above the arrow. For optimal development, social ecologies should have a low level of structural and direct forms of violence. Moreover, interventions to promote peace can be tailored to the particular set of challenges posed by varying geohistorical contexts. For instance, children and youth growing up in socially unjust geohistorical contexts may associate peace with emancipatory agendas and not so much inner peace (Christie et al. 2008). Below we describe in more detail the social ecologies and foundations that support a path to peace.

Foundation 1: Healthy Human Development

Whether or not children are on a peaceful developmental trajectory is largely a function of foundations and social ecologies. In socioecological contexts marked by resource scarcity, inequity, and inefficiencies, the primary task is to cobble together a foundation that supports healthy human development (foundation 1). Under these conditions, interventions for healthy human development typically target prenatal care, nutrition programs, and the development of caregiver skills that can result in physical, cognitive and socioemotional gains (Kagitcibasi et al. 2009), though admittedly these programs are small steps in the face of structurally driven inequalities.

The task of building foundation 1 is not limited to low-income countries. In recent years, income inequality has surged in high-income countries, and efforts to level the playing field are ongoing (e.g., through early childhood programs such as Head Start in the United States). From a global perspective, the rapid growth in many developing countries over recent decades has resulted in a substantial reduction in poverty and inequality, despite increased inequalities within many countries (Rodrik 2014; Behrman and Kohler 2014).

Foundation 2: Interventions for Emotion Regulation and Healthy Primary Relationships

In some geohistorical contexts, the focal task is to restore children's primary relationships within the family and community. For instance, for child soldiers a process of disarmament, demobilization, and reintegration (DDR) into their families and society is required (Betancourt et al. 2013a). This process and its cultural construction is most evident in a number of African countries, where purification rituals are used to exonerate child soldiers. These rituals serve to protect former child soldiers from the revenge of their victims' spirits and help reintegrate former soldiers into society (Honwana 1997).

For children in war zones or post-war contexts, interventions often target the child's emotional well-being. For example, following highly disruptive events, practices such as expressive arts and play activities are commonly used to ameliorate stress, distress, and trauma in young children. Researchers and practitioners agree that the key is to adapt interventions to the child's capabilities and to acknowledge the child's interpretation of reality without superimposing an adult-centered resolution of issues (Lacroix et al. 2007).

Another example of an intervention aimed at promoting emotional well-being was implemented during the Israel-Lebanon war (Sadeh et al. 2008). For a group of children, aged two to seven years, who displayed severe stress reactions, an experimental cohort was given toy puppies. The children were asked to protect and care for the puppies whenever they themselves felt anxiety and distress. In comparison to control groups, the children who received the toys showed significant reductions in stress reactions, up to three weeks after the end of the war. Sadeh et al. (2008) conclude that *Huggy Puppy* is a cost effective intervention for young children experiencing highly stressful circumstances.

Similar approaches have been applied in the wake of natural disasters. Dugan et al. (2010) reported that children aged four years and above, who presented with severe symptoms of distress following Hurricane Katrina, were able to regain a sense of control and safety through the use of toys and role-playing. Similarly, following the Pakistan earthquake of 2005, children engaged in art-based activities and communicated their feelings, an activity that reportedly facilitated the healing of emotional trauma (Ahmed and Siddiqi 2006). In a related study following the earthquake in Taiwan, 8- to 12-year-old children who were exposed to art and play activities scored significantly lower on anxiety level and suicide risk than did children in a control group (Shen 2002).

Foundation 3: Social Skills and Prosocial Orientation

In relatively peaceful contexts, interventions are often designed to enhance children's skills in managing interpersonal conflicts constructively. Not surprisingly, conflict resolution skills are often emphasized in programs. For example, Vestal and Jones (2004) provided evidence for the effectiveness of a 40-hour teacher-training course in conflict management and problem solving with preschool children. Following the program, children exhibited increases in prosocial behavior and used fewer forceful solutions to solve interpersonal problems than children whose teachers were in a control group that did not receive training. In another intervention, teachers were offered a series of seven one-hour training sessions that targeted socioemotional problem solving and positive communication strategies for students in kindergarten and first grade. Posttest results yielded significant decreases in verbal and physical aggression in children who participated in the program (Heydenberk and Heydenberk 2007).

In high-income countries that are status-quo powers and occupy the top of the global economic hierarchy, peace in children is often associated with efforts to promote harmonious relations through school-based programs that foster socioemotional development. Most of these programs emphasize some combinations of self and social awareness, self-regulation, relationship skills, and responsible decision making (Greenberg et al. 2003). To a large extent, foundation 3 and its implications for programming to enhance a prosocial orientation are based on findings from research in high-income countries.

Foundation 4: Fostering an Orientation toward Intergroup Peace and Social Justice

When children are embedded in social ecologies characterized by intergroup conflicts and episodes of violence, the intervention of choice is to bring together groups in conflict and work toward improved relations. One example is the program Media Initiative for Children Respecting Difference, a preschool program developed to address the problem of segregation and hostility that marks the daily experiences of children (aged 3 and 4 years) in Northern Ireland. The initiative incorporates nationwide televised cartoons with messages of inclusion along with numerous activities focusing on tolerance and respect for diversity. Parents and community agents take part in the workshops, and toys and materials are sent into the homes to ensure continuity. A large-scale random control trial showed that the intervention resulted in increased empathy, prosocial behavior, and social problem solving in children. The intervention has been extended down to two-year-olds and up to the age of seven (Connolly 2011).

In other contexts characterized by deep fault lines between identity groups, interventions typically focus on encouraging children to develop empathy for the other. Stephan and Finlay (1999) reviewed a number of school-based programs that have been designed to encourage empathy and improve intergroup relations in children. Examples include:

1. The "jigsaw classroom" in which children from various identity-based groups are brought together to work in an interdependent fashion to achieve a common goal.
2. Dialog sessions in which members of various social groups seek to understand each other's viewpoint on a range of issues.
3. Applications of the "contact hypothesis" (Allport 1954; Pettigrew and Tropp 2006) in which equal status groups are brought together and engage in cooperative actions aimed at common goals in a context supported by institutional authorities.
4. Multicultural education programs that typically include instructional materials describing various ethnic groups and encourage perspective taking.

Although Stephan and Findlay (1999) emphasize the mediating role of empathy at the individual level of analysis, there also is evidence that the establishment of antibias norms in the classroom contributes to the improvement of intergroup relations (Verkuyten and Thijs 2013).

Many of the interventions discussed thus far focus on the harmonious feature of peace which emphasizes the development of competence or skills in inner, interpersonal, or intergroup peace. The notion of the child as an active agent of social change in pursuit of more egalitarian societal arrangements is largely missing from these constructions. Yet children's development of a "critical consciousness," by which is meant their awareness of inequalities, takes place in early childhood. Moreover, there is evidence that children are able to engage in praxis (i.e., they can take action on perceived inequities as early as four to five years old). For example, in one study that took place in Canada, kindergarten children learned that their principal thought they were too young to be included in a school-wide event. Their exclusion prompted them to survey other kindergarten classes and petition the principal to allow their participation (Vasquez 2004).

Simon (2010) cites a number of instances of social activism among children (typically between 8 and 11 years old), which range from protest over the lack of activities from which to choose during recess to desegregating the male and female seating arrangements in the lunchroom. In most of the instances cited, the children involved in activism were learning about social justice in the classroom.

The importance of nurturing the child's sense of social injustice combined with a nonviolent orientation is most apparent in geohistorical contexts that regard the notion of "peace" as suspect. For instance, in South and Southeast Asia, Latin America, and parts of Africa, the term "peace" is associated with pacifism and oppression under colonial rule (Montiel and Noor 2009). Imperial powers used "divide and rule" policies that left in their wake interethnic fault lines and authoritarian regimes that persist to this day (Noor 2009). Under such conditions, the pursuit of a sustainable form of peace is associated with democratization movements, economic prosperity, and rule of law (Montero and Sonn 2009). Intergroup power differences in other parts of the world, such as the Middle East, are also ripe for the development of emancipatory agendas. The zero-sum, existential, and seemingly intractable nature of Middle East conflicts (Bar-Tal 2007; Coleman 2003) underscores the importance of generational change in which children and youth develop a sense of agency and exploit the power of nonviolent approaches to social justice.

As a general principle, children growing up in deeply divided societies are likely to develop oppositional social identities. Hence, the path to peace means somehow negotiating social identities in ways that are more inclusive and tolerant.

Similarly, identity-based conflicts remain prominent in contexts marked by genocides, such as in the former Yugoslavia (Simic et al. 2012) and Rwanda (Staub et al. 2005), where the path to peace involves identity issues combined with reconciliation processes to restore intergroup harmony. Intergroup reconciliation is also a crucial concern in South Africa—a country that has undergone a democratic transition with the dismantling of apartheid but which continues to grapple with transitional justice (Hamber 2009), especially in the economic sphere (Marais 2001).

To date, little attention has been given to children's social activism, perhaps due to the faulty assumption that children do not engage in praxis or perhaps because activism by children is often misinterpreted as negative behavior (Simon 2010). For instance, Norton et al. (2005) described the refusal of a seven-year-old child to sit on a dirty rug with classmates. While school authorities interpreted the child's refusal as a behavior problem, closer examination revealed that the refusal was because the child's family had limited access to laundry facilities. As Norton et al. (2005:121) put it: the child's resistance to the policy "makes visible the realities of poor children who have different life experiences than children and/or teachers with money."

Directions for Future Research

In this chapter, we suggest that there is a sequence of foundations that build upon one another and culminate in a *peaceful* child who has internalized the values of nonviolence and social justice: healthy human development (foundation 1) undergirds healthy primary relationships (foundation 2), which in turn provide the scaffolding for the child to engage in prosocial behavior toward others (foundation 3), followed by a peace and social justice orientation toward out-group members (foundation 4). Although research efforts have identified many of the variables that contribute to each of these foundations, the links between foundations are tenuous. Of particular importance for the development of peaceful children are linkages between the prosocial child and the peaceful child: How is the development of a prosocial orientation related to the child's competence and skills in extending the scope of prosocial actions to those who fall outside the child's identity group?

In reference to interventions that specifically target foundation 4 (peace and social justice orientation), research evidence underscores the importance of designing programs that increase the child's positive attitudes toward others and reduce intergroup bias and aggression as well as socially exclusive practices such as gang membership.

Another issue is the question of multiple pathways to peace. We have proposed one path, based on our consensus and extant research, much of which originates in the West. A potentially fruitful program of research would be to identify other pathways that are more nuanced and varied, as a function of the geohistorical contexts in which children are embedded.

We also have suggested that sustainable peace requires the pursuit of both relational harmony and equitable well-being. There is a fair amount of scholarly inquiry into the antecedents of relational harmony, especially in research on conflict resolution skills in children. However, there has not been a commensurate amount of research on children's awakening sense of social injustice and internalization of the value of equitable well-being for all. Emphasis on relational harmony runs the risk of implementing interventions that pacify children who are embedded in socially unjust circumstances. Thus an important research question arises: What kinds of social ecologies foster the development of a critical consciousness and tendency toward nonviolent social justice activism in children?

In addition to exploring the development of critical consciousness in children, it remains unclear whether the child's developing sense of social justice is related to peace. To what extent are the constructs of equitable well-being and relational harmony orthogonally related? Do they have similar antecedents and consequences? Does emphasis placed on one affect the other and if so in what direction and to what extent? What are the moderating and mediating variables for each of these constructs?

There also are gaps in the research literature in terms of the relational harmony dimension of peace. While there has been some research on children's acquisition of conflict resolution skills to maintain relational harmony, there is a paucity of research on the development of forgiveness in children and the skills involved in restoring harmony in relationships. Finally, what are the neurobiological mechanisms associated with empathy, a capacity which underlies the pursuit of relational harmony and equitable well-being for all? Related research questions include distinctions between the neural signatures associated with cognitive versus affective empathy, intragroup versus intergroup empathy, and relational harmony versus equitable well-being.

A practical question also arises: Why should a society value and invest in children's acquisition of a peaceful and socially just disposition?

Conclusions

It seems unlikely that societies will support research and intervention programs designed to encourage children to be peaceful unless there are strong indications of societal benefits. At present, we do not know the societal benefits of interventions that increase the likelihood of children developing competencies and skills to create, maintain, and restore harmony and equity in relationships. For any discussion of societal benefits, a requisite question arises: How can the measurement of *peaceful* child development be improved so that programs intentionally designed to encourage the development of peaceful children can be meaningfully evaluated?

Some examples of measurable and beneficial societal outcomes that could be examined include violent behavior within the family as well as cooperative and helping behaviors. In the school context, indices of peace could include the degree to which there are reductions in aggressive behavior, both verbal and physical, decreases in bullying behavior, and an overall change in the cascade of negative outcomes including school failure, dropping out, and engaging in crime. A positive cascade might include an increase in empathic responses during early childhood followed by higher levels of sharing, cooperation, and helping behavior in school settings along with increases in achievement, school attachment, attendance, leadership activities, and school completion. Effective interventions aimed at enhancing a peace and social justice orientation should increase positive attitudes toward others, reduce intergroup bias and aggression as well as socially exclusive practices such as gang membership.

A carefully designed benefit to cost assessment of research and intervention programs is needed. Costs include the private and public resource costs, including the time costs for service providers, family members, and others. Costs will increase as trained personnel and targeted components are added to intervention programs, but so, too, could the benefits. With explicit cost-benefit ratios, the case for incorporating justice and peace interventions might well be strengthened.

Finally, our proposed model (Figure 15.2) reflects an agentic perspective that places the child at the center of efforts to create harmonious relations and long-term changes in the access and distribution of resources necessary for equitable human well-being. By so doing, we are advocating research and intervention programs that target healthy human development and fully engage children to be part of a long-term solution. Our approach also encourages children to listen to their awakening sense of social justice and take action to promote harmonious relations within the family and beyond. This kind of approach supports and encourages children to become an integral part of the process of transforming societies in ways that create a sustainable peace, at home, in the community, and on the global stage.

Program and Policy Implications

16

Interventions

What Has Worked and Why?

Cigdem Kagitcibasi and Pia R. Britto

Abstract

Early childhood interventions are implemented to make a difference in people's lives, but demonstrating how they *have* worked is a challenge. Because many programs reported in the literature are conducted in high-income countries, results are not representative or balanced. This chapter reviews the evidence obtained from a range of early childhood interventions designed to reduce violence and build peace, and the outcomes that were achieved in children and parents. Classic longitudinal as well as more nascent early childhood interventions are analyzed using a broad framework. These interventions focus on young children and families and are associated with peaceful outcomes at individual, family, and community levels. The mechanisms by which benefits contribute to the peaceful outcomes are unclear. However, at child and family levels, these outcomes are predictors of reduced violence and a culture of peace in adulthood. It is suggested that early experiences pave the way to positive outcomes later in life, and thus early interventions are important. Programmatic and policy-level strategies are proposed to link peacebuilding with early childhood behavior, and a call is made to improve the direct measurement of peace promotion outcomes.

Introduction

Promoting peace requires concerted action. Most early childhood interventions do not focus on peacebuilding and are not implemented by peace studies scholars, yet because such interventions promote skills and abilities linked to peacebuilding (e.g., reduction in aggression and violent behaviors), they have significant implications for peace.

Our basic premise in this chapter is that certain developmental pathways are conducive to peaceful orientations and peacebuilding. These pathways involve, for example, better executive function as well as increased communication skills, social competency, and empathy. Early childhood interventions can promote these pathways and, in turn, contribute to peace. Indeed, most early childhood interventions have implications for enhanced cognitive and socio-emotional development, which are child-level predictors of peace, as manifested in a child's ability to solve problems, to express emotions appropriately, and to show empathy. In this chapter we seek to make such implications clear so that pathways between early childhood interventions and peacebuilding can be mapped. This approach utilizes a "micro" concept of peace, considered mainly at the individual, interpersonal, and family/group levels.

Early childhood interventions are important and necessary for two basic reasons: (a) global inequalities exist in children's environments and opportunities, and (b) the period of early childhood is critical for human development (see, e.g., Steele et al., this volume). Overwhelming evidence of this has been provided by psychologists and child development specialists as well as neuroscientists, economists, and policy scientists. Traditionally, early childhood interventions serve two populations: the child and/or the adult caregiver (Britto et al. 2011). Though some would argue that all quality early childhood interventions involve parents, many center-based programs focus solely on the child. Here we consider early childhood interventions that involve parents and include a brief discussion of work involving children and institutional (preschools and schools) interventions, examining both home- and center-based interventions. We review early childhood interventions that are associated with intrafamily peacebuilding and violence reduction and the resulting outcomes for children, and draw implications for practice and policy.

We begin with a discussion of the conceptual frame used in our analyses of evidence and then provide an overview of the early childhood interventions and associated peacebuilding outcomes. We present a background to the interventions and their evaluations and examine the present state of affairs in early intervention research and applications. Implications for practice and policy are posited. Since most of the research stems from the United States, and reports of experience from the rest of the world (especially from the Majority World[1]) are limited, these findings are not generally applicable in all settings.

General Framework for Early Childhood Interventions

Early childhood interventions have existed for many years in North America and Europe; however, research on their long-term effects is not abundant in the literature. In the Majority World, demonstration of long-term effects has also been limited, but this situation is improving (Britto et al. 2013; Engle et al. 2011; Young 2002:195–218; Kagitcibasi 2007; Kagitcibasi et al. 2001, 2009; Kirpal 2002).

---

[1] Majority World refers to the majority of the world's population that live outside high-income Western countries.

Early childhood interventions include a range of programs and services which aim (a) to enhance the development and well-being of children during the early years of life and (b) to improve their family environments. These interventions encompass a range of programs across several dimensions, all of which need to be considered with regard to a program's goal-setting, scope, outcomes, and potential for going to scale and/or impacting policies. These dimensions include (Britto et al. 2011):

- age of the child (e.g., infancy, toddlers, preschool ages, extending into school ages),
- focus area (e.g., health, attachment, protection, violence prevention, education, the empowering of mothers and enhancement of their social capital, the engaging of fathers to be more active in child rearing),
- generation being served (e.g., children and/or parents),
- modality (e.g., home-based, center-based),
- structure (e.g., home visits, group meetings like the Mother Child Education Program in Turkey,[2] or one-on-one programs like the Nurse-Family Partnership Program[3]),
- duration, ranging from short-term to very long-term interventions,
- sponsorship (e.g., government, nongovernmental organizations, private for profit groups), and
- level of engagement or partnership with other relevant sectors (e.g., local government agencies versus national or international partnerships).

Given this complexity, we provide a framework within which the results presented in this chapter can be understood. We begin with a brief overview of the history of early childhood interventions and evaluations before discussing the conceptualization of outcomes associated with reduced violence and peacebuilding. Different studies are reviewed that have been able to evaluate outcomes longitudinally, compared to those that have more immediate-term outcomes predictive of peacebuilding. When outcomes are measured in early childhood as compared to adulthood, the association between outcomes and impact on peace tend to be less straightforward; this has implications for programming and policy.

Historical Background

Most early childhood interventions, and the subsequent research to evaluate these interventions, have been conducted in the United States with varying outcomes. Varied interpretations and policy recommendations followed, resulting in extended debate. Three stages of evaluation research in the United States can be identified (Kagitcibasi et al. 2009): The first was carried out in

---

[2] http://www.acev.org/en/ (accessed June 14, 2014).

[3] http://www.nursefamilypartnership.org/ (accessed June 14, 2014).

the 1960s during President Johnson's "war on poverty" initiative, particularly under Project Head Start. Expectations were unrealistically high: from raising IQs to decreasing poverty. The relatively meager findings during this stage led to great disappointment. Over time, initial gains from the intervention programs diminished, causing a serious setback. Only limited short-term evidence was available; however, on this basis, conclusions were drawn and policy recommendations made to discontinue investment in early education (Cicirelli et al. 1969; Smilansky and Nevo 1979).

Over the next two decades, the next wave of evaluation delivered a more positive outlook through the reporting of delayed gains and longer-term encouraging effects, such as lower school dropout rates, less grade repetition, and fewer referrals to special education (Berrueta-Clement et al. 1984; Lazar and Darlington 1982). Favorable effects on better school performance and social adjustment for at-risk children were generally accepted, and long-term risk prevention effects were noted (Campbell and Ramey 1994; Ramey and Ramey 1998; Reynolds et al. 1998; Yoshikawa 1994; Zigler et al. 1992).

A third stage in the 2000s added a comparative perspective, aiming to arrive at generalizable conclusions. Meta analyses (e.g., Blok et al. 2005) or comparisons of many programs (e.g., Young 2002: 145–194) were used. Recent reports on longer-term outcomes of a number of well-known American intervention research projects were also published: the High/Scope Perry Preschool Project (Schweinhart et al. 2005), the Chicago Longitudinal Study (Reynolds and Ou 2004), and the Abecedarian Project (Campbell et al. 2002). These studies reported longer-term school-related benefits (e.g., lower rates of school dropout and lower referral to special classes), higher educational attainment, and better overall adjustment in adulthood. Similarly, in a meta-analysis of sixty home-based intervention studies, Sweet and Appelbaum (2004) reported significant benefits. However, Blok et al. (2005), while corroborating cognitive gains, found low levels of gains in the socioemotional domain.

Outside of the United States, there are few evaluations of early childhood home- and center-based interventions. Two noteworthy studies should be mentioned. First, the Turkish Early Enrichment Project demonstrated overall sustained gains in cognitive development and school-related issues (e.g., better school performance and school adjustment, higher educational attainment, better cognitive functioning) as well as socioemotional benefits that carry over into later parenting and family skills (Kagitcibasi et al. 2001, 2009). Second, the Jamaica Study demonstrated long-term gains for early stimulation and nutrition interventions into adulthood, with respect to positive family functioning and higher economic earnings (Grantham-McGregor et al. 1991a). A compilation of research from the Majority World (Young 2002) provides reviews focused on the quality of group-based child care in early interventions and policy recommendations (Young 2002:195–218; Kirpal 2002). European research with ethnic minorities has yielded variable outcomes related to mother-child interaction (van Tuijl et al. 2001).

Outcomes Associated with Peace

Peacebuilding is the focus of our broad conceptual framework within which early childhood outcomes (in terms of cognitive, social, and emotional functioning) are considered, primarily at the level of the family. These outcomes are predictive of positive social functioning later in life. We define peacebuilding as the skills and processes needed to promote better interpersonal relations, resolve conflicts, and establish harmony. A wide range of dimensions are linked to peacebuilding, such as importance of identity, sense of belonging, respect for diversity, and sense of citizenship. These dimensions are not considered in the present discussion. Here, we focus on a specific set of individual orientations that have been measured, during the years of early childhood, as constructs of emotional, social, and cognitive development.

We hypothesize that executive function or the ability to control impulses can help inhibit inappropriate reactions to frustration and express appropriate emotions. Executive function is linked to a child's ability to solve problems, which is achieved by using information appropriately and consciously inhibiting impulsive behaviors (National Scientific Council on the Developing Child 2008; Garon et al. 2008). For example, children with higher executive function skills are less likely to act impulsively and react violently or aggressively. Furthermore, research has shown that the ability to suppress impulses can be seen as early as the first year of life (Kochanska et al. 1997).

Another set of outcomes is linked to empathy, perspective taking, and moral reasoning. These outcomes cut across the domains of emotional and cognitive development and are characterized by feelings of concern and a desire to alleviate distress in others (Knafo et al. 2009; Young et al. 1999). These aspects can, again, been seen in the first few years of life (Vaish et al. 2009). In keeping with a holistic conceptualization of child outcomes, behaviors expressed through aggression and bullying (a common form of violence in childhood) must also be considered. In children, even as early as three years of age, bullying and aggression have been noted in group settings, such as in preschool settings (Monks et al. 2005; Ostrov et al. 2004; Vlachou et al. 2011). Resolving behavioral problems, addressing aggression, helping children build conflict resolution skills and learn positive, empathetic, and constructive responses to difficult situations are all linked to violence reduction. Taken together, these outcomes offer insights into a conceptualization of early childhood development in relation to peacebuilding. Socialization promotes both the cognitive and the socioemotional steps that contribute to greater social competence and better interpersonal relations, both of which impact peacebuilding

The third dimension of our framework concerns the longitudinal nature of the outcomes from an intervention. Taking a life-course perspective, where early childhood is the foundation for later skills, abilities, and competencies, we examine the point in time at which life-course outcomes are measured. The evaluations reviewed fall into two categories: longitudinal studies of longer-term outcomes and an assessment of short- or immediate-term outcomes. For the most part, longitudinal studies have not specifically focused on peacebuilding or violence reduction. However, these studies permit adult outcomes to be measured that derive from interventions delivered early in life. The more immediate- or short-term evaluation studies, by contrast, examine outcomes that can be more readily linked to peace promotion, measured earlier in life.

Overview of the Literature

Longitudinal research with a "life span" perspective, though not common, has made its mark in the field of early childhood intervention. The importance of longitudinal studies lies in the comprehensive nature of long-term follow-ups, which cover a broad range of outcomes.

We begin with a discussion of three well-known interventions that were conducted in the United States: the High/Scope Perry Preschool Project (Schweinhart et al. 2005), the Chicago Longitudinal Study (Reynolds and Ou 2004), and the Abecedarian Project (Campbell et al. 2002). Designed to promote better cognitive functioning and long-term achievement, all three interventions targeted at-risk groups for cognitive development, educational attainment, and low levels of social participation and adjustment. Risks that were considered included delinquency and substance abuse in adolescence and young adulthood as well as social disadvantages associated with minority status, poverty, and discrimination. These projects aimed to promote cognitive and school-related benefits for children in disadvantaged contexts; they differed, however, in methodology and evaluation assessments. Although the methodology in some of these studies has been criticized (e.g., for small sample sizes), they have nonetheless shown that early enrichment and support can bring about long-term benefits. As such, they have led the way to investments in early childhood, a sensitive period of human development.

The High/Scope Perry Preschool Project studied long-term effects of an enriched preschool environment. In early adulthood, key findings were that High/Scope participants attained higher educational and economic status than the control group, had less involvement with crime, and a higher percentage of women participants achieved stable families. Later findings, through the age of 40 years (Schweinhart et al. 2005), demonstrated that these gains were sustained over time. The well-known calculation of cost-benefit ratio, 1 to 7, helped draw attention to the long-term economic benefits of center-based early childhood education as an effective model of intervention. Other studies have shown similar marked returns (e.g., Gertler et al. 2013; Kaytaz, unpublished).

A significant time-related finding from the High/Scope Perry Preschool Project was that some of the initial gains declined slightly during middle childhood, only to emerge again during adolescence and early adulthood. This finding points to the timing of the intervention effects. As mentioned earlier, this problem was encountered in the initial evaluations of Project Head Start, where the emergence of delayed gains rendered the original evaluations premature. Delayed effects have also been noted in other evaluations. Thus, the trajectories of gains must be calculated throughout the developmental span. From these three projects, this is evident only in the Abecedarian Project, where growth curves are examined in the cognitive domain (Campbell et al. 2002).

The Abecedarian Project involved long-term delivery of intensive multimodal intervention. It had a rather complex design with interventions at different developmental periods: infancy through early childhood only (preschool age intervention); school age intervention; combined preschool and school age intervention; and a no intervention control group. The Abecedarian Project was followed by Project CARE (Burchinal et al. 1997), which also included home visits together with center-based intervention. Evaluations of the Abecedarian Project point to gains in cognitive development, school achievement, and occupational status. However, social developmental benefits were more limited, exhibited mainly in lower levels of teenage pregnancy and substance abuse. Delinquency was not affected. Benefits from the preschool plus school age intervention surpassed the preschool age intervention; however, no advantage was seen over the school age intervention alone (Campbell et al. 2002).

The Chicago Longitudinal Study (Reynolds and Ou 2004) included a preschool intervention program with parent involvement. Family support was provided along with postprogram school support. The evaluation of the Chicago Longitudinal Study showed benefits in high school completion, low rates of special education and grade repetition as well as low crime rates.

Another large-scale intervention study conducted in the United States, the Infant Health and Development Program,[4] began in 1985. It has accompanied nearly 1,000 low birth weight, preterm infants from birth through the age of 18 years. The aim of the program is to enhance the cognitive, behavioral, and health status of low birth weight, premature infants so as to reduce later developmental problems. The program has had significant effects on cognitive and social development and lower risky behaviors, as compared to heavier birth weight infants (McCormick et al. 2006).

Moving beyond a discussion of U.S. interventions, we now turn to programs that have been implemented in the Majority World. The first program, the Turkish Early Enrichment Project (TEEP), addressed overall development as well as cognitive and achievement outcomes into adulthood; its interventions focused on children as well as on mothers and the family. The original four-year study (1983–1985) involved both center-based, preschool environmental enrichment as well as home-based mother training in an experimental

---

[4] http://www.socio.com/eipardd04.php (accessed June 14, 2014).

design (Kagitcibasi et al. 2001). Mothers were trained to support the over-all development of their preschool-aged children, including preparation for school. At the end of the original study, benefits were found in all spheres of development, cognition, school adjustment, school performance, and social acceptance by peers; in addition, higher levels of autonomy and less aggression were measured. In the tenth year of the program (1993), the first follow-up was conducted at the stage of adolescence: sustained benefits were found in cognitive development, school achievement, school attainment, socioemotional development, and social integration. Mothers and families continued to show benefits from the program as well, in terms of better family relations and increased intrafamily status for participating mothers. The second follow-up, carried out in young adulthood, revealed long-term benefits in educational attainment (including university education), cognitive performance, occupational status, and social participation for those young adults who had participated in the educational preschool program, or whose mothers had been trained, or both (Kagitcibasi et al. 2009). These results substantiate positive youth development into adulthood and better social integration—strengths that are conducive to peacebuilding. Based on these demonstrated benefits, TEEP led to the establishment of Mother Child Education Foundation (AÇEV), which has been implementing the Mother Child Education Program (a continuation of TEEP) in large numbers throughout Turkey and abroad.

The second program, popularly known as the Jamaica Study, has had a strong influence on the early child development literature. This study examined the impact of nutritional and psychosocial stimulation on stunted children between 9–24 months of age. Two years later, results showed that the strongest effects were achieved for children who received a combination of nutritional and psychosocial services, compared to children who received nutritional services only, psychosocial support only, or the control group (Grantham-McGregor et al. 1991a). Long-term positive results on adult functioning, achievement, and reduction in risky behaviors were also noted. Other research on the effects of early childhood intervention also point to similar gains related to health, cognitive development, and family relations (Grantham-McGregor et al. 2007; Hines et al. 2011; Walker et al. 2007, 2011). All of these benefits are relevant for peacebuilding.

From Projects to Programs and Policies

To date it is unclear how the benefits that children receive from early childhood interventions contribute to the creation of peaceful societies. From the longitudinal programs discussed above and select short-term programs presented below, possible programmatic and policy-level strategies can be proposed to link peacebuilding with early childhood behavior.

Implications of the Exemplary Studies

As discussed above, the U.S. studies, TEEP, and the Jamaica Study are examples of high-quality early childhood interventions. They share a number of common features, such as working with at-risk children, the involvement of parents (to varying degrees), the use of experimental designs, and the evaluation of long-term effects of the intervention. Importantly, they all demonstrate gains as a result of the early intervention. Most benefits concern school-based achievements, with some measured effects on occupational status. These benefits correspond well to the aims of the studies, which focused on better educational performance. In addition, social benefits were observed, such as better acceptance by peers, less crime, and reduced substance abuse.

In this sense, it may be claimed that these interventions were successful. The main viewpoint from these studies is that the early years of childhood hold particular significance in human development and that interventions conducted during this period can make a difference over time. These programs demonstrate that the lives of young children can be enhanced and that the benefits gained in one area of development can transfer to other areas as well as to other people in the family and the community. Younger siblings, for example, benefit from better parenting, even when the mother-support intervention focuses on an older child; peers also benefit and learn from a child's peaceful orientation (Kagitcibasi 2007). This point is particularly relevant for peacebuilding. Even though "peace" per se was not a direct goal of these studies, the gains achieved in cognitive, educational, and socioemotional areas had implications for peace. As young people develop higher cognitive skills, attain higher education, and are better integrated into society, they can expect to avoid risks and pursue more peaceful lifestyles.

Similarly, enhanced family and interpersonal relations can be generated, particularly through better communication skills, as exemplified by the mothers who participated in TEEP (Kagitcibasi et al. 2001). Thus it follows that intrafamily dynamics can be improved through such programs. Indeed, one of the significant side benefits from TEEP was better spousal relations and an increased status of the woman in the family (Kagitcibasi et al. 2001). A systemic approach, rather than one focused on the individual, would therefore be more appropriate in terms of devising intervention programs as well as in evaluating their impact. This is because changes in one element (member) of the family system can be expected to influence changes in the others and, in turn, the whole system.

Evaluations of effective interventions point to the potential value of engaging groups of mothers. By creating an awareness of a mother's significant role in enhancing their child's cognitive and socioemotional development, mothers become empowered and this contributes to the building of self-efficacy and social capital. Group engagement offers the promise of contributing to stronger and lasting effects as groups provide their members with support as information is exchanged and experiences are shared. The sense of belonging to a group coupled with the feeling of group support helps mothers persist in implementing more positive and "modern" parenting styles, sometimes over the objections of their traditional social environments (Kagitcibasi et al. 2001). Clearly, the potential of group engagement applies not only to groups of mothers but to fathers as well.

Short-Term Evaluation Studies

Several studies can be used to examine how peacebuilding (however measured) can be linked to early childhood. These studies are taken from a systematic review of the multidisciplinary literature over the past decade—a review that aimed at identifying different programmatic approaches that have been effective in reducing violence and promoting peace. An extensive set of search terms included, but was not limited to, early childhood and home-based parenting programs, which were used to search online databases across the social and natural sciences. The resulting articles were then screened according to PICO (population, intervention, comparison, and outcome) criteria, yielding a set of 64 papers. For the purposes of the present discussion, we have selected studies that used home-based and/or parenting programs and which measured child outcomes in areas associated with peace to permit comparisons to the early childhood interventions presented above (see Table 16.1). One criterion used to select papers was that child outcomes measured in the study must be linked to the conceptual framework for peacebuilding.

The articles fall into three categories based on their goals: (a) prevention of behavior problems (e.g., aggression), (b) improvement of intrafamily dynamics toward peaceful resolution of conflicts, and (c) implementation in contexts of war. These three categories are linked with our definition of peacebuilding, as they incorporate conflict reduction and promote harmonious relationships.

Prevention of Behavior Problems

In this category, we found three interventions. Two targeted the parents of toddlers (Toddlers without Tears and Early Head Start) and one focused on preschoolers (1-2-3 Magic). Four of the corresponding papers addressed reduction in behavior problems (Bayer et al. 2010; Bradley et al. 2003; Hiscock et al. 2008; Love et al. 2005). All of the interventions were conducted in high-income countries (Australia, Canada, and the United States) and were implemented through an existing health or community-based system.

Toddlers without Tears (Bayer et. al. 2010; Hiscock et. al. 2008) is a parent anticipatory guidance program delivered through the universal primary care system in Victoria, Australia, where health visits are scheduled at frequent, almost monthly, intervals for the first 24 months of a child's life. The take-up rate is over 90%. An intervention consists of three sessions which address unreasonable expectations, harsh parenting, and lack of nurturing parenting. The first session is part of a regular scheduled home visit, when a child is 8 months old; mothers receive literature on normative child development and ways to encourage language development. The next two sessions are group sessions at 12 and 15 months of age. Parents attend 2-hour group sessions aimed at discussing ways to develop warm, sensitive, and responsive parenting and encouraging desirable behaviors. The intervention is delivered by trained intervention nurses. The control families receive the normal treatment available as part of the health system, which covers child behavior problems but does not address parenting in early childhood. At 18 and 24 months, no differences were noted in children's behavioral outcomes (i.e., as reported by parents, externalizing behaviors were similar). Differences between intervention and control groups were, however, noted: less harsh parenting and less unreasonable expectations were exhibited by the intervention parents. The authors of the study conclude that the dose of this universal parenting program in primary care is insufficient to impact child behavior, although it has a modest impact on parenting behaviors.

1-2-3 Magic is a community-based service that offers a brief psychoeducational parenting program to parents of three- to four-year-old children in Canada (Bradley et al. 2003). The program focuses on promoting positive parenting behaviors and reducing parental yelling, hitting, and critical comments. Developed in a hospital setting, the program is delivered by trained community workers in community centers. The intervention strategy uses video-training complemented by facilitated group discussion. To strengthen learning, parents are given handouts after each of the three sessions. Even though the duration of this intervention was brief (three 2-hr group sessions, with a final follow-up meeting), it had immediate and continued effects (measured one year later) on reducing child behavior problems.

The Early Head Start program, in the United States, is a comprehensive second-generation federal program that focuses on improving child outcomes while strengthening families. It targets low-income families with infants and toddlers. Evaluation of the program was carried out across 17 program sites, serving over 3,000 families. Because of the wide range of program sites, specific implementations varied slightly; however, all programs were either home based, center based, or mixed home and center based. Here we focus on findings linked to peacebuilding, when children were three years old (Love et al. 2005). Results indicate that the children who participated in the intervention displayed higher emotional engagement with the parent, lower aggressive behavior, and more sustained attention to play objects compared to the control group. Parents who participated in the intervention demonstrated more emotionally supportive behavior and less harsh punishment toward their children, compared to the control group. The results appeared to be the strongest for programs that offered a mix of home-visiting and center-based services and which fully implemented the performance standards early.

Table 16.1 Overview of experimental evaluations in six early childhood interventions and their outcomes with implications for peace.

Program (country)	Toddlers without Tears (Australia)	1-2-3 Magic (Canada)	Early Head Start (U.S.A.)
N	733	70	3001
Target population	Parents of children 8–15 months	Families with preschool children	Participants from low-income families
Intervention	Anticipatory parental guidance	Parenting groups to prevent behavior problems and support effective discipline	Child development and strengthening families
Delivery setting	Health clinic	Community centers	Home based, center based, and mixed
Delivery format	Home visit or group session	Group sessions	Home visit and center-based care
Components	Individual counseling, printed materials, group discussions	Video and facilitated discussion	Individual counseling and parent education
Dosage	Three sessions: one home visit and two 2-hr group sessions	Three 2-hr group sessions, once a week; a final booster meeting 4 weeks after the last group session	Varied across the 17 sites Duration of enrollment: Home based: M = 22 months Center based: M = 1,400 hr/child Mixed: M = 23 months
Implementer	Trained nurse	Community worker	Varied: child care providers, community home visitors
Outcomes and findings	No impact on child outcomes; minimal impact on parenting, favoring intervention; decrease in self-reported harsh parenting and unreasonable expectations	Reduction in child problem behaviors, favoring intervention	Children exhibit higher emotional engagement with parent, sustained attention with play objects, and lower aggressive behavior, favoring the intervention
Reference	Bayer et al. (2010); Hiscock et al. (2008)	Bradley et al. (2003)	Love et al. (2005)

Table 16.1 (continued)

Program (country)	Parental Mediation (Canada)	Family Foundations (U.S.A.)	Huggy Puppy (Israel)
N	48	169	292
Target population	Families with young children	Families expecting their first child	Families in refugee camps
Intervention	Parental mediation of sibling disputes	Co-parental and spousal relationship, parental mental health, parent-child relationship, and child outcomes	Stress reduction post-conflict
Delivery setting	University based	University	Refugee camp
Delivery format	Parental training program	Groups	Individual child counseling
Components	Individual counseling sessions	Manualized parenting and couples counseling	Toy; psychosocial counseling; parental follow up
Dosage	Two sessions, 1 week apart	Eight sessions	One session
Implementer	Researcher	Researcher	Researcher
Outcomes and findings	Children felt empowered to solve conflicts using the mediation strategies, favoring the intervention	Reduction in child behavior problems and enhanced social competence, favoring the intervention	Significant reduction in child stress reaction, favoring the intervention
Reference	Siddiqui and Ross (2004)	Feinberg et al. (2010)	Sadeh et al. (2008)

Intrafamily Dynamics

Sibling conflicts constitute one of the foremost expressions of aggression in intrafamily dynamics and often require parental mediation to resolve the conflict. In this category of interventions, we found two programs. A short-term intervention program, Parental Mediation, focused on building skills and examined its impact on resolving sibling disputes (Siddiqui and Ross 2004). In this study, 48 families in Canada participated in two mediation training sessions, 1 week apart, whereby their children participated in the second session. Results of the content analyses of qualitative data from maternal diaries between the two sessions, observation of parent-child interaction, and parental interviews indicate that the intervention group mothers used mediation strategies, and that these strategies were favored by both mothers and children. Furthermore, children from the intervention group felt empowered to resolve conflict through the mediation strategies, in particular in the interaction between younger children and their older siblings. These are useful skills for peacebuilding.

A second program dedicated to family harmony and peace, Family Foundations in the United States, focused on improving the co-parental and spousal relationships, parental mental health, and the parent-child relationship, leading to child outcomes (Feinberg et. al. 2010). The program reached 169 couples who were living together and expecting their first child, and consisted of eight interactive sessions. These classes sought to strengthen the relationship between the couple, by enhancing their awareness of areas of co-parental disagreement around child rearing, and communication skills to manage disagreement and conflict. Three years later, results indicate that the intervention had a positive effect in terms of reducing behavior problems, particularly for the boys, and improving social competence for the children of the intervention family. The intervention also reduced parenting stress and the likelihood of using physical punishment. These results make a strong case for understanding the dynamics of family relationships as a pathway in the promotion of positive child outcomes linked with peacebuilding.

Implementations in Contexts of War and Conflict

The third category of interventions is associated with contexts that involve conflict, as there is an immediate need to implement interventions to alleviate psychosocial stress and trauma and promote long-term peace. The external validity of programs implemented in nonconflict situations to conflict situations is limited. Therefore, we also considered programs implemented in conflict areas to understand the implications for peacebuilding.

The intervention targets children aged two to seven years. Implemented in a refugee camp in southern Israel to help children deal with the stress of war (Sadeh et al. 2008), this cost-effective intervention consists primarily of giving a child a soft toy dog and explaining that the toy needs to be comforted by hugging it. Parents are asked to encourage their child to hug the soft toy after the counseling. Results of the intervention showed a significant reduction in the level of children's stress. A higher level of attachment and play with the soft toy was associated with better outcomes. This type of intervention provides insights into potential pathways for peacebuilding and may limit factors linked with aggression and depression later in life.

Engaging Fathers

Developmental scientists have known for many years that fathers play a central role in the development of their children. Thus, it stands to reason that peacebuilding efforts must also include the active participation of fathers. A recent systematic review of father engagement in early childhood interventions suggests that while few interventions focus on fathers, the results of involving fathers in parenting has beneficial impact on child outcomes and the caregiving environment (Panter-Brick et al. 2014a). Despite this recognition, interventions that target fathers have been sporadic and limited in scope. In addition to the disproportionate attention on mothers, there are practical difficulties in reaching the fathers which must still be resolved.

Current work with fathers, conducted in different locations, offers promise to remedy this situation. One such program is being implemented by the Mother Child Education Foundation (AÇEV) in Turkey and elsewhere. Preliminary evaluations of this father support program, which grew out of TEEP and the Mother Child Education Program (see above), show positive outcomes related to peace, such as better intrafamily and community relations as well as better relations with others of different ethnic or religious affiliations.[5]

Other programs have had significant impact on men's fathering role, even though this was not an explicit goal of the program. For example, in the Integrated Basic Education and Skills Training Program, underskilled and/or nonnative English-speaking young men are assisted in acquiring and sustaining employment in the state of Washington.[6] Such interventions can contribute to peacebuilding both in the family setting and beyond. However, studies are needed to analyze the pathways that underlie this process.

Implications of Short-Term Evaluation Studies for Peacebuilding

Inquiry into early childhood and peacebuilding is in its early stages. Only a limited body of literature addresses this relationship. In our review, we selected 64 studies from the literature, of which only seven measured child outcomes

---

[5] As reported by A. Kocak in an internal report (Evaluation of the Father Support Program, 2004), prepared for the Mother Child Education Foundation (ACEV).

[6] Washington's I-Best by J. Kerr: Paper presented at Transatlantic Forum on Inclusive Early Years, January 20–22, 2014.

in family-based interventions for nonclinical populations. Despite this small sample, the following implications can be drawn.

First, based on the programs that we reviewed, it appears that a strong service system, which includes equal access and training level of service providers, is required to implement effective programs. Most studies were implemented through an existing health or community-based system. By finding an entry point into a system, a program can be operationalized based on existing structures (e.g., service providers, locations or settings for service delivery). Partnering with government agencies or public institutions is likely to be valuable for all intervention programs. Such collaboration promises to contribute to the sustainability of the programs and to increase their potential for impacting policies.

Second, the degree of impact of the program appears to be linked to the dose of the intervention, and possibly with the age of the child. In line with the former, the Early Head Start program demonstrated the strongest impact when a mix of home-visiting and center-based services was utilized and when programs were fully implemented (Love et al. 2005). With respect to a child's age, two interventions were examined: Toddlers without Tears, for children under two years of age (Bayer et al. 2010; Hiscock et al. 2008) and 1-2-3 Magic for preschoolers (Bradley et al. 2003). While other factors may not have been reported (e.g., measurement of outcomes) or examined that could be linked to the results, we used a developmental perspective to analyze these results, given that the dose was fairly similar. Results were noted for older children, which could suggest that peacebuilding behaviors are easier to measure in older children. Alternatively, the higher cognitive competence of older children might also have been a contributing factor. These studies have implications for using a clear theoretical perspective on change to inform the intervention model. Studies which focused on family dynamics (Family Foundations, Feinberg et al. 2010; Parental Mediation, Siddiqui and Ross 2004) addressed relationships between family members through the intervention. These interventions provide insight into the reduction of violence in the home, as they were successful in reducing parenting stress and providing strategies for conflict resolution. Furthermore, the Parental Mediation intervention (Siddiqui and Ross 2004) positively impacted younger siblings in the family by empowering them to resolve conflicts with their older siblings in a peaceful manner.

Other intervention research concurs with the importance of the familial context. For example, interventions that have attempted to decrease conflict in families have tended to lessen harsh parenting and violence, especially involving the father (e.g., al-Hassan and Lansford 2010; Cowan et al. 2009). All of these studies are relevant to peacebuilding and early child development, as they validate the contextual approach to promoting change and provide guidance for future family-based programs. On the basis of this evidence, we may surmise that peacebuilding may require interventions that address the entire family.

Questions and Challenges

Early childhood research is limited by the lack of direct measurement of peace promotion outcomes. Conceptual links have been created between outcomes of better executive function, empathy, better communication, social skills, and reduced aggression and peacebuilding, because of the predictive links between these behaviors in early childhood and later adult social functioning. However, this conceptualization needs to be supported empirically in diverse contexts.

The conceptualization of peace is important (see the Foreword, this volume), in itself, since the very nature of peace permeates scholarship focus on the possible connections between early childhood and peacebuilding. Child development experts, psychologists, and others involved in early childhood interventions make use of individual and interpersonal levels of analysis. Accordingly, effective interventions involve the enhancement of individual socioemotional development (e.g., empathy, social competence, positive self-worth) so that more positive child outcomes and interpersonal relations, together with individual competence, better social adjustment, and success, can be achieved. Work with more specific reference to peacebuilding has mainly examined violence reduction and conflict resolution, again within the context of more direct person-to-person relationships. Yet peace is a far more encompassing concept that requires a broader set of linkages between outcomes and societal functioning. At this level, peace is contextual by definition. In particular, conceptualizations of peace in terms of structural violence, as advanced by Dawes and van der Merwe (this volume), emphasize the context but not the interpersonal level of analysis.

Can we address peace, construed as a macro concept, using a micro approach? Or are we "psychologizing" if we view early childhood as a possible path to peace?

Scholars who study phenomena such as "honor cultures," poverty, war, and conflicting economic-political interests tend to ask this question. A satisfactory answer requires sound empirical evidence regarding the micro-macro linkages. In this chapter, we have endeavored to present such evidence, but we admit that it is not extensive; assumptions were needed regarding the relevance that positive outcomes (evidenced in the evaluations of the interventions) have for peace. For example, we assume that benefits created by early childhood intervention (e.g., higher cognitive performance, school attainment, educational achievement, better social adjustment, less crime and delinquency, higher earnings) lead to more peaceful outlooks on life.

Some interdisciplinary perspectives on peace also point to the need to consider interacting multilayered factors. For example, intersections of individual orientations (e.g., tolerance vs. hatred) and institutional or social structural factors (e.g., social norms and legal or educational systems) are often examined from multidisciplinary perspectives, in particular, in peace education (e.g., Bar-Tal 2013; Bekerman and Zembylas 2011; Noddings 2012). What we add here is a "developmental stance": Early experiences pave the way to later outcomes and thus early interventions are important. Although our approach may be seen as micro, we strongly endorse a contextual perspective. This is clearly evident in our focus on caretakers or parents and the home environment as the key to the enhancement of peaceful orientations in the growing child as well as peaceful relations and values in the family and beyond.

Over the past two decades, research into early childhood has demonstrated its value for social and economic development. Until recently, linking the formative years of life and economic returns was considered far-fetched. However, rigorous analyses by economists have shown the strong association and high returns on investment in early childhood. As we embarked on our analyses of the connection between early childhood intervention and peace, we began to chart a new direction in the literature linking early childhood with peace studies, akin to the early processes that linked child development to macro economics. We are at the stage of our examination where hypotheses are being generated and tested to a limited extent. Preliminary results appear to be in the direction of predicting an association between early childhood interventions and building a culture of peace. However, the analytical distance still needs to be travelled to produce credible findings that will unequivocally link what we do with young children and families to building peaceful societies.

17

Linking Peacebuilding and Child Development

A Basic Framework

Mohammed Abu-Nimer and Ilham Nasser

Abstract

This chapter addresses debates in the field of peacebuilding, with a focus on conflict resolution and peace education. Strategies in conflict resolution and peace education which can be applied as mechanisms to promote peace-oriented behaviors in young children are shared. Peace education studies conducted in the early years of life are reviewed and a call for investment in education programs that promote healthy children in peaceful communities is advocated. This chapter encourages dialog on best methods and strategies to utilize the knowledge in peacebuilding and conflict resolution in early childhood development.

Introduction

According to the seventh Secretary General of the United Nations, Kofi Annan, three factors must exist for a state to prosper: peace and stability, economic development, and rule of law. There is a need to create this environment of peace and sound governance as well as promote economic development to build nations and sustain them.[1] In this chapter, we examine ways to transform knowledge accumulated from the field of peacebuilding into developmental pathways in early childhood, the period of rapid growth when building a peaceful foundation is critical yet possible.

---

[1] Kofi Annan in a recent public presentation on peacebuilding in Africa (Initiative for Change Annual Conference, Caux, Switzerland, on July 24, 2013).

Early Child Development: Influences and Debates

In the early childhood development field, there have been few documented studies conducted to investigate the connections between childhood as a critical period of growth and peacebuilding and peace education. In addition, there is no clear evidence of the role that caregivers (parents, family members, and caregivers from day-care centers and preschools) play in instilling values such as peace and conflict resolution in the children under their care. There is, however, evidence for the opposite: parents have an impact on children's understanding of wars (Deng 2012). In communities where physical or cyber bullying exists at home or in schools, or in cases where military occupation and/or policies trigger or perpetuate violence against ethnic and national groups, the need for peace education and the development of a peaceful agenda in early childhood is critical. The initial goal of such an agenda must be to protect the rights of children, especially the fulfillment of their basic needs (in particular, the need for food, shelter, safety, and security).

Thus far, a body of knowledge in child development research confirms that creating environments which are supportive, secure, and stimulating in the home and early childhood settings has a huge impact on the healthy development of the young brain. Those conditions are also critical for learning and the development of cognitive abilities (Fox et al., this volume). Recent accumulated knowledge suggests an individual is shaped by internal, physical, as well as external sets of social and environmental factors. The nature-nurture debate has been settled by recent advances in brain research; the early childhood years are understood to be complex and dynamic, affected by multiple layers and actors (Preskill et al. 2013; Carter and Porges, this volume; Keverne, this volume).

Nevertheless, traditional Western theorists who are inspired by the work of developmental theorists such as Piaget, Erikson, and others continue to focus on the individual while others, such as ecological theorists, focus on the contexts of growth and the holistic development of the child. According to ecological theorists such as Bronfernbrenner (1979), the child operates within multiple contexts and influences, starting with the home, school, and community and extending to distal influences such as historic and political events. In addition, the individual is constantly interacting with people who, in turn, exert direct and indirect effects on the individual through their interactions within the different systems (De Abreu 2000). Examples of mental health issues and cultural revolutions after World War II in Europe and the Great Depression in the United States illustrate the power of context on an individual's development. Despite advances in the neurosciences and increased evidence for the biological and genetic bases of growth and behavioral patterns, we are still looking at a field that is impacted by complex and fragmented layers—one in need of connectors, such as family variables and relationships, to ensure healthy childhood development (Preskill et.al. 2013).

Whether a person is motivated by internal or external forces or whether it is our biological makeup (including brain functions and hormones) that impacts our behaviors, education plays an undeniable role in shaping and forming the citizens of tomorrow. Education can provide spaces for establishing those connectors between the multiple players in the life of the young child. It can play a key role in changing minds and hearts and in providing options that are not necessarily available at home or in the community, especially in conflict areas. Such a claim has been supported by influential philosophers in education and psychology, such as Dewey (1938) and Vygotsky (1978), and their writings on the power of education in creating a new generation of productive citizens and the emphasis on learning with others. Gardner's multiple intelligences theory (Gardner 1983), and its emphasis on the multiple ways that people of different minds and cultures express their intelligences, adds to this assertion.

Two major questions remain: What are the most influential factors that influence children to choose nonviolent behaviors and embrace a peaceful way to address conflicts? Are peaceful behaviors innate and biologically motivated (for details on oxytocin and its impact on infants, see Carter and Porges, this volume), or are they learned behaviors?

As an emerging field of academic practice, peacebuilding can offer direction and guidance to reaching states of peace and stability in various communities. In addition, it addresses knowledge and skills required to promote peace in early childhood settings. In this present discussion, we are not ignoring the existence of destructive and violent behaviors in childhood, but rather choose to focus on the area of peacebuilding and peace education for the purpose of this volume.

A Peacebuilding Framework

As a working definition and for the purpose of this chapter, peacebuilding is used as a broad conceptual term to include theories, processes of conflict management, resolution, transformation, nonviolence strategies, and peace education. Thus, in this context, peacebuilding refers to any form of intervention carried out in response to a perceived conflict situation. Such a broad definition includes activities aimed at prevention of conflict, settlement, and management of violent and crisis situations, as well as processes aimed at reconciliation after the signing of an agreement (or postconflict reality). (For further definitions of peace, see the Foreword, Leckman et al., and Britto, Gordon et al., this volume.)

In educating for peace in formal and informal education settings, it is important to clarify the framework that guides the peacebuilding process. A number of principles serve as basic assumptions in the field of peacebuilding, and these should guide all intervention programs—home- or school-based (assuming that early years expand into formal schooling)—in promoting the development of social emotional skills in children:

- *Conflict is an integral part of human life.* This assumption asserts that human differences (both natural and constructed) constitute a base for conflict to emerge. Conflict is defined as a situation in which one or more parties perceive their goals to be incompatible. If conflict is inevitable whenever humans live together, the question then becomes: How can conflicts be addressed constructively and nonviolently?
- *Conflicts can be resolved in nonviolent ways.* Research and experience from the field of conflict resolution provides ample evidence to suggest that conflicts on various levels (individual, family, community, ethnic, and international) can be settled and resolved without necessarily resorting to the use of violent force. Similarly, the field of peacebuilding has generated enough knowledge and evidence to argue that the deployment of violence in resolving conflicts may actually perpetuate violent conflict, producing a reality of winners and losers, and causing a large degree of human and structural destruction.
- *Cooperation is more effective and less costly than avoidance, competition, or accommodation in resolving conflicts.* The field of conflict resolution relies on facilitating and creating constructive engagement between disputing parties by utilizing cooperative tools instead of their existing competitive modes of interaction.
- *Addressing the root causes of a conflict is a necessary step in resolving it.* There are a number of deep-rooted conflicts that are generated and sustained by inadequate and unjust structures or systems. The cause of many conflicts is rooted in and perpetuated by these systems (legal, social, political, economic). Effective conflict resolution processes and frameworks require ways to address these systems and construct alternatives.
- *Conflict resolution processes should address the asymmetric power relations among parties.* The imbalance of power among conflicting parties is often one of the major factors or causes for generating conflicts; it is also a major factor in perpetuating a reality of violence. Thus conflict resolution processes ought to be based on the assumption that all parties to the conflict should feel empowered in the process of resolution and should challenge the power differentials maintained by systemic inequities.
- *Conflict resolution can bring about structural social and political changes* (Abu-Nimer 1999). Processes of peacebuilding are aimed at generating new conditions under which all parties feel that their goals and objectives have been met. Such change in perception among the parties cannot be sustained without adjusting and, in some cases, replacing existing structures. Thus one of the necessary outcomes of conflict resolution is the change in systems (such as social, political, economic, and legal).

- *Safe spaces for dialogical learning must be generated when conflict resolution models are implemented.* In any given conflict relationship, safe spaces are essential to break the cycle of violence and dehumanization that characterizes relationships between adversaries. Constructing these dialogical spaces is a crucial step in building new relationships across conflict divides.

Based on the above and borrowing from some of the main ideas in peacebuilding, one can advocate for an early childhood development and education agenda and corresponding programs that accept conflicts as part of life and promote collaboration instead of competition in early childhood settings (Crawford 2005). Very often, and in some cultures, avoidance of conflicts is preferred and encouraged; in still others, the context and macro systems do not allow for the avoidance of political and social conflicts (Deng 2012). Training caregivers to "deal with" and address conflicts as part of life is a crucial step forward. There are curriculums and programs that teach children how to address conflicts; when scaled up, they might become more impactful and measurable (for examples of peace education programs, see Nusseibeh as well as Kagitcibasi and Britto, this volume).

Promoting Peace Education in Early Years

Peace education is defined by UNICEF as "the process of promoting the knowledge, skills, attitudes, and values needed to bring about behavior changes that will enable children, youths and adults to prevent conflict and violence, both overt and structural; to resolve conflict peacefully; and to create the conditions conducive to peace, whether at an intrapersonal, interpersonal, inter-group, national or international level."[2] Peace education is based on a philosophy that teaches nonviolence, love, compassion, trust, fairness, cooperation, and reverence for the human family and all life on our planet. Some of the associated skills include communication, listening, perspective taking, cooperation, problem solving, critical thinking, decision making, conflict resolution, and social responsibility.

Introducing peace education to children as early as preschool age can be a powerful conflict and violence prevention tool; it has the potential to save many communities from a great deal of suffering and victimization. When accompanied by child-centered pedagogy, peace education is an effective tool in the promotion of peace in communities (Connolly and Hayden 2007). Integrating peace education values and practices at this early age can break both the cycle of violence and habituated system of conflict that have been transmitted between generations. In the area of peacebuilding and human rights, the development of a peace education research and practice agenda (formal and informal)

---

[2] http://www.unicef.org/education/files/PeaceEducation.pdf (accessed May 23, 2014).

has already provided support to the assertion that education is an essential tool for conflict prevention (Banks 2010; Gartrell, 2012). Sociopolitical and cultural contexts are important in addressing issues related to implementation of peaceful strategies and practices that are sound and responsive to the specific needs of varied communities around the globe.

Investment in early childhood education and the training of early childhood caregivers is an investment in peace and human rights; development and education creates possiblities for economic prosperity and empowers individuals and groups (Britto and Kagan 2010). The introduction and further development of peace education curricula and materials offer one way to counteract violent conflicts and destructive behavioral patterns in young children, such as bullying, which is becoming more prevalent in schools in industrialized as well as developing countries (Sharp and Smith 2002). Peace education (e.g., nonviolence, communication, negotiation, peer mediation) can be used as a preventive tool as well as an intervention in conflict and in postconflict contexts for both adults (parents and teachers) and children (at home or in school settings).

In the United States, formal and informal curricula for peace programs have been developed for early childhood education around topics of pluralism, multiculturalism, and social justice. Examples include the peace education curriculum developed by the United States Institute for Peace and Anti-Bias curriculum[3] developed for early years and the initiative developed by Arigato International[4] on ethics education for children. Unfortunately, many of these programs are often not available for children in war or conflict zone areas. In addition to the lack of resources to invest in such programs, politicians, security forces, and even community leaders are often suspicious of the topic or of the implementing agency. Regardless, it is clear that comprehensive and integrated peacebuilding strategies in educational systems require the engagement of children in their early childhood years. Page (2000) argues for reframing early childhood education and its curricula to become more future oriented. She argues that the field of early childhood has made huge strides forward by adding global, environmental, and peace studies to its agenda: "Because of isolation, these have lacked reference to underlying methodology that emphasize their relative values and shared concerns" (Page 2000:2).

As part of a curriculum focused on peace education, systematically investing in the integration of conflict resolution values, skills, and narratives in formal and informal educational systems can be an effective strategy to counter violence in school environments as well as in society in general. Since new knowledge on the human brain asserts the continued development of an individual's brain well into the third decade of life, there is hope that, even in situations of adversity, schools and other proper intervention programs may be able to repair damage done earlier in life (Shonkoff and Phillips 2000). To

---

[3] www.usip.org/publications (accessed June 14, 2014).

[4] http://www.arigatouinternational.org/en/ (accessed June 14, 2014).

do so, governments need to integrate conflict resolution and peace education in their formal and informal curriculum. Special programs have to be designed and energy must be invested in raising new awareness among children in early stages of development.

When politicians hesitate to transform their educational systems to reflect the new reality that emerges from a peace process, children in schools and pre-schools will continue to grow up with old perceptions and habits of the conflict (e.g., children in deeply divided societies such as Northern Ireland, Cyprus, Iraq, and Israel-Palestine). There are many stories of white and black, Catholic and Protestant, Israeli and Palestinian individual peace makers who have been changed by their experiences of meeting their enemy from the other side. Such inspiring stories are important in spreading a sense of hope and the possibility of peaceful coexistence among the divided communities. Evaluation of such dialog and encounter programs provide clear evidence that meeting the "other" in a safe educational setting changes negative perceptions and forms new, positive attitudes toward the "other," especially on individual levels of interaction (Hammack 2011; Abu-Nimer 1999; Maoz 2004). Sustainability of such attitudinal changes, however, remains an elusive goal. Although, the symbolic importance of these peace education programs should not be underestimated, it is equally important for peacebuilding programs and practitioners to examine ways in which their efforts can have collective and systemic impact.

Theories of Conflict Resolution

In designing peace education programs for early childhood, there are various ways to classify the theoretical frameworks utilized by experts to explain causes of conflicts and their resolution processes. Regardless of the typology, it is clear that conflict resolution is an interdisciplinary field that draws its theories from a number of disciplines (e.g., psychology, sociology, education, political science and international relations, and communications). Below we attempt to capture a few theoretical streams in the field.

Basic Human Needs (BHN) theory is one of the most developed theoretical frameworks in the field. This approach assumes that violent conflicts can be prevented, and in many cases resolved, if human structures and systems are designed in ways to respond to the generic and universal human needs of all people. John Burton, a scholar and diplomat who applied this principle to conflict resolution theory, argues that conflict emerges when individuals and groups are deprived of their basic needs. In this framework, the only way to resolve these conflicts is to provide venues and alternatives to satisfy these unmet, frustrated basic human needs (Burton 1990a, b). BHN theory assumes that there are needs beyond the universal human physical needs, such as security, identity, and development. Burton suggests the use of analytical problem-solving tools to understand and devise alternatives that will satisfy deprived sets of needs causing conflicts, so as to overcome the dynamics of power politics (or competitive power paradigm) that generate conflicts and block their resolution. There have been many critiques of the BHN theory, especially regarding the criteria in defining the number and scope of "generic" basic human needs (Avruch and Black 1987). In addition, as a theory, it has not been widely tested. Few conflict resolution practitioners or policy makers have adopted the analytical problem-solving tools or framework as a way to address conflicts.

A second set of theoretical frameworks can be classified around principles and assumptions of misperception and communication. Scholars and practitioners in this area see conflicts generated as a result of communication and perception problems. Thus if obstacles to clear communication are removed, conflicting parties will be able to communicate more freely and solve their problems (Broome 1993). Misperceptions are created as a result of conflict socialization processes and dynamics which can perpetuate animosity, hatred, and fear of others. Conflict resolution practitioners in this category invest a great deal of effort in designing and carrying out processes that establish trust and build sustainable human relations among conflicting parties and their communities. Regardless of the level of intervention (individual, community, or state) the emphasis is on correcting the negative image of the other, diffusing negative feelings toward the enemy, and establishing proper and open communication channels to address current and future conflicts (Kelman and Cohen 1976; Kelman and Fisher 2003; Fisher 1997, 2005). Dialog is one of the main processes of intervention that can be associated with this theoretical framework. Scholars and practitioners in the field have both conceptualized and applied this process of peacebuilding as a tool to address many negative conflict dynamics symptoms, such as dehumanization, stereotyping, and belief in the use of violence (Abu-Nimer 1999). The theoretical roots of this framework are well articulated in the contact hypothesis tradition of social psychology, constructed in the late 1950s (Sherif and Sherif, 1953; Hewstone and Brown, 1986). Interest-based negotiation is another significant part of this theoretical construct in explaining the causes of conflicts and their resolution (Fisher and Ury 1983). The main assumptions underlying this approach include:

- Conflict is a product of perceived incompatible goals or interests.
- By focusing on interests instead of positions, conflicting parties will discover common ground to build their agreement.
- Emotions (e.g., anger, fear) are factors which block cooperative negotiation processes and thus need to be controlled.
- By following problem-solving steps, conflicting parties can creatively generate alternative options that were unavailable to them when they were locked into positional bargaining.

Such a process is utilized in many training and capacity-building projects implemented in local and international settings (Sri Lanka, Mindanao, Philippines, Egypt, Israel, and Palestine) by organizations such as Search for Common

Ground,[5] Harvard Negotiation Project,[6] Creative Associates International,[7] and others.

A third set of theories of conflict resolution can be classified around structures, resources, and development. Scholars and practitioners in this theoretical tradition place more emphasis on the role and function of tangible, material resources and concrete structures that determine the distribution of such resources (Galtung 1969; Kriesberg 1998). Galtung's structural violence concept has been central in generating debates and guidance for many of the intervention processes in this area. Institutional building, governance, and other policy changes are just a few of the techniques that are often explored in resolving conflicts especially in the post-agreement phase. South Africa, Northern Ireland, and Israel-Palestine are three examples of conflicts where we see efforts to transform economic, political, and governance structures in their post-agreement phase. Since the early 1990s, the field of peacebuilding has witnessed a good number of research studies that have attempted to capture the dynamics and conditions (which influence rebuilding) of fragile states and communities which have emerged from a long history of violent conflicts and whose leaders have signed political agreements. When examining the above theoretical frameworks in the context of early childhood education, both researchers and practitioners lack clear answers to several pressing questions that emerge: What is the most developmentally appropriate theoretical approach in integrating conflict resolution in early childhood? What are the effective conflict resolution tools that can be applied in early childhood years across cultures? When working with parents and families, should practitioners apply the same frameworks utilized with children? How should socialization agents respond to the contradictions between these conflict resolution frameworks and the existing educational systems and frameworks?

Conflict Resolution Research

The theoretical approaches discussed above provide one of the more salient entry points for a discussion on the role of human development and childhood in peacebuilding. Across the theoretical traditions of conflict resolution, only a few studies focus exclusively on the biological basis of behavior and its role in conflict resolution methods (McCarthy et al. 2010). In the broader conflict literature, however, there are studies that examine the biological causes of violence and aggression (Lorenz 1966; Wilson 1975; Dawson 1996). For many of these studies, biological deficiencies (e.g., hormonal imbalances) were identified as leading factors in explaining aggression (especially sexual offenses). A

5   https://www.sfcg.org/ (accessed June 14, 2014).

6   http://www.pon.harvard.edu/category/research_projects/harvard-negotiation-project/ (accessed June 14, 2014).

7   http://www.creativeassociatesinternational.com/ (accessed June 14, 2014).

classic argument in this category focuses on the assumption that anxiety and fear are part of the human condition with particular genetic and neurological functions in their evolutionary process (Ehrenreich 1997; Carter and Porges, this volume; Keverne, this volume). New knowledge about biological explanations for behavioral aspects of the child in early developmental phases can have implications for the type and scope of peace education and conflict resolution frameworks and skills that are introduced in formal and informal education. Such exploration is missing from both fields of peacebuilding as well as early childhood education. Such explanations are often located on a particular side of the nature-nurture or biology-culture debate. Indeed, one perspective on the development of conflict resolution is as an alternative to the more realpolitik versions of "human nature," which advance a hierarchical power and deterministic (and pessimistic) view of the natural world and human relations. As mentioned above, one can argue that conflict resolution itself emerged in response to such determinism as a direct challenge to the power politics of the Greek historian Thucydides: "The strong do what they can and the weak suffer what they must."

The discussion on the role of culture, as well as religion, in conflict resolution is, of course, robust and diverse. For example, some approaches (e.g., the BHN theoretical approach) do not view culture as relevant to a conflict resolution process that is concerned with universal, generic human needs (Zartman 1993). A second perspective recognizes the relevance of culture but only as one variable among many, in a still fairly instrumental approach to conflict resolution (Bercovitch 1996; Cohen 1991). Still another views cultural variation as fundamentally significant to the narration and analysis of conflict, and its subsequent resolution (Avruch 1998; Avruch and Black 1987, 1991; Lederach 1995; Galtung 1996). Among these three views of culture, conflict, and conflict resolution, one might identify a sort of descending order of resonance with biological perspectives on behavior. For example, within the theoretical tradition of the BHN approach, one might find greatest resonance with biological explanations of behavior and their relevance to conflict resolution; this resonance decreases, however, with the second approach and arguably disappears with the third.

While much research has been concerned with explaining the causes of violence, aggression, and war, a serious gap exists in addressing the applicability of these various biological explanations to collective forms of violence, as well as to the capacity of these theories to be translated into concrete tools to help resolve interpersonal or intergroup conflicts. In other words, there has been little connection made to collective and macro-level conflicts involving nations or even small groups. The issue of whether knowledge accumulated from the neurosciences, regarding the biological bases for violence and conflict, has implications in the design of intervention programs in conflict resolution or prevention is relevant, pressing, and timely.

Strategies in Conflict Resolution

As indicated above, early childhood peace education has to be based on certain conflict resolution principles and frameworks. What, then, are the specific processes and tools that need to be integrated into a framework for early childhood education for peace? In general, conflict resolution processes are strategies that aspire to empower people to deal, address, and manage their conflicts. Regardless of the approach, it is assumed that a process is more effective when there is a high level of willingness to engage with each other. In addition, face to face interactions among conflicting parties are a preferred form of intervention, especially if they are willing to meet. The use of a third party in resolving conflicts must be determined by the conflicting parties themselves; the process becomes more effective if the third party enjoys a high level of legitimacy and credibility. There are many conflict resolution tools that exist in the field, such as problem solving, mediation, negotiation, dialog, and reconciliation processes, all of which rely heavily on people's ability to interact, sympathize, and rationally think about resolving conflicts. As we review these methods and tools, it is important to examine whether they are applicable in the context of early childhood development. A child-centered approach and engagement in developmentally appropriate practices is assumed, as indicated earlier.

Joint problem solving is a process which has been utilized by many practitioners and in many contexts. The process of problem solving can be summarized in six steps:

1. Identify the problems and issues.
2. Analyze and understand the nature of the problems (e.g., issues, parties, power).
3. Jointly generate options.
4. Evaluate options according to set criteria.
5. Select agreed upon options (agreement).
6. Implement the agreement.

Mediation is another process of intervention that requires the use of a third party to assist conflicting parties in communicating properly and identifying areas of common agreement. Mediators are different from arbitrators in their inability to decide for the parties on best solutions for their conflict. Mediators are committed to impartiality and have no invested interest in the outcome of the process. Mediation processes are applied on all levels and areas of conflict (interpersonal, family, community, ethnic, and interstate). In fact, mediation as a subfield of conflict resolution has been one of the most researched and practiced, leading a number of studies to conceptualize and improve mediation processes. In response to some critique, a transformative mediation process has been developed which allows parties to resolve their disputes in ways that build deeper relationships and prevent future conflicts (Bush and Folger 1994). Mediation processes have proven effective not only in assisting parties to resolve their conflicts, but in raising awareness about the value of nonviolent communication and the pursuance of peaceful means in conflict resolution. This can be seen in the growth of peer mediation as well as restorative justice programs that have been developed and implemented in elementary and middle schools all over the world. In the United States, many elementary schools have integrated peer mediation programs into educational curricula as well as formal activities available to students (Johnson and Johnson 1996; Schrumpf et al.1997; Amstutz and Mullet 2005; Cremin 2007).

Negotiation processes are another set of intervention strategies. Similar to mediation, parties explore common interests that underlie their bargaining positions. An effective negotiation process is one that produces an agreement between the various parties that satisfies their interests and provides them with proper channels of communication to express their concerns and desires. There have been many critiques leveled against this process of conflict resolution, including its lack of attention and inability to manage strong emotions or injuries as a result of the conflict or the cultural factors that influence the capacity and willingness of parties to engage in such a process (especially relevant for parties not comfortable with Anglo, European, or American urban- and business-oriented settings). This critique extends to the inability of interest-based negotiation processes to address significant power imbalances between conflicting parties. The capacity and willingness of parties to engage in interest-based negotiation and collaborative mode of interaction can be obstructed or fail to begin because the powerful party to a conflict may have little incentive to engage constructively in such a process.

Dialog processes constitute another path of conflict resolution intervention. Dialog or encounter frameworks in conflict resolution are processes that have origins in contact hypothesis theories from social psychology. The process of meeting the other in a safe setting encourages open and honest conversation about conflict issues, misperceptions, and other dimensions of conflict relationships. The dialogical process requires a qualified facilitator who is able to construct a safety net; this opens up a safe space for participants to take risks and expose their feelings and perceptions of the other. Such a safety net is the product of a gradual process of trust that is built through careful adherence to communication guidelines, positive role modeling by the facilitator, discovery of the commonalities among participants, and step-by-step confrontation of conflict issues. There are at least two types of dialog processes. One places emphasis on education or raising awareness as a primary objective of the process of engagement. The other places additional emphasis on the need to act and confront social injustice (Abu-Nimer 1999). Both types of dialog require participants to be committed to the process and to adhere to a defined set of conditions (e.g., respect, participation, avoidance of judgment). Dialogical tools are powerful tools that can transform participants of a dialog process if they permit themselves to engage seriously and fully in the program. However, in protracted conflict systems, due to the impact of cycles of violence on cognition and information processing of participants, very few individuals might actually allow themselves to delve in and explore their own perceptions and image of the other. Dialog tools include critical self-reflection, self-observation, deep listening, compassion, reframing, sensitivity to emotion and hurt, and the capacity to separate the issues from the person. According to Bohm (1996), when participants engage in dialogical relations they are able to discover their interconnectedness and nurture their human fellowship.

Reconciliation processes constitute another form of conflict resolution interventions and have been implemented on interpersonal as well as small and large group levels. The process of reconciliation aims to restore broken relationships between conflicting parties. In the last two decades the concept has emerged as a central theme in peacebuilding, especially in the discussion of postconflict dynamics. Lederach (1997) has proposed a model for reconciliation that is based on personal, structural, and societal transformation. In this approach, reconciliation is manifest in building new relationships between conflicting parties based on values such as mercy, compassion, truth, justice, and equality. Only through such deep and comprehensive change can deep-rooted conflicts be transformed.

To institutionalize an agenda of peace education in early childhood programs, we need to integrate and infuse the above methods into curriculum materials as appropriate for children and the context surrounding them and their families. These strategies exist in conflict resolution programs in the United States and a few other countries, but they are not part of the formal educational structures; if they are, they are sporadic and have not been measured for impact.

Attempts at implementing these strategies in early childhood intervention programs suggest some limited success, in particular in programs that rely on infusing these strategies in everyday life events at school, especially in primary grades (Crawford 2005). A study by Sandy and Boardman (2000) measured the impact of applying a conflict resolution program (Peaceful Kids Conflict Resolution Program) in U.S. preschoolers (ages two to six years): children who participated in the program scored higher on self-control, assertiveness, and cooperation and lower on aggressiveness and socially withdrawn behaviors than their peers in control group. In another study conducted in seven states in the United States, Maxwell (2007) suggests that conflict resolution (especially mediation processes) can contribute to self-discipline and self-regulation in early childhood years, and that programs which promote mediation and problem solving can decrease challenging behaviors in early childhood settings. A third and more longitudinal study (since the 1980s), on the growth of sociability and cooperation in young children three to six years old, suggests increasing playful and child-centered pedagogies rather than designing specific programs on conflict resolution (Broadhead 2009). In another study with toddlers, conflict resolution skills were found to be utilized by toddlers, especially during play interactions (Ashby and Neilsen-Hewett 2012). This suggests that we need to be even more intentional in providing opportunities and creating spaces for young children to practice these strategies through, for example, play, sociodramatic activities, and music instruction (McLennan and Pecaski 2012).

These studies certainly provide clear and promising empirical evidence on the effect and value of conflict resolution programs in early childhood on an individual level. However, further research on the effectiveness of these methods in raising children in more peaceful communities is very much needed, especially in various global contexts.

Conclusions

Education provides the means to address conflict resolution and offers an avenue for peaceful values to be instilled and reinforced. When peace education is integrated systematically at all levels, individuals not only gain an understanding of the meaning of peace, this understanding will grow and deepen. In addition, skills related to the management of conflict can be learned and honed, yielding more peaceful and collaborative ways of resolving conflict in their lives. For early childhood development, it is imperative that a peace education agenda be set and that peaceful values are integrated into preschool intervention programs.

The current research agenda of the peacebuilding field needs to expand its capacity to explain the impact of new knowledge from biological and neuroscience research on conflict perceptions and behaviors. Additional insights from this new body of knowledge will certainly have consequences on the design and implementation of peace education programs. However, peace education programs need to be aligned with the new knowledge on brain development, biological bases of behaviors, and neuroscience research. The intensity and scope of intervention programs may be affected by recent scientific developments and to date this has not been taken into consideration by peace educators or by others.

Similar gaps exist between the application of accumulated knowledge in early childhood developmental research and the peacebuilding field (both theory and practice). Thus we need to find ways for practitioners to adjust their models of conflict resolution so as to respond to the needs and contexts of early childhood developmental pathways, including biological factors.

The link between these three areas—biology, early childhood development, and peace education—is still in an early stage. If we are to advance the human capacity to solve our conflicts peacefully, a number of central agencies should be involved in the process of systematically connecting knowledge and practice from these three areas. Formal and informal education systems are essential areas in which such capacity can be built and developed. However, unfortunately, educational systems are often neglected and marginalized in terms of resources and priorities, especially in low-income and conflict contexts.

In the current national and global structures and institutions, continual investments are made to resolve conflicts by primarily targeting adults. The results are less than adequate: we end up moving from one crisis to the next. Putting out the fires of violence around the globe is, indeed, an important intervention and act of peacebuilding. However, addressing the root causes of violence requires longer-term investments in peace education in all of our systems (legal, social, political, economic, educational, etc.). Transforming the global culture of violence can only be accomplished when children are enabled to learn and practice values and skills inherent to peace education, starting in their earliest developmental phase. Such education would advance the use of violence to become a universal taboo.

18

The Power of Media in Peacebuilding

Lucy Nusseibeh

Abstract

Given the complexity and intractability of present-day conflicts, this chapter discusses the potential role that positive media can play in peacebuilding. Problems associated with group identity are examined and the potential for media to strengthen issues surrounding the core identity (self-esteem and self-worth) of an individual is analyzed. The view is taken that educational media can enable individuals as well as large groups (nation, tribe) to become less vulnerable to malevolent manipulation. Examples from Palestine and Northern Ireland are presented to demonstrate the effect that age-appropriate educational media has on the building of secure attachment and prosocial behavior in young children. It is suggested that age-appropriate educational media can also promote global citizenship. Consideration is given to how media programs for children can be reinforced by programs for parents/caregivers and communities, and recommendations are offered on how these might be expanded. To achieve maximum effect, these programs are reliant on input from international and academic communities. A model is presented to illustrate how groups can progress from an existence marked by active conflict (where large group identity is under threat) to one of peaceful coexistence (where groups are connected and relate with mutual respect), and the role that media can play in this transition.

Introduction

Media is often (and perhaps rightly so) perceived as a force for evil—one that aids and abets violence and war through varying degrees of propaganda (obvious or not) and dehumanizes individuals, thereby aggravating conflicts. Here I evaluate, by contrast, the potential, positive role that media can play in counteracting negative stereotypes and dehumanization, and discuss whether this offers a way to reduce violent conflict and create pathways to peace.

I begin with an examination of the role of early childhood development in the formation of attitudes that lead to violence. Thereafter, an assessment is made as to whether media interventions might function as an effective tool to contain the development of such attitudes. Examples from Palestine and Northern Ireland are used to explore potential links between early childhood development and work with the media. Throughout this chapter the hypothesis is put forth that media can be harnessed to contribute to peacebuilding in today's world, where globalization has increased the complexity of violence and armed conflict.

Complexities of Conflict

The Classical Approach to Conflict

One of the more standard ways of viewing conflict, violent or otherwise, is to envision it as a curve that follows a fairly predictable linear path: it begins with a point of latency, rises as conflict escalates to a peak where hurt is inflicted and a stalemate reached, declining thereafter when there is a de-escalation of conflict, followed by dispute settlement and ending with postconflict peacebuilding. This linear curve implies a progressive path that inevitably leads to talks, conflict resolution, and peace. Although setbacks may occur, the underlying assumption is that a solution will be found based on the interests of the protagonists. Nowadays, the complexities of war and armed conflicts defy this classic view and its implied classic solutions.

Among these complexities is an increasing level of intractability. It is no longer—if it ever was—reasonable to assume that protagonists prefer peace to war. Vested economic interests (via globalization and often linked with international crime) can create as well as prolong a conflict (e.g., to achieve financial gain). Protagonists may use mass media, which may be under their control, to maintain and or manipulate conflict. As Kaldor states, "waging wars becomes more important than winning them" such that "wars tend to spread and to persist or recur, as each side gains in political or economic ways from violence itself rather than 'winning' " (Kaldor 2013:2; see also Keen 2012).

Another example of complexity is the threat of violence, which seems to be much more pervasive and embedded in all levels of society than in the past, when sharper distinctions between fighters and nonfighters existed. For instance, the deliberate targeting of civilians, as opposed to fighting between armed combatants, has increased markedly: civilian fatalities in wartime have climbed from 5% at the turn of the century to more than 90% in the wars of the 1990s (UNICEF 2014). This pervasiveness reflects a continuum of conflict, from urban violence to terrorism to war, that lacks clear distinguishable characteristics.

If we are to explore potential pathways to peace, we must analyze the causes of war. However, these are numerous and highly complex as well as elusive or, at best, unclear. National interests blur with economic, tribal, or religious considerations. Each seems to have its own particularities that need to be studied separately if we are to discover the specific cause behind a conflict and learn how best to resolve it.

Identity Politics and Manipulation of Identities

In addition to vested interests and the pervasiveness of violence and war, including structural violence,[1] which complicates the search for pathways to peace, there are many issues related to identity politics. Part of the problem seems to be associated with the way they are used to manipulate and prolong conflicts. According to Kaldor (2013:3), "wars are often fought in the name of identity (ethnic, religious, or tribal)....Perhaps most importantly, identity politics is constructed through war. Thus political mobilization around identity is the aim of war rather than an instrument of war, as was the case in old wars." This is not to say that identity is the cause of war, or necessarily even one of the causes; identity is, however, a constituent that can be constructed via war. Identity issues may thus be manipulated to prolong war and conflict so that the promulgators can, for example, make more profits in our globally interconnected world. Part of this manipulation may include whipping up existing (or latent) hatred connected to issues of identity. This may happen via chosen glories or traumas, which play important roles in specifying the identity of a large group. "At times of stress, when the group's identity is threatened, an inactive chosen trauma can be revived through propaganda or hate speech and may be used by leaders to inflame the group's shared feelings about themselves and their enemy (or enemies)" (Volkan 2004:49). Volkan emphasizes the importance of identity in relation to manipulation of levels of violence in conflict and explains that "manipulation of large-group regression and its accompanying large-group rituals in the service of maintaining, protecting, and repairing identity may create an atmosphere ripe for unspeakable, seemingly inhumane acts of violence" (Volkan 2004:50).

Thus identity—whether genuine or constructed, distinct or blurred—across large groups (e.g., tribes, nations)—may be a central component in present-day conflicts of all kinds. Because identity is a product of belonging to a large group, it may also play a role in negative stereotyping and intergroup aggression.

Using Erikson's interpretation of identity (i.e., the sustained feeling of inner sameness within oneself, evidenced by the individual's inner working model

---

[1] For further discussion on structural violence, its normalization, and its broad impacts on young children, see Dawes and van der Merwe (this volume).

of him/herself), Volkan (2004) states that the larger identity, in which an individual is placed, is intimately connected to his or her personal core identity. As a result, serious threats to large group identity (e.g., shared helplessness and humiliation) are perceived by members of that large group as *individually* wounding and *personally* endangering, psychologically speaking. Further he explains how threats to the abstract psychological creation of large group identity produce shared anxiety; this may lead to societal regression among members of the large group. Societal regression is characterized, for example, by the loss of individuality, the extensive use of projective mechanisms that lead to a sharp division of "us" versus "them" mentality, and a sense of entitlement to do anything necessary to maintain the shared group identity (Volkan 2004). Societal regression, therefore, tends to include violence, both intragroup and intergroup.

Volkan describes *large group identity* as an "abstract psychological creation," and this abstract creation may be a factor that leads to concrete physical aggression, via the profound connection to the vulnerable individual. Thus the question becomes: If individuals are less vulnerable (e.g., through early childhood interventions), will this affect large group identity in a positive way? Consider, for instance, an idea put forth by the Mother Child Education Foundation (Anne Çocuk Eğitim Vakfı): grassroots changes at the family level contribute cumulatively to create change in communities and societies. If the links between core identity formed in childhood and large group identity are visceral enough to make people perceive threats to the group as threats to themselves as individuals, then perhaps one potential way of stopping these patterns is to strengthen that core from the very beginning of life. Perhaps if there were a strong enough core identity in an increasing number of individuals, reinforced by other similarly sturdy core identities within the large group, a stronger and more resilient core would emerge in the large group. In turn, the large group would be less vulnerable to fear and manipulation and would not need to engage in conflict or war over perceived threats to the large group identity. Alternatively, to what extent is it possible to regard another large group with respect and without fear if one's own group feels weak and vulnerable?

The Importance of Secure Attachment

Just as it generally does in societal development, early childhood development may play a role in conflict. It would be interesting to examine whether this could be influenced positively so as to address the many and varied forms of violence (societal, structural, urban, interstate or intergroup war) that make up the complex nature and changing patterns of conflict. Such an approach could involve working outward and upward from within civil society, utilizing the input of caregivers and the local community. It would focus on early childhood programs designed to build resilience and resistance to manipulation and aggression, so that children would be equipped to withstand perceived and actual threats to the large group identity. In this way, there would be restraints on both inter- and intragroup violence. This implies a blurring of boundaries between what is psychological and "real," but connections may be more important than boundaries.

Peacebuilding presents difficulties that are both psychological and real: real in the sense that there are extreme physical dangers and discomforts associated with war and violence; psychological in the sense that violence permeates the invisible and unconscious as much as (or even more) the conscious. In addition to causing trauma, often on multiple levels (Srour 2005), (mis)perceptions and polarization can occur, often in the form of myths or demonization across hostilities. In particular, the unconscious defense mechanisms of splitting and projection (often unconsciously) permit an internal conflict to be externalized and projected to a location outside the self (e.g., *we* are good, *they* are evil; *we* are victims, *they* are perpetrators; *we* are peace loving, *they* are aggressive). More importantly, just as individuals utilize defense mechanisms, nations and large groups mobilize social defenses to protect themselves against unbearable feelings and unconscious anxieties (Menzies Lyth 1959). These defense mechanisms lead to processes of dehumanization and demonization, as each side projects all the evil qualities they cannot own themselves onto the other side; this, in turn, makes any form of violence seemingly acceptable as "self-protection" against "others." Therefore, unconscious processes may tend to reinforce fear and negative stereotyping and encourage a retreat into the "secure" perception of "us versus them" and the apparent safety of the large group. This can be exploited by manipulative leaders, especially through the use of media.

Recent developments seem to indicate that one way to build a strong core identity, and thus a strong sense of security, is through a secure attachment base (e.g., Ainsworth and Bowlby 1991; see also Hinde and Stevenson-Hinde, this volume, and Hinde 2011). If secure attachment in early childhood linked with recognition can lead to a capacity for empathy, it might also be linked to large group identity in ways that could contribute to overcoming prejudices and negative stereotyping. To counteract present-day leaders who stir up hatred and exploit prejudices that contribute to current conflicts, future interventions that target early childhood development might be able to spawn leaders capable of rising above traditional "us versus them" prejudices, thus encouraging others to do so as well. Recent research indicates the importance of secure attachment to leadership; secure attachment contributes to better relationships as well as better leadership throughout life (Reichard and Paik 2012). This does not exclude the possibility that a secure individual may be unscrupulous, manipulative, and uninterested in peacebuilding. It simply implies that a secure base is a necessary condition for peace-seeking leaders.

The Role of the Media in Peacebuilding

An Example of Role Models

A recent peace-teaching film, *Beyond Violence*, directed by Irris Singer (2012), analyzes how two individuals become able to take a stand against violence as well as the norms of their societies. It is a psychopolitical exploration of the background of two former fighters, an Israeli and a Palestinian, who became leaders in the movement "Combatants for Peace." These two "peacebuilders" visit schools and other institutions on the opposing side of the conflict to promote the humanization of the other. Both men went through the "normal" rites of passage within their two conflicted societies: the Palestinian was sent to prison, the Israeli served in the army. The Israeli took part in killing a group of Palestinians as part of his duty as a soldier. Both experience an awakening. For the Palestinian, this occurs via lengthy debates with his prison guard (who ends up convinced of the Palestinian position). For the Israeli, a film that he sees one evening sparks the realization that he is a killer.

What emerges in the film, for both the Palestinian and the Israeli, is the recognition that it is possible to transform to a self-aware individual—one willing to see their enemies as human. This ability is associated with the strong, secure attachment that each had to their parents, as well as the constant recognition and support from them. Attachment seems to be the key element that enables them (both in terms of human awareness and courage) to go against their communities and explore ways to actively build peace. This ability holds, even after the ten-year old daughter of the Palestinian is killed (apparently by a random Israeli shooting into a Palestinian school playground), undoubtedly an event that could have made it easy for him to turn away from any effort toward peace.

In the film, interviews with the protagonists and others are designed to teach and to promote discussion. The film attempts to reach Israelis and Palestinians living in the middle of the conflict who are interested in peacebuilding and to serve as a base for further exploration into the question of how this can be achieved against all the odds.

Beyond Violence is an example of how media can be used as a pathway to peace. It is also a very effective tool for teaching peacebuilding to adults. However, media is a broad term that can take many forms, including print media (e.g., books, newspapers), mass communications media (e.g., TV, radio), and various forms of social media. By nature, media is pervasive. If certain elements of early childhood development contribute to the potential of an adult to be peaceful, or even become a peacebuilder, then it would seem to make sense to try to harness the power of the media to support this process. During the launch of the Early Childhood Peacebuilding Consortium in September 2013, UNICEF asserted that media holds a transformative potential to reach many different groups at once to communicate messages and strategies that promote peacebuilding.

Opportunities to Promote Prosocial Behavior in Young Children

In addition to reach and amplification, media has the power to influence (for better or for worse) individuals through the delivery of age-appropriate messages. It can provide role models for children, caregivers, and the general community and create heroes and heroines who are nonviolent and who work toward peacebuilding, modeling reciprocal respect and dignity. By showing positive images, the media can help people to recognize and reflect positively on themselves. This can be as simple as showing children positive images of themselves. For instance, in a Palestinian context, where children normally see Palestinians portrayed by media as victims or perpetrators, the Sesame Workshop depicts them as agents for good. In response, the children perceive themselves as such (Cole 2008). According to Cole (2008:359): "The positive sense of self in media comes through finding your own place, your own likes and dislikes and your own culture, hearing them from others."

For many years, the Sesame Workshop has led the field in developing clear age-appropriate educational media material to address issues of self-esteem and relationships, as well as more standard cognitive educational issues. From the outset of their pioneering work on educational media in the United States in the late 1960s, Sesame Workshop has based their programs on integrated action research to ensure age-appropriateness and to ascertain the correct understanding of the messages they attempt to convey. In the beginning, the message targeted race relations in the United States. Subsequent research showed that children who viewed programs with mixed race characters were more able to identify with these characters, contributing therefore to a prosocial impact. Much of their work was aimed at building self-esteem (i.e., the secure base or the strong core identity) (Morrow 2006). Although the cognitive skills taught by Sesame Workshop assist the building of self esteem, longitudinal research has shown the sustained influence of the early Sesame Street programs in prosocial behavior beyond cognitive skills. For instance, evidence shows that boys who watched Sesame Street were less aggressive at age 16 than those who had not seen the programs (Morrow 2006). This may seem far removed from pathways to peace in an intractable conflict; however, more direct work on peacebuilding in Israel/Palestine, Kosovo, Northern Ireland, and at the global level has yielded positive results.

At the Global Summit on the Use of Educational Media to Promote Respect and Understanding on May 30, 2002, Charlotte Cole (Vice-President for Education at Sesame Workshop) summarized their approach:

> First comes having a positive sense of self. Second, comes having a knowledge and awareness of others, and recognizing the similarities and differences between you and others. Third, comes recognizing the impact of your own actions on other people, and how what you do affects people both in your local community and in your global community.

In relation to peacebuilding, the second and third steps can be problematic, as stereotyping (including very harsh negative stereotyping) seems to be present as of a very early age, and stereotyping tends to allow dehumanization. These areas, however, have been shown to be positively influenced by the media. For instance, the Shara'a Simsim/Rehov Sumsum series, produced by Sesame Workshop (then Children's Television Workshop), was established in 1996 (soon after the signing of the Oslo peace agreement in 1993), with the vision and strong hopes of contributing to the peacebuilding of the young generation in the region from the outset. In preparation for the series, research conducted by Sesame Workshop and Bar-Tal (1996) showed that Palestinian and Israeli children possessed ugly stereotypes (e.g., "dirty," "he wants to kill me") of each other as young as three years old—the same age that Bowlby found evidence of empathy and mutual recognition of self and others in securely attached children.

Subsequent research, particularly in Northern Ireland, has shown how very early negative (e.g., sectarian) stereotyping begins in young children. Connolly et al. (2002) found that "the general picture is that the majority of children in Northern Ireland are introduced to and become aware of various cultural and political events and symbols as of the age of three years."[2] This happens when the child is not even fully aware of the meanings of these. By the age of five or six years (essentially the age at which they start school and encounter a much larger community), children identify with particular communities and express sectarian attitudes: children know, for example, which flag is theirs as well as its colors.

Connolly's findings show a marked increase in stereotyping once children attend school, implying a powerful influence from the community or large group. By the time children reach school, peacebuilding work (e.g., breaking stereotypes, building self-esteem), whether in the home or at a national or international level, takes on the nature of damage control. According to Cole (2008), the depth of negativity expressed by very young children in the studies suggests the need to take action to counter the messages they are receiving at school.

Evidence from work with children and media (e.g., Sesame Workshop in Israel/Palestine and Kosovo, and Early Years in Northern Ireland[3]) indicates that negative stereotypes in children can be changed, even when inter- or intragroup relations have not changed. Research on three Sesame Street projects suggests that "these media interventions are making an impact and that such projects are strongest when they are child-relevant, age-appropriate so as to provide direct and explicit messages" (Cole 2008:364). The program Early

---

[2] van IJzendoorn and Bakermans-Kranenburg (this volume) indicate that the in-group/out-group approach seems to be present by as early as 14 months.

[3] See the online description "About Us" on the website of Belfast: Early Years: http://www. early-years.org/ (accessed June 6, 2014).

Years in Northern Ireland has produced short television spots to promote inclusiveness among young children in Northern Ireland, and there is evidence of their positive impact.[4] The Sesame Stories program has been especially effective in promoting peer-to-peer prosocial attitudes. Researchers discovered that children exposed to the series, when compared to those in a control group, "demonstrated significant increases in moral reasoning skills when asked to make judgments about situations that reflected the series' prosocial content. They concluded that their data support the use of Sesame Stories as a vehicle to promote positive moral reasoning (Cole 2008:362). Although the researchers pointed to a ceiling effect in their research on these projects and the fact that there was more impact on the children who had already shown prosocial tendencies, "the comparison of children who viewed Sesame Stories with those who did not demonstrates that, on the most basic level, the program successfully presents prosocial messages. The measurable increase in moral reasoning with respect to contexts that were specific to those modeled in the program is clearly an important first step" (Cole 2008:364).

What is it about these interventions that make them work? Sesame Workshop goes to great lengths to make certain that the message is "child-relevant, age-appropriate" and it does so in various ways:

- by building a "curriculum" that develops the messages and characters in detail,
- by engaging in formative research from the very beginning of production and testing episodes with groups of children and adults, adjusting when necessary, and
- by taking care never to allow any images that model inappropriate (e.g., dangerous or aggressive) behavior.

Sesame Workshop uses an entire team (which usually includes people from the target geographical area or those involved in the focal point) to build a curriculum and analyze every aspect of the series, especially what might or might not be appropriate. Great attention to detail is given to ensure that programs will have a prosocial impact. Research is organized both before and after production,[5] and professional expertise, experience, and imagination (as well as new knowledge) is used to try and achieve this goal.

Despite this, it is not always clear how a particular issue should be addressed. Potential points of tension between media interventions and the realities of conflict may exist. For instance, there may be a point of tension between the promotion of prosocial behavior and the dismantling of stereotypes, which must be done in ways that do not clash too jarringly with these stereotypes;

---

[4] See the Executive Summary of Findings from the Media Initiative for Children in Belfast. http://www.atlanticphilanthropies.org/sites/default/files/uploads/mifc-exec-summary.pdf (accessed June 6, 2014).

[5] http://www.sesameworkshop.org/what-we-do/our-research-model/ (accessed June 6, 2014).

otherwise the program may risk backfiring completely, as in the Shara'a Simsim/Rehov Sumsum series.

In their attention to detail, Sesame Workshop takes great care to base their programs on reality, so that what the child sees on the screen is within their (and their caregivers') frame of reference; this enables children (and caregivers) to understand and act on the program. In the case of Israel and Palestine, this meant that the series made in 1996 showed children going on occasional visits to each other's streets during this first "peace process" series. However, reflecting and working with reality is not easy in the context of an ongoing conflict, or even an ongoing postconflict. As the coordinator for outreach materials for the Palestinian team, I witnessed constant debate: Many wanted very much to promote mutual respect (between Israelis and Palestinians) by making this a prominent goal. Others (specifically on the Palestinian team) felt strongly that too much emphasis on "respect for the other" (in this case Israel) and a portrayal of more contact than actually existed would lead to outright rejection by adult viewers, who would then not allow their children to watch the programs. This matter was particularly sensitive for outreach (printed) material that was developed to be "evergreen" (i.e., popular and easily accessible); this material was subject to closer scrutiny than the television programs. In these materials, mutual respect and coexistence could only be promoted by positioning the Israeli muppet (or child) with the Palestinian muppet (or child) in a somewhat diluted, for instance, international context.

Even diluted portrayals of coexistence were not possible for the second series of these programs. The Shara'a Simsim/Rehov Sumsum series had to adapt as reality changed. The violence which disrupted the peace process in 2000 destroyed many forms of human connections: there were no more street visits in the next round of the Sesame materials, only stories. These narratives were shared across the cultures of Israel, Jordan, and the Occupied Palestinian Territories via the next series of "Sesame Stories" (Salamon 2002), which sought to humanize and demystify Israeli and Palestinian identity through separate but analogous stories (Lemish and Götz 2007). Interestingly, research showed that this, too, had a strong prosocial impact (Bernard van Leer Foundation Program Staff 2007).

This "separate story" approach may offer a more realistic model for breaking negative stereotypes during conflict. It demonstrates how media can raise awareness of multiple narratives and encourage curiosity about others, without creating resistance, which the more direct approach might provoke.

Empowering Children and Their Parents
to Become Global Citizens

In addition to counteracting negative stereotypes, media can be used to promote positive outcomes. This is exemplified by an ambitious multimedia project conducted by Sesame Workshop, Panwapa, which seeks to "foster a foundation for global citizenship and community activism in young children" four to seven years of age.[6] Founded on the principles and findings of the Global Summit on Promoting Respect and Understanding among Children through Media, Panwapa is a social networking site that reaches a global, multicultural audience. Accessible through the Internet, it is accompanied by a DVD and a board game. Panwapa was designed to be used in schools; thus it also addresses teachers and caregivers. Research from the program has shown that it has had significant impact on generating knowledge about, interest in, and empathy toward children from other parts of the world (Lee and Cole 2009).

Panwapa encourages children to engage in interactive games and tasks with peers from around the world. In addition to promoting self-esteem, awareness, and appreciation of individual differences (by exploring various needs and wants of children in their own and other situations), Panwapa promotes a sense of agency and awareness of impact. It has been successful in promoting positive outcomes due to the attention that was given to the educational goal.

Through a careful blending of reality and fantasy, new media can be used to encourage children to reach out and connect with others whose lives are very different from their own. It is not perfect; Panwapa inadvertently left out a connection point for Palestinian children and thus could not be used in schools in the region.[7] Yet apart from this design flaw, it demonstrates how a multimedia approach can be used to build global citizenship by developing connections and interests between young children in diverse countries and cultures.

Internal Reinforcement

To build a secure base, media work intended for children also needs to be geared toward parents and caregivers. Reaching these people is very important as they provide (or fail to provide) the environment within which a child is able to develop a secure attachment. Since attachments develop by the age of three years—the same age as the negative stereotypes seem to develop—caregiver support is warranted. Research by Feldman et al. (2010:310) among Israeli and Palestinian children suggests that a child's "ability to handle conflicts is learned at home through mechanisms of participation and observation, participating in

---

[6] Panwapa: Social Networking for Children. California Learning Resource Network. Modesto: California Department of Education. http://www.clrn.org/weblinks/details.cfm?id=5105 (accessed June 6, 2014).

[7] Panwapa seems to have been prepared with insufficient participation. This led to an unfortunate flaw in relation to its distribution and use among Arabic speakers. It was designed in a multilingual manner with Arabic as one of the languages used but unfortunately left out a place for Palestinian children to connect.

parent-child conflict and observing the conflicts between parents." In addition, research into the prosocial impact of the Shara'a Simsim/Rehov Sumsum series concluded that "effective interventions need to build on children's general moral reasoning skills" (Cole 2008:362).

One possible pathway for peace via early childhood development may be realized through an internally reinforcing system that offers mutual support for children, caregivers, and the community, with the goal of building secure attachments. Reinforcement between children, caregivers, and communities has been shown to contribute to the success of early childhood development projects throughout the world (Connolly and Hayden 2007), even in very violent situations. Evidence from a wide variety of programs in the field, including various approaches that have been attempted in different places (e.g., Albania, Colombia, Chad, urban Baltimore and Los Angeles, as well as post-conflict northern Ireland—countries and cities at different stages and with different "types" of conflict, internal blood-feuds, kidnapping, internal and external tribal warfare), all indicate the need for triadic mutual reinforcement. In particular, results from these programs emphasize the importance of (a) providing safe space for children, (b) offering support for caregivers and parents, and (c) being responsive to the needs of a community, providing support when appropriate. Work conducted by the Mother Child Education Foundation, for example, suggests that parents can be instrumental in building peace when they engage in early child development programs. Their interventions brought together mothers (then separately fathers) from various cultural backgrounds and engaged them in group sessions focused on their children. Even when hostilities broke out external to the intervention, mothers/fathers chose to continue meeting; this has been interpreted to indicate increased prosocial behavior (for further details, see Kagitcibasi and Britto, this volume).

Reinforcement through Various Forms of Media

Media programs have the potential to contribute to triadic mutual reinforcement by delivering information aimed directly at children, as well as directly or indirectly to parents/caregivers and the wider local community. This could contribute to increasing the sense of security and reducing negative stereotypes within the large group. Part of the integrated approach taken by Sesame Workshop includes the production of outreach materials to reinforce their television and radio programs. Workshops with caregivers or schoolteachers are also organized to maximize the use of these materials, which include printed activity books and magazines (Fisch and Truglio 2000). Printed materials are particularly useful in conflict settings, where basic supplies such as electricity may be minimal and unreliable. Printed materials are easily accessible, long-lasting, and generally cheaper to produce and deliver.

Ways in Which Media Could Promote Peacebuilding

Dedicated educational channels in key global languages can be used effectively to promote positive early childhood development practices at caregiver and community levels. In the English-speaking world, there are a variety of educational media programs for very young children and ample resources (online and in print) for families to access when questions or concerns arise. In the Arabic-speaking world, the only available educational media program directed specifically to Arabic-speaking children is produced by Sesame Street. Programs offered on satellite channels are either violent (Cartoon Network, Space Tunes), mostly imported/translated, or religious in nature: Tuyour al-Jenne is a religious channel that is very popular with children because of its songs; however, the songs also encourage religious extremism and martyrdom. There is a great need to expand access to dedicated educational channels globally, with requisite participation and cultural appropriateness.

Social media offers another means of providing essential discussion and support for caregivers and communities. However, for some major languages (e.g., Arabic), this platform does not yet exist. Social media offers an interactive interface for users and provides a unique opportunity to share life experiences through transmedia storytelling. It is, however, contingent on being connected to the Internet. For example, by focusing on early childhood development in a camp or conflict zone, a narrative can be transferred to inform; questions can then be posed and answers collectively explored while interacting with experts. This permits individuals (i.e., those directly involved as well as others further removed) to follow virtually real-life settings so as to increase understanding and encourage engagement. Currently, the Mother Child Education Foundation is developing an app that will permit parents to access the foundation's programs.

Teaching films are effective in helping caregivers and preschool teachers build secure attachment and self-esteem in children by modeling correct childcare practices in situations of violence (e.g., during bombing raids or prolonged curfews, where both fear and boredom are paramount, and where caregivers may be equally as afraid as the children). A pilot series has been created by Sesame Workshop and the Institute of Modern Media in the Occupied Palestinian Territories. Its programs address the problems internal to Palestinian society and has been widely used by the Palestinian Ministry of Education. Other areas of conflict could also benefit from teaching media, and this potential remains to be realized.

Combining education with entertainment offers an additional approach. Radio soap operas, for example, that promote good child-rearing practices via drama or telephone counseling programs have met with success (more anecdotal than researched) in the Occupied Palestinian Territories. (Radio is often more accessible than television in these areas, as it can be operated without electricity.) Radio soap operas have been used successfully to promote active nonviolence and youth community engagement. In the series, each episode ends with a cliff-hanger, so as to encourage the listener to return; this is also an effective way to integrate and address many real-life situations without coming across as being too didactic. Consider, for example, a romantic story, where the "focal" character must confront various difficulties, such as a traumatized child or a particular instance of violence in the community. The appeal of the story and identification with the character can help bring a discussion of these matters into the general discourse, thereby raising general awareness. It can also help build internal support for those directly involved in looking after young children, encourage engagement and action, and offer a way of overcoming victimhood. Radio soap operas have been used successfully to promote peace in Burundi and other African countries. In the Palestinian context, various soap operas have been produced to promote nonviolence over violence and to address the need for community engagement and community building, as a way of managing the frustrations and oppression of the prolonged Israeli occupation. The audience clearly has understood these messages: at the anecdotal level, writers of these soap operas receive continuous, grateful, and positive feedback, with requests for more. While these soap operas are aimed at youth and adults, they can become an excellent way to bring discussions about the pros and cons of different methods of child-rearing into communities, thereby contributing to community support for building self-esteem and breaking stereotypes.

Interactive therapy via media: Television and the Internet can support the delivery of live and recorded therapy sessions. This approach was used during the attack on Gaza in 2009/2010: a therapist, present in the studio, discussed specific problems with an audience, some in person and some by phone. This type of programming needs to be expanded to other areas of conflict. For instance, in the Arab-speaking world, broadcasts into refugee camps could permit questions from refugees themselves to be voiced to local psychotherapists. In addition to delivery via television and the Internet, radio sessions may be warranted where electricity is unreliable.

Integrated Support System of Partnerships between Universities, Practitioners, and the Media

Returning to some of the initial issues inherent in current conflicts, it must be recognized that some people have vested interests and will exploit conflict to exact a gain. Given the increasing interconnectedness of our societies, it would seem that effective buffers could be created to reduce or eliminate the impact of vested interests. Improving the conditions for early childhood development on a local, community level could be enhanced by efforts from the international community. To this end, an integrated support system between international organizations, universities, and practitioners would be helpful—one dedicated to increasing the awareness of work with early childhood development and its overall importance to our world. Research based on partnerships between universities, practitioners, and media outlets (a reinforcing triad) could provide support through constant monitoring of media messages and their impact (Connolly and Hayden 2007). The academic community, for instance, would continue to research various aspects of early childhood development, publish this research as widely as possible, as well as analyze and evaluate the impact of early childhood development interventions in contexts of violence and war, so as to build a positive feedback loop. This loop could be reinforced by the media, which in turn would feed into awareness-raising campaigns taken on by governments and intergovernmental agencies at global and local levels.

One way to start would be via awareness-raising campaigns of early childhood development and basic parenting/caretaking needs at global and local levels. These would be followed by multicultural, inclusive approaches (including promotion of human security) via high-profile stakeholder conferences between, for example, representatives from the United Nations, academia, NGOs, policy makers, media, social entrepreneurs, etc. Such campaigns could support the creation of multiple narratives at the community level through, for instance, bilingual or multicultural schools (e.g., several bilingual schools now exist in Israel, including one in East Jerusalem).

The complexities that surround peacebuilding and pathways to peace cannot be overemphasized, especially in conflict situations where multiple levels of trauma among adults as well as children are compounded by horrendous physical deprivation and suffering (Srour 2005). Recent news describes the horrible living conditions for inhabitants of Homs, Syria, who have been under siege for the past 18 months; these people have had to survive on eating grass since no other food sources are available. Under such conditions, does it make sense to think of ways to create enough security for children to withstand trauma? To resist the negative stereotyping and see both their own group and the other as they are in their complexity? To grow into adults, who can reject the ideals of violence and domination in a conflict; who will instead be the ones to show an alternative and lead based on reciprocal respect for human dignity? To what extent can programs—even massive mutually reinforcing communications (or other) programs—which support early childhood development actually have a positive influence on a regressive large group identity or structurally unequal and oppressive conflict? Especially, since "ruining the family system and child-parent relations is a crucial expression of severe societal regression" (Volkan 2004:74). When physical violence is constantly and unavoidably present, will all the early childhood development work be able to create a strong enough base to withstand it?

In the model that follows, I explore one possible way: via a mutually reinforcing systemic approach that focuses on early childhood development and media—a system envisioned to bring people and countries out of prolonged violent conflicts and into security and peace.

To ensure basic human rights and human security, peacebuilding needs to be encouraged at multiple levels: top down as well as bottom up. Peacebuilding is rooted in the idea that a secure base must be provided in early childhood to the greatest extent possible; this allows an individual to develop sufficient self-esteem, which in turn equips the individual with the courage to reach across identity boundaries and act inclusively, so as to build local and global multicultural communities based on reciprocal respect and dignity. At the community level, support is needed from the larger global level, and this can be reinforced by media. Otherwise, communities will remain essentially isolated and therefore vulnerable to vested interests.

Pathways to Peacebuilding: A New Model

Using the following illustrations (see Figures 18.1–18.4), I present a model of a potential pathway to peacebuilding. Figure 18.1 depicts a situation that is marked by pervasive and prolonged conflict: two large groups are shown that are at odds with each other. Within each group, children, caregivers, and communities live in isolation and are thus unable to support each other. Within each group, conflict may also prevail. The identity of each large group is not at all stable and is extremely vulnerable to outside perturbations. There is no possibility for groups to accept each other: fear and aggression prevail, leaving the groups locked in conflict. Aggression is manifested against everyone. Despite the presence of international organizations (top of figure), not much can be done, outside of humanitarian efforts, to influence the conflict. In fact,

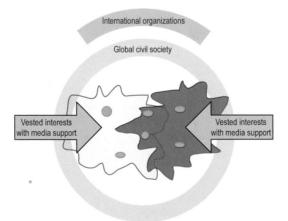

Figure 18.1   Pervasive and prolonged conflict exists between two fragmented groups (yellow and red shapes). Circles/ovals represent children, community, and caregivers. Vested interests, supported by media activities, negatively impact the identities of these groups, which are locked in continual conflict. International organizations are unable to alleviate the conflict and are themselves often subject to the violence.

representatives from international organizations may themselves fall victim to the conflict (e.g., via kidnapping, piracy, terrorism). A very high level of vested interests exists that feeds into and off of the conflict, locking it into place. Often these interests fuel the propaganda and demonization of the "other," thus exacerbating hostilities—often through their use of media. Global civil society (in particular, NGOs and academia) is, in general, not actively engaged.

Figure 18.2 depicts initial steps that are undertaken to counteract conflict and initiate the process of building peaceful communities. Early childhood interventions are implemented to engage children, caregivers, and the community, creating the opportunity for mutual reinforcement in each group. In particular, age-appropriate educational media contribute to the building of self-esteem. The dismantling of negative stereotypes is amplified, which has a positive impact on the groups. International organizations are able to support and reinforce work at the community level (e.g., through awareness campaigns) as an integrated support unit. This work is reinforced through U.N. resolutions, charters, and (national and local) laws that promote specific practices, related to early childhood development, needed to create a secure attachment base. Such laws would specifically protect very young children, their caregivers as well as their community in support of creating a conducive environment for children to be raised. The academic community is active in assessing the impact of programs, laws, and campaigns. The positive feedback loop between academia, communities in conflict, and international organizations permits an evaluation of what works best. Educational media programs are implemented to reinforce

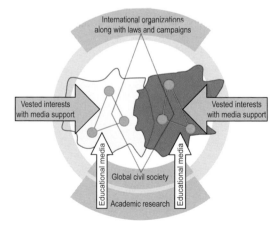

Figure 18.2 Initial steps are taken to counteract conflict between the two groups (yellow and red shapes). Early childhood interventions (supported by international organizations, global civil society, and academia) have a positive impact on the children, caregivers, and community (circles), softening the lines of group identity and lessening the potential for continued conflict. Educational media reinforces these efforts. Vested interests and associated media are still present, but their influence is mitigated by new campaigns and laws.

356   L. Nusseibeh

these efforts. Conflict is still present at the level of the large group identity, but
its impact is less because communities are more secure. As a result, there is
less splitting and projection between groups, less violence among the protagonists, and less overflow onto the global community; protagonists become more
connected to global civil society. Vested interests are still present and may
indeed increase (e.g., media use for negative propaganda), as efforts are made
to maintain hold over the conflict. Nonetheless, their impact is reduced by the
campaigns and laws promulgated by the international organizations.

Figure 18.3 shows the onset of peaceful coexistence between the communities that were once at odds. Supported by mutually reinforcing early childhood
development programs and aided by age-appropriate educational media, children, caregivers, and the local communities form an interlocking secure base.
This base enables a large group identity to be created that is whole, strong,
and secure. Because of this, a group's identity becomes stable enough to withstand outside threat and/or violent acts without retaliation. This allows a group
to view itself on par with other groups—a recognition that leads to less aggressive acts against other groups. The interlocking secure core will continue
to expand and gain strength if it is firmly protected by laws, campaigns, and
early childhood developmental programs and reinforced by age-appropriate
educational media. Academic research provides a crucial role by assessing the
impact of programs, laws, and campaigns, thus permitting adjustments to be
made when warranted. As the two communities grow stronger, they become
more connected to global civil society. However, the two communities are still
separate and very much defined by their own large group identities. Residual
violence is present, as vested interests may be successful in penetrating the

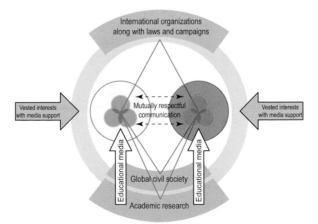

Figure 18.3   The beginnings of peacebuilding: two communities (yellow and red
shapes) move toward peaceful coexistence. Early childhood interventions and age-
appropriate educational media enable children, caregivers, and the community (circles)
to coalesce and form a secure group. Impact from vested interests and their supporting
media diminish, leaving the two groups to form stable self identities.

space that surrounds the communities. However, in contrast to the situations depicted in Figures 18.1 and 18.2, this does not impact the cohesion and solidarity of a community's large group identity. Vested interests may still employ media to penetrate into a community, but their chance for success is lessened because of the positive countereffects created by educational media. As self-identities gain stability and strength, communications between the large groups begin to develop positively: perceptions of each other become less tainted by fear and mistrust. This positive development in communications creates its own virtuous cycle: knowledge and equity increase in both groups so that each group is able to view itself as well as each other without prejudice.

Figure 18.4 shows peaceful coexistence. Large group identity has developed and is so secure that each group can now perceive itself as belonging to a larger community. The confining and divisive aspects of large group identity, which caused fear and aggression earlier (cf. Figures 18.1 and 18.2), no longer affect the communities. Age-appropriate educational media continue to reinforce and amplify this development. The two groups, which were originally engaged in continual conflict, are now so secure that they are able to fully recognize each other's humanity. This enables them to imagine and employ creative solutions to join together and connect progressively to a securely based, interconnected global human community. Vested interests can no longer penetrate and project mechanisms that produce "us versus them" mentality because the communities are linked. The media that support vested interests have less impact than ever. International organizations continue to support the process as does the academic community. Global civil society has been integrated into the support

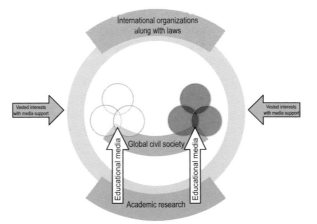

Figure 18.4 Peaceful coexistence: children, caregivers, and community (depicted as circles) have attained secure, mutual existence; the two groups (yellow and red) can now be viewed as belonging to a larger group embedded within the global civil society. Educational media, early childhood interventions, international organizations, and academia support this process. Vested interests and their support media are unable to penetrate this secure, peaceful coexistence.

framework, but it no longer needs to be as visible due to the strength and inter-connections of the communities, which enables secure human beings.

Conclusions

Media has the potential to break stereotypes and encourage prosocial behavior. Especially during early childhood, it has the potential to deliver clear messages that are age-appropriate to support the development of prosocial behavior. Based on extensive action research and expanded use of technology, prosocial media programs can and should be developed to reach children throughout the world. In this way, media can contribute substantially to enabling a bottom-up approach to peacebuilding. Positive educational media will always confront a background of negative media and ongoing conflict as well as trauma and vested interests in prolonging conflict and deepening trauma. Still, with suffi-cient global awareness and support, media can be used to move our societies in the opposite direction: it can provide the muscle for forging a possible pathway to peace.

To support this process, further enquiry will be needed into the mechanisms and potential of age-appropriate educational media, and the following ques-tions are offered as a guide:

- What is the best way to measure the impact of television shows on children?
- How can social media be used to engage children and families, in view of the increasingly available technology (e.g., mobile phones and apps)?
- How can different types of media be used to reach those most in need (i.e., those in refugee camps or conflict areas)?
- In very young children (e.g., as of one year of age), are there ways that media can be used to develop an overarching human identity (as op-posed to a group identity)?
- How can a multicultural approach be developed in key conflict areas?
- Are there ways that media can be used to protect the most vulnerable in conflicts (e.g., by reducing stress or providing some form of support buffer)?

First column (top to bottom): Mohammed Abu-Nimer, Gary Gunderson,
Geraldine Smyth, Olayinka Omigbodun, Jacqueline Bhabha, Lucy Nusseibeh,
Olayinka Omigbodun, Cigdem Kagitcibasi
Second column: Rima Salah, Ilham Nasser, Jacqueline Bhabha,
Mohammed Abu-Nimer, Cigdem Kagitcibasi, Gary Gunderson,
Mikiko Otani, Rima Salah
Third column: Pia Britto, Anwarul Chowdhury, Mikiko Otani, Jim Cochrane,
Geraldine Smyth, Pia Britto, Anwarul Chowdhury, Lucy Nusseibeh

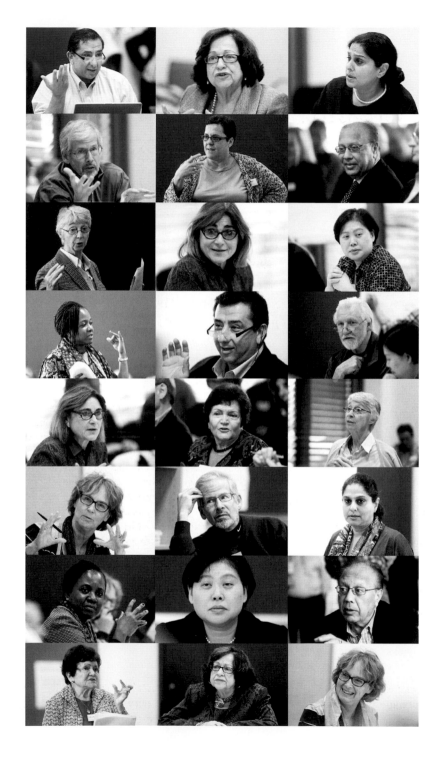

19

Creating Effective Programs and Policies to Reduce Violence and Promote Peace

Pia R. Britto, Rima Salah, Mohammed Abu-Nimer,
Jacqueline Bhabha, Anwarul K. Chowdhury,
Gary R. Gunderson, Cigdem Kagitcibasi,
Lucy Nusseibeh, Olayinka Omigbodun,
Mikiko Otani, and Geraldine Smyth

Abstract

The focus of this chapter is on the social and biological underpinnings of child development and its contexts to create effective programs and policies that will reduce violence
and promote peace. It addresses a range of issues emanating from fields of education,
media, religion, psychology, and cultural studies. The emergent themes address interconnected pathways and multilayered perpsectives, across a range of disciplines, that
form a link between formative childhood and peace, including strengthening families
and building resilient communities. The primary theme underscores that the well-being of children is fundamental to peace. However, knowledge of the association between early childhood and peace needs to be expanded. While much is known about
promoting peace, evidence is lacking on whether formative childhoods constitute a
potential path to peace. Further research, coordination, and partnerships are needed
between disciplines and sectors engaged in peacebuilding and early development. In
addition, a perspective on human securities, rights, and capacities is needed to support
this work—one that encourages individual capabilities, cultural and community assets,
and an emancipatory vision and inclusive practices.

Introduction

Peace is a desired state of being, at personal and societal levels. Virtually every
language in the world has a word for peace, albeit with varying nuances and
emphases. Its universal appeal, however, is also its greatest challenge, both in

its varieties of definition and cultural association as well as in its achievement and aspiration. The existence of childhood constitutes another universal reality. The mosaic of humanity, with all its differences, is united through a universal process of life course development from the time of conception. Research evidence clearly indicates that the earliest years of life constitute a critical foundation to human development. Evolutionary biologists have concluded that of the 27 protohuman species which evolved on Earth, only *Homo erectus* has survived, in part due to the six-year period of early childhood, which allowed their brains to adapt to the environment and survive (Walter 2013). The paradox of early childhood is also clearly recognized: this period of great opportunity is also a period of vulnerability. A succession of challenges lies between the desired vision of healthy holistic development and the realities of the world. What is required to engage these challenges is thoughtful, contextually sensitive, concrete action at several interconnected levels.

This chapter addresses the overarching question: How can new knowledge emanating from biological and social sciences about child development and its contexts be used to create effective programs and policies that will reduce violence, increase human security, and promote peace? It attempts to address how peace can be more than an abstract term that can take shape and form in every aspect of our daily existence. It presents a road map that emphasizes the agency, both actual and potential, of the child, families, and communities to create change by linking sound research, knowledge, experience, and positive concrete action to programs and policies. Critical questions include:

- What are the operational constructs of peace and violence that can be linked to the theory of change and life course perspective (including early childhood through adolescence), drawing on multidisciplinary knowledge?
- What are the realities of contexts and characteristics of knowledge change agents, including children, families, communities, practititoner, policy makers, that shape and influence the multidirectional transfer between knowledge, policies and programs?
- What are the principles that we should consider when new knowledge is adapted for use in very diverse contexts?
- How can micro and macro levels of this issue be linked, from early childhood to peace, locally and globally, and what lessons can be learned from best practices of similar initiatives?

To address these questions, we engaged in rich discussions at this Forum, which are summarized in this chapter. To some questions, we agreed upon answers. Other questions are still open, in part because of the complexity of the principal constructs of "formative childhoods" and "peace." The dialog that occurred between disciplines and sectors during the course of the Forum was akin to a laboratory for testing ideas and experimenting with the correlation of different epistemological frameworks, different scientific modes of enquiry, and cross-fertilization of ideas and knowledge. While this innovative Forum revealed both the potential and challenges of knowledge and expertise sharing, it also exposed the need for deeper and further exchange to address the complexity of issues embedded in this topic, within and across disciplinary fields as well as across the sectors of academia, practice, and policy making.

Conceptual Framework

What Is the New Knowledge of Early Childhood and the Culture of Peace?

Knowledge, as referred to in this chapter, spans a range of scientific disciplines, inclusive of, but not limited to, anthropology, economics, political science, developmental psychology, law, peace studies, gender studies, education, ethics, philosophy, theology, and biobehavioral sciences, together with those pertaining to more applied fields of inquiry such as communication, group dynamics/organizational behavior and conflict resolution, peacebuilding, and the creation of a culture of peace. Using this broad base of perspectives, we sought a conceptual frame of reference that would bring together key constructs of peace and early childhood with the research, policies, and practice that inform them, and the translational processes and relationships which can contribute to necessary change.

Peace

Definitions of peace tend to limit it when it is contrasted with war and violence. Violence itself is a complex construct that covers the spectrum from individual to collective, direct to structural, episodic to chronic; it also has different focuses of concentration (e.g., gender-based, physical, psychological), from bilateral ethnic conflicts to all-out war between states and state blocs. In our conception of peace, we elected to make peace and the understanding of peace itself the starting point and sought to explore its inner and outer meanings, substance, and texture. In understanding peace as a positive experience and generative construct, we sought to define it above and beyond the absence of war and violence, personally, socially, and ecologically.

Peace, however, is a complex and indeed contested construct. The multiple definitions of peace highlight components and characteristics, depending on the vantage point of formulation. Furthermore, an additional challenge to defining peace emanates from the opponents of peace, who dispute its very value or dismiss it as "soft" or unrealizable. Our perspective on peace draws on its universalizable aspects, on its potential for universal appropriation and operationalization, and for approaches across the life course. Human beings, individually and collectively, are a central feature of this conceptualization. Through this definition, we recognize multiple elements of peace, including the internal, external, personal, and collective aspects and freedom of choice to pursue what is meaningful with opportunities to support the development of the person's full potential and life chances. We also include those factors and active contributors to peace, understood as a basic right for all and constitutive of humanity.

> Peace is an opportunity, including internal awareness, which allows human beings, individually and collectively, to pursue their lives in a meaningful way to their fullest potential, and contributing to the realization of universal human rights, freedom justice, and oneness of humanity.

Early Childhood

The actualization of this definition is linked with a life course perspective of human development, the foundational stage of which is early childhood. Our conceptualization of early childhood draws on the traditional definitions but then expands this in congruence with the purpose of the chapter.

Continually burgeoning evidence from childhood studies demonstrates one clear conclusion: the earliest years of life can be critical for a child's subsequent holistic development across various domains of functioning and well-being (Britto et al. 2013). Early childhood is understood as the first years of life, until the transition to primary school has been completed. It encompasses the child and their environment. With respect to the child, holistic development is recognized as vital and inclusive of all domains of physical health and well-being: motor, social, cognitive, emotional, spiritual, and moral development; language, literacy, and communication; self-identity, cultural developmental flourishing; as well as a comprehensive approach to learning and access to life chances. With respect to the context, multiple layers are involved, ranging from the most proximal—such as families (including nuclear, extended and nontraditional)—to the most distal (including global settings, e.g., international laws, global belonging, ecological relationships, influences, and impacts) (McCartney and Phillips 2006; Shonkoff and Phillips 2000).

The neurosciences are demonstrating the importance of plasticity of the brain early in life. While the specific timing and issues linked with irreversibility or reversibility of outcomes are still contested and not fully understood, there are areas where evidence has provided clues to the foundational significance of the early years for the future life course. For example, biobehavioral research has indicated that early-life bonds impact our neurobiology in ways that have a multigenerational impact. In particular, the oxytocin system, involved in the process of bonding and nurturance early in life, is demonstrably associated with capacities for trust, empathy, and reaction to stress (see Carter and Porges, this volume). Scientists and peace theorists alike emphasize that while there is not a direct causal association between biology and peacebuilding, physiological systems and bodily reactions play a central role in influencing personal agency and motivation as well as in the dynamics of social inclusion and (pro) social behavior. In addition, the individual and collective capacities to generate and engage in trust is a crucial step in peaceful relations. Other work has demonstrated that specific capacities for empathy, self-regulation, and cognitive control relate to brain and neurological functioning and develop during early childhood (van IJzendoorn and Bakermans-Kranenburg, this volume). They are considered to be important in enabling apposite response to social cues, in the promotion of mutual understanding and tolerance, and in the reduction of violent and unconstrained reactions.

Gaps remain in our understanding of the association between early childhood and peace, in that limited research has been conducted to develop and test this hypothesis. Yet the conceptual links between biobehavioral and psychological outcomes early in life are predictive of and aligned with adult social functioning and behaviors associated with resilience and the capacity for positive development (Kagitcibasi and Britto, this volume).

Policies

Policies are vehicles for large-scale action. There are a range of policies that address peace in official government, civil society, and international communities (e.g., UN conventions and norms on human rights, behavior in war, peacebuilding codes). Seldom are these policies coordinated. Most policies on peace emanate from the perspectives of postwar settlements, military securitization, and conflict reduction mechanisms. This must be expanded to include human security, with its emphasis on the individual, and the ongoing development of international policies geared to social peace and justice that bring the particular needs of children, women, and families and social justice to the fore (both within states and for those who are stateless). Given this range and unevenness, we present a general conceptual framework for policies.

For the purpose of our work, we define progressive policy as a statement of action, supported institutionally, that pays attention to and is inclusive of values of majority and minority perspectives, including those of fragile groups and populations. Policies are important because they aim to ensure access and equity while maintaining good quality programs and strategies across the regions and the populations they address. Policy provides guidance for meeting needs while addressing development and progress. Typically, policies consist of four components: (a) vision (including goal objectives and impact), (b) programs and strategies (the mechanism for achieving the vision of the policy), (c) governance (the respective interrelated roles and responsibilities of the key stakeholders), and (d) finance and resourcing (to ensure sustainability). Policies need also to be socially sustainable (i.e., owned by families and society) and politically sustainable so that they can survive across political transitions and differences of ideology and power structures. This angle is particularly important because in many conflict situations, due to the threat and danger to human life and physical and emotional fragility, the civic and social infrastructure needs to be rebuilt through structural policy development, implementation, monitoring, and realignment.

Peace, Early Childhood, and Policy: What We Know and What Are the Challenges

There are several areas of knowledge that we are attempting to link in this chapter. First, we wish to link micro-level issues, such as child development, to the macro level of peace. Safety and security present one of the biggest implications for this conceptual linkage. At the micro level, they are expressed in biobehavioral models of safety whereas at the macro level they appear as national and human security, stable order, and the rule of law. There are a few constructs that allow for such linkages, although the path between them is still marked by major knowledge gaps and policy fissures. For example, safety is a concept and reality that can be understood and measured across the spectrum of sciences, from biological to social. However, the properties of safety, when conceptualized at the level of biology and the individual, might be viewed as possessing different properties when viewed under the respective rubrics of "the rule of law," "human security," and "the responsibility to protect." In essence, there is a thread running through ideas of safety from individual to societal levels that has the potential to link the reality of safety and security (secure attachment) in early childhood in its contexts to the wider reality and manifestations of human security and peace. However, the challenge in the identification of the nature and characteristics changes according to the varying unit of analysis from "one" to "many."

Second, meaningful linking of the micro to the macro requires greater cohesion and synergy between disciplines. Given the current situation of high levels of specialization and limited platforms for multidisciplinary research and exchange, achieving consensus or knowledge integration is a challenge. What could be envisaged is a sequential multidisciplinary effort that would take the results from one or more disciplines and link them with a subsequent set, as in a chain, thus allowing the micro and macro to be connected. For example, one might explore how to preserve and develop the necessary building blocks of security in infancy and childhood into social structures enabling adolescents, youth, and young adults to flourish and realize fundamental aspirations and goals. Excellent work on the development of pre-primary and primary education needs to feed into a more sustained social engagement with secondary and tertiary education, with skill development, with gender, class, and other forms of safety and justice. Such a platform needs to be established.

Third is the process of "translating" knowledge of early childhood and peace into policy action (discussed in greater detail below). Translation is more than just a repository of information; it is a way of framing the issues for the intended audience. Our perspective on translation stresses a necessary bidirectionality, by emphasizing that knowledge needs to move not only from science to policy and practice (or from scholars in neurosciences and child sciences to peace studies, legal and public policy scholars) but also in the other direction, if there is to be optimal positive impact on childhood and peace through policy change.

Fourth, research in peace and family has produced evidence that when macro conditions of conflict and war exist, especially for a sustained period, they leave a destructive and developmentally harmful impact on children and their families. However, when macro conditions facilitate stability and nonviolence, children and families are able to experience a context of security and safety that promotes growth. Such links between macro policies and micro human development exist already and need to be used further to promote peace.

Theory of Change: The Well-Being of Children Is Fundamental to Peace

New knowledge and evidence from basic biology to social sciences indicates that optimal interaction between the developing child and context is important for positive development and well-being. Evidence has recognized that environment is as much a part of our endowment as our genes, so both context and biology are important for early development, with implications for the life course. The theory of change underlying our work is that development occurs across the life course, and we recognize the first two decades of life as being formative. With respect to sensitive stages, we focus on early childhood as foundational for continuing development. Taking a life course perspective, with early childhood at the start, we present two dimensions of our theory of change:

1. Children have to be protected to promote peace.
2. Children, even young children, have a voice and agency in promoting peace.

Positive overall human development, and the provision of secure parenting and communities of belonging, particularly in formative early childhood, helps build pathways to peace, though without guarantee, given the myriad of factors and variables involved.

The Convention on the Rights of the Child,[1] an almost universally ratified human rights treaty, provides a legal framework for understanding the first dimension of the theory of change, that of protecting the child. Several of the articles address our first dimension (i.e., children's right to survival, development, and protection):

> Article 6: "States Parties shall ensure to the maximum extent possible the survival and development of the child."

---

[1]   http://www.ohchr.org/en/professionalinterest/pages/crc.aspx (accessed June 6, 2014).

Article 2: "States Parties shall take all appropriate measures to ensure that the child is protected against all forms of discrimination or punishment on the basis of the status, activities, expressed opinions, or beliefs of the child's parents, legal guardians, or family member."

Article 27: "States Parties recognize the right of every child to a standard of living adequate for the child's physical, mental, spiritual, moral and social development."

Positive well-being and healthy development of young children, starting *in utero*, has been linked with protective, safe, responsive, supportive, and stimulating environments. Despite nearly universal ratification of this landmark convention, 200 million children (i.e., over one-third of the world's children living in low- and middle-income countries, under the age of five years) do not achieve their developmental potential (Engle et al. 2007). This is a stark, challenging figure. Inadequacies in the environment due to a wide range of conditions are responsible for this dramatic gap between rights entitlement and realization.

As per our theory of change, two arguments corroborate the claim that connects the rights and support and protection of children with the promotion of peace and the active work of peacebuilding.

The first concerns social injustice and economic disparities, which contribute to and maintain "structural violence" (Galtung 2008). Children suffer from structural violence when they do not receive adequate stimulation, support, and protection during the most sensitive periods of growth. Thus, their opportunity to develop specific skills and capabilities associated with later functioning and flourishing are compromised. Remediation later in life is often costly, and reported success in such area compares poorly with that of children whose infancy was structurally peaceful in this sense. Early childhood is the phase of life when the most rapid gains are made across all domains of development. Neurobiology has demonstrated the rapid proliferation of neuronal development in the first few years of life that set the foundation for later skills and capacities. Brain architecture is built in a bottom-up sequence, with each stage requiring the adequate development of earlier capacities. Early childhood is the foundation to life and impacts adult functioning and well-being. Given that social and economic disparities are perpetuated by differences in adult capacities and opportunities, assuring all children of the right start and support in life helps to narrow social inequity and economic exclusion—thereby eliminating the factors that maintain the cycle of structural violence.

Second, the new generation of wars being fought in the name of identity (ethnic, national, or religious) rather than ideology has had a more direct and lethal impact on noncombatants and civilians—not least, children—compared to the earlier generation of wars. Social identity theory has demonstrated that development, formation of prejudice and stereotypes, and awareness of differences between self and others occurs as early as three years of age (Connolly et al. 2002). The emergence of "social self," or the development of a sense of self as a member of a particular group, starts to occur early in life (Ruble et al. 2004). Parenting socialization patterns have been shown to influence this early identity development. Case studies from conflict and postconflict environments, such as those of Palestine, Northern Ireland, and Chad, have shown that early childhood development provides a unique entry point for transcending existing divides and refocusing attention to positive models for development (Connolly and Hayden 2007). Other media-based models, such as Sesame Street and Early Years programs, have demonstrated success in reducing stereotyping in children and promoting inclusiveness among children (Abu-Nimer 1999; Nasser and Abu-Nimer 2007).

Expanding on the second dimension in our theory of change (i.e., when children and youth have a voice then they have the potential to be agents of peace), the Convention on the Rights of the Child asserts:

> Article 12: "States Parties shall assure to the child who is capable of forming his or her own views the right to express those views freely in all matters affecting the child, the views of the child being given due weight in accordance with the age and maturity of the child."

Children should be invited to participate in developing policies and programs, beyond the tokenism of their superficial presence in front of adult audiences. Although inviting young children to participate in such a process may be outside the realm of possibility, indications of a child's agency are noted early in life. Such agency needs to be encouraged. Early childhood interventions are the first microcosm of society for children (Astuto and Ruck 2010): not only are they contexts for development, they are deeply embedded in and are part of larger societal, cultural, and macrostructures and systems (Carretero 2011). Through participation in these programs, not only will the well-being of children and families be improved, children will also learn to participate in society, mature in their social and civic capabilities, and become effective agents of change, thus contributing to the common good.

Novel Approaches to the Use of Knowledge for Policy

Knowledge can be effective in the promotion of peace—a peace driver. Knowledge that promotes inclusion, justice, and equality emphasizes commonalities and provides analyses of root causes of violence and fear of differences; this will build social cohesion and provide resources for peace and peacebuilding. We recognize, of course, that knowledge is a necessary but insufficient condition for change. However, knowledge in concert with open attitudes and practices can be an important resource for peace, especially when combined with positive and hands-on experience (Head, Heart, Hand). Paulo Freire's groundbreaking educational work in actively connecting knowledge and action for justice (conscientization and praxis) has proven effective in Latin America and other contexts of the Global South.

We may need to question claims about the "newness" of knowledge, regarding early childhood development, neuroscience, and peace testing; that is, whether it is "new" or simply "new validation" of existing knowledge. Furthermore, we may need to reflect on how far such new, validated knowledge can be asserted as universal. All knowledge applicability needs to be tested within and across specific contexts related to existing knowledge and traditional praxis. With these provisos in mind, we now take a reflective perspective that draws on research and briefly describe six approaches to using knowledge for policy. We note that these six approaches are not mutually exclusive. While they extend the field in using knowledge to inform policy, they are also exploratory given the newness of the exploration of the relationship between early childhood, peace, and peacebuilding.

Global Citizenship and the Culture of Peace

In early childhood, traditional domains of development have emphasized functioning in areas linked with school, education, and learning success (e.g., physical health, motor, social, emotional cognitive, moral, spiritual and language development, and approaches to learning). However, the new world order calls for expanding this framework toward understanding the importance of functioning as a global citizen, because the changing nature of the world (environment, technology, connectivitiy, mobility, etc.) is also shaping dramatic changes in education. The United Nation's report on education places global citizenship as one of three priorities for the world community.

Global citizenship requires a transformational change, toward enabling children (and adults) to think and act in ways that forge more just, peaceful, tolerant, and inclusive societies (see the Foreword, this volume). It is no exaggeration to assert that the foundation for global citizenship is laid during childhood, where children learn compassion and empathy, toward both their own groups and others, together with the understanding, values, and skills which they need to cooperate in resolving the interconnected challenges of the twentry-first century. Global citizenship entails not only preparing children for the world of the future but also education for peace and sustainability.

The concept of the culture of peace (see the Foreword, this volume) derives its essence from the assertion in UNESCO's Constitution that "since wars begin in the minds of men, it is in the minds of men that the defenses of peace must be constructed." This very profound expression establishes emphatically that peace, in its most comprehensive sense, is secured through the individual mind. In this context, it is believed that the flourishing of the culture of peace will generate a mindset that is the prerequisite for the transition from force to reason, from conflict and violence to dialog and peace. In 1999, the United Nations adopted the Declaration and Program of Action on a Culture of

Peace—a monumental document that transcends boundaries, cultures, societies, and nations. The principle underlying this program is that peace cannot be gained by government action alone (for further discussion, see the Foreword to this volume).

As stated earlier, early childhood is a vital formative phase for identity and life development. Therefore, in thinking through the implications of the growing interconnectedness of the world, we need to prepare children to live and succeed in a reality that will be influenced both by their immediate family, community, or town as well as by what happens in regions and ecosystems around the world. The tenets of the culture of peace rest on a person's capabilities for respect, nonviolence, justice, and equality—underlying values and orienting attitudes that can be encouraged as early as three years of age.

Ecological Paradigms of Nested Systems Overlaid by Networks of Association

One of the most cited and used ecological paradigms to explain human development was developed by Urie Bronfenbrenner in 1979. According to this ecological systems theory, children develop in four levels of a nested system: the *microsystem* (e.g., family), the *mesosystem* (two microsystems in interaction), the *exosystem* (external environments which indirectly influence development), and the *macrosystem* (the larger sociocultural context). For early childhood, the microsystem, as the most proximal context, has the most significant direct influence on development; the more distal the context, the more indirect its influence.

In the context of globalization, however, and in what has already been noted about the nature of *structural* violence, we need to ask what is actually distal. In light of current technological advances and interconnectedness, nested systems are now affected by the interference of networks. No longer are contexts of the macrosystem distal. Certainly within the microsystem of the developing child, contexts are viable and dynamically interactive entities (see Figure 19.1).

Women's networks (e.g., local women's panchayats in India) embody the most basic intelligence of a neighborhood. These social networks, through tangible services of food and intangible services of support and encouragement, help new mothers and never allow babies to be left unattended. These complex associations extend across an array of actors including government, faith, health, media, philanthropy, and civil society groups. This intricate associational ecology overlays the traditional nested systems to connect levels in more direct and potentially meaningful ways to socialize children for peace and to promote basic rights for children. In relation to early childhood and peace, this ecology of human associations brings a complexity to understanding the influence of proximal and distal contexts with respect to children's development because of the fluid and dynamic nature of human systems.

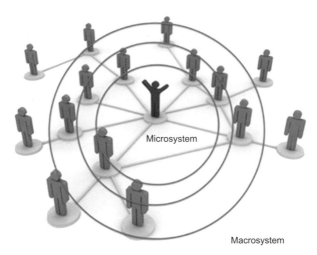

Figure 19.1   Nested systems and networks: social ecologies of development.

Capabilities-Based Approach to Practice, Policy, and Programs

Studied factors which drive conflict include poverty, certain political and religious ideologies and practices, as well as aspects of new technology and identity "mania." These have been known to generate tension and conflict in community for several reasons. First, they are easily manipulated and mobilized in ways that can bring individual persons and communities to behave like a mob and commit acts of violence and revenge. In such situations, individuals can lose their capacity to think intelligently, confront problems, and resolve conflict cooperatively. These factors also increase fear and insecurity. Differences between groups, in particular decisions regarding who belongs to the in-group versus the out-group, fuel conflict and violence. "Us versus them" differences take on several forms: One is that of negative difference (i.e., "We are not like them"), which can lead to polarization and dehumanization. "Us versus them" issues also form a dominance hierarchy (i.e., "We are better than them"). This in turn can heighten insecurity, fear, and threats, making violent outbreak more likely and magnetic in attraction.

Peacebuilders, policy makers, and practitioners need to take early childhood into account when intervening in societies. Social, cultural, economic, ecological conditions, and systemic structures are essential. The promotion of secure childhood and sustainable peace benefits from approaches that encourage human capabilities as well as cultural and community assets, including emancipatory vision, inclusive participatory decision-making processes, and promotion of human security and human rights.

We start with a straightforward approach of resolving the "us versus them" tension, using the work of Sherif (1966), who demonstrated in a field experiment that intergroup competition and conflict creates negative stereotypes and hostility. In contrast, under certain conditions, intergroup interdependence and cooperation can lead to positive intergroup attitudes. In this study, called the "Robber's Cave," 11-year-old boys in a summer camp were organized into two groups. They played competing games with desirable rewards for the winner group. Such competition and conflict created in-group cohesion but also frustration and intergroup hostility. The researchers then introduced critical events that required the two groups to work together, making them interdependent. For example, when their bus broke down, both groups had to push it or face not getting back to camp. One group acting alone could not succeed. Such episodes involving the embrace of "superordinate" goals by both groups enabled them to appreciate the need to be interdependent and cooperate. Cooperation further engendered positive attitudes toward the other group and reduced prejudice.

On a more complex level of systems and structures, we consider that child and health assets may be a way of realizing peace assets. In this regard the role of religious communities as a resource for peace comes into view. In many parts of the world, some of the largest institutions, built on an earlier generation's moral vision, are hospitals. Thus, in many countries in Africa, faith-inspired hospitals provide between 40–70% of healthcare. Many also have networks of primary care and prevention programs extending into surrounding areas (Gunderson and Cochrane 2012). These institutions are almost always among the largest in their community and only compete with the most established institutions of higher education in the number of employees, capitalization, and budget. Most do relate to caring for children and often participate actively in governmental prevention strategies, including violence-related ones. These religiously initiated health systems are lightly and loosely connected to each other and are easily convened. Harnessing the capability of health assets and making them available across boundaries is considered an innovative approach to policy (Cochrane 2012).

Extrapolating from this, religion can also play a role in intensifying violent conflict, just as it can work to inspire and sustain the vision and practice of peace. Care is needed when speaking abstractly about "religion," whether as a driver of conflict or peace. People who live in religious communities do not see themselves belonging to a "Religion" but rather to a community of religious vision and practice that is not a separate compartment of their lives, but interwoven with their world view (in its transcendent and immanent aspects), their traditional and changing ethos, and relationships to those both within and beyond their own context in ways that are increasingly plural and differentiated. In such complex layered forms of organization, the formal and informal, sectarian, and communitarian dynamics are embedded in traditions and can sometimes be locked into ethnic and national identities while also freely floating as global phenomena. The major religious traditions, and even most of their subsidiary currents flowing within them, precede nation-states by at least a thousand years, just as they predate the earliest steps toward organized scientific discovery. The relationship between faith, reason, and religious experience is negotiated variously by different world faiths. So, too, the ways in which people of faith or religious communities relate to the domains of science, history, secularity, society, modern states, and intergovernmental organizations are not homogeneous, but rather differentiated and dynamic. The relationship is continually under fresh interpretation and renegotiation, as remains the case today. It is surprising to many that religion in both novel and very traditional forms remains a potent force in human affairs. It is more helpful and more in tune with reality to think of the structures of faith and religious organizations as fluid, dynamic, and complex.

For our purposes, religions, faith, spirituality, and service can be approached in terms of their potential role in transforming people and promoting peace—encouraging the human capacity to open to meaning, sharing, healing, forgiveness, and new hope. So, too, are their organized forms of care and social justice toward those who are suffering and abandoned. Our purpose here is not ideological debate, but to see ways whereby spiritual wisdom and solidarity embodied in religious assets and agencies can contribute to peace and be drawn into creating and sustaining strategies for advancing generations of healthy and whole children who themselves advance the hopes of human peace. Every faith tradition, organized enough to have a newsletter and website, is porous and constantly in dialog with many other bodies of thought, belief, ritual, and faith. Faith traditions hold open space for questions as well as answers, and in some cases the tradition of questioning and reflecting on the need for inner and outer transformation is more useful than its more time-bound answers. Many academic institutions founded by religious traditions (e.g., Harvard or Cambridge) protect space for critical inquiry and philosophical research in which respect for disciplinary boundaries needs to be properly informed, including the social sciences, law, and ethics relevant to peace developed. It is not surprising that forces operate within and through religious channels to fight for the past and against competing groups. However, religious traditions are malleable, usually from within, and nearly always have positive deviants, even within the most conservative-appearing streams. All of the top ten to twenty religious groupings have long histories of varied thought and perspective that offer up a treasure trove of alternative views and language that skilled, artful, and appreciative partners can engage as resources for developing new knowledge and science; this, in turn, may create the grounds for surprising partnerships. It is helpful to see the institutional complexity that has grown out of the religious streams as multilithic and fluid. Even within highly structured institutions, such as the Catholic Church, there is a wide range of compliance and scope for variance, even within a council of bishops, social service and health organizations, and its thousands of educational institutions. So, too, in the world of Islam, there are many variants; different geographical cultural locations and language traditions show different manifestations of Islam whether in the Arab regions, the Indian Sub-Continent, Iran, or Indonesia. This is also true in the nontheistic traditions such as Buddhism. The fluidity and differentiation offer opportunities to engage with ancient, new and newly relevant knowledge to form new partnerships to advance the link between early childhood development and peace.

There is a positive role for meaning-making and value-sustaining human associations as creative and supporting partners with research and government. There are obvious tensions to be expected in the relationship, as in all partnership arrangements, although this is less significant vis à vis action for the earliest years of child development, which the relevant science considers of the highest priority.

Media and Education, in Addition to Family, Are Powerful Channels to Promote Peace through Early Childhood

Two approaches to peace considered in our discussions were education and media, for a variety of reasons, including their salient influence on early development. Given the life course approach that we adopted, education was considered in the broad sense and inclusive of all levels, from early learning opportunities to higher education. With respect to early childhood education, identity development and global citizenship—guiding principles of integrating "diversity and pluralism" in all early childhood education—should be integrated into existing curricula on oneness of humanity, commonalities, and similarities. Addressing these identity issues in early childhood is crucial for "life skills," adaptability, and peace. This is an essential part of the capacity to survive in the world. Equally important is the education of educators. One of the greatest challenges to achieving global citizenship involves the lack of capacity of educators, limited curricula, restricted pedagogies, and learning materials. A critical skill for educators engaged in peace education is listening, which is also a core skill that needs to be developed in children (see Abu-Nimer and Nasser, this volume).

Successful media approaches to reach children include children and youth radio and television (see Nusseibeh, this volume). These have been successful in changing attitudes and behaviors. However, there is far too little good media for children, which leaves open space for those who want to manipulate it as a conflict driver, especially media programs that expose children to a culture of violence and legitimize structural and institutional forms of violence (e.g., weapons, killing, fear of others.) Another powerful media tool for building public awareness is campaigns. Through the multiple technological applications, even in low resource areas, such campaigns can be disseminated beyond traditional means of posters and flyers to more effective technologies of television public service announcements during popular shows, bumper stickers, radio spots, transmedia, and multimedia. For the media to be effective, however, it needs to be treated as a stakeholder from the inception of the process. Media literacy is an important component of peacebuilding as it builds self-awareness and awareness of others and reduces bias and stereotyping, thereby building resistance to propaganda. Media literacy means knowing how the media works: how emotions and images can be manipulated as well as how to work actively with media. Media literacy is a two-way concept: it is both protective and proactive. Protective skills, insofar as children are taught to analyze media content and read between the lines; understanding the messages behind the images can help children become less vulnerable and fall less easy prey to negative influences. Children must be taught to read, listen, watch, and interact with an active critical approach, not simply a passive receptivity. It is particularly relevant in relation to stereotyping and bias. Proactive insofar as children are also taught to work creatively: not as technicians, but in regard to content so that they can produce their own media messages. By encouraging greater awareness of the various forces in society (e.g., media owners, businesses, special interests), media literacy programs encourage civic engagement along with open-mindedness.

Redefining Translation of Knowledge

The identity and function of knowledge change agents and multipliers is context specific. When it comes to translating knowledge, sensitivity to context is paramount. Thus, it is important to be able to identify those within specific contexts who act as doorkeepers of knowledge or who function as change agents in knowledge formation or who can create multiplier effects (see Figure 19.2).

Those who generate, "consume," and translate knowledge are often one and the same, operating interchangeably according to a different identity and role according to need. For example, when science is informing policy, scientists are the generators and policy makers are the consumers; when policy

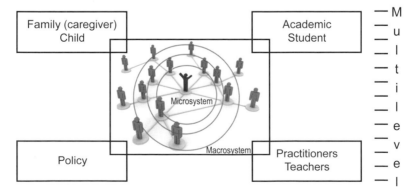

Figure 19.2 Knowledge change agents and multipliers: generators, consumers, and translators.

informs science, policy makers are the generators and scientists are the consumers. Regardless of role, to ensure meaningful translation of knowledge into policies, dialog and conscious efforts for understanding one another's sphere of work and expertise between scientists, policy makers, and practitioners is needed. Such interaction should be bidirectional. Furthermore, the translator is not a neutral conveyer of information. The translator's identity, attitude, and ability to understand and communicate information effectively is critical. There is a danger of oversimplification of information and not understanding the complexity of the interactions involved in the relationships between knowledge generators, translators, and consumers.

The challenge is how to make knowledge available in such a way as to make sense and be convincing to those who will apply it. "Translation" works best if there is joint work by scientists and policy makers, involving bilateral information sharing, so that the latter will develop "ownership" of that knowledge and its application. Thus we can avoid the cultural imposition of certain models or policies in educating children for peace or in applying new knowledge. A science-practice-policy process is more likely to be achieved this way, and endeavors are more likely to be sustained over time.

It is important to take note of "good examples" in the field and make use of the experience accumulated rather than "reinventing the wheel." Examples need to be drawn from the non-Western "Majority World" as well as from the Western contexts. The former may present socio-economic-cultural environments similar to those where new interventions or policies will be introduced.

One strategy of peacebuilding is to bring knowledge to society by "spreading the message" through non-experts into mainstream culture. For this purpose, knowledge about relevant parameters has to be translated into "common and easy language." One example for a successful translation of complex scientific results might be the various television productions, or "infotainment," from astrophysics, which are used to explain our universe in fantastic pictures and easy language. This translation process should not be performed by scientists (or politicians) but by using the creative potential of musicians, artists, bloggers, young students, etc., because they know what they would like and understand. This process can itself be seen as peacebuilding because it exemplifies transparency and provides a model for communication between different groups and joint problem solving.

Universal Principles and Adaptations to Contexts

Knowledge needs to be applied to programs and policies across a range of settings and systems. To this end, our discussion focused both on the universal principles identified in the literature and adaptations to contexts. When abstracting universal themes, it is important to consider the process and content. The focus of the intervention dictates the application of universal principles.

Interventions may focus on the child, family (mothers, fathers, etc.), and community as well as at a systems level. In the latter category, an additional area of focus is whether the programs are targeting physical, psychological, social, or spiritual goals. Programs impact different levels of the individual: knowledge (Head), attitude (Heart), and practice (Hand). Principles for adaptation to contexts include a bottom-up approach, strengths from the community, learning from resources within communities, and realizing that every community has its resources and ways to sustain programs. Adaptation requires partnerships and reciprocal learning. Another way to view developing and developed regions and countries, and to refer to them, is as Differentially Resourced Regions: each has its own strengths and weaknesses. Finally, approaches should reflect the cultural and societal context. Below, we include a strong case study example where cultural adaptation was sufficiently addressed.

The Immersion Approach to Peacebuilding: National Youth Service Corps in Nigeria

On May 22, 1973, the Nigerian government established the National Youth Service Corps (NYSC) to foster national unity and promote understanding among the youth. The establishment of this program followed the Nigerian civil war between 1967 and 1970, which was fought along ethnic lines, with one ethnic group killing those from another. This program was supposed to be one of the tools to bring about healing in postcivil war Nigeria by developing a united, strong, and self-reliant nation.

The purpose of the program was primarily to enable the youth of Nigeria to develop attitudes of selfless service to the community, oneness and unity in a nation that is extremely diverse in terms of culture, religion, and socioeconomic backgrounds. Some of its objectives include phrases such as: "providing opportunities for higher ideals," "development of common ties that promote national unity and integration," "removal of prejudices, elimination of ignorance and confirmation first hand of similarities among ethnic groups of Nigeria," and "development of a sense of corporate existence and common destiny for the people of Nigeria." The modus operandi is as follows: NYSC takes graduates from tertiary institutions (universities, polytechnics and colleges of education) in Nigeria, who are less than 30 years of age, and has them spend one year living and working in a place and culture that is different from their own. Diversity in the corps members assigned to live and work together is ensured, allowing experience with a different culture and language for a sustained period of time. Following the year of service, corp members are encouraged to seek employment in different parts of the country.

Several thousand young Nigerians have embarked on this program since 1973 and the operators of this program describe successes, such as an unprecedented increase in interethnic marriages and a change in attitude of host communities as a result of community development projects. Other outcomes described are the unification of corps members from various ethnic backgrounds through healthy sporting activities and the subsequent relocation of corp members thereafter, who choose to live in parts of Nigeria other than their own area of origin.

In recent years, NYSC has come under increased pressure from the public, who have called for it to be dismantled. This came about after several corps members were killed in the Northern part of Nigeria as a result of the Boko Haram terrorist activities.

Recommendations

One of the goals of this Forum was to examine novel approaches to translating knowledge into concrete action. We have briefly described six such approaches; however, we did not present the action steps, as implementation of those novel approaches requires multiple actors and creative thinking in the actual context. Therefore, here we present a few recommendations for several actors engaged in early childhood and peace that are linked with the creative approaches presented in the previous section. The discussion also leads to the identification of several gaps, which are presented as recommendations for future examination and engagement.

For Academics

- How do we measure peace? We do not have a comprehensive measure to capture the results of evaluations of peacebuilding programs at the institutional level. Indicators and evaluative measures need to be gathered from grounded theory and practical research on peacebuilding. How do we think about peace in its unquantifiable realities? How can we begin to correlate the inner and outer, the personal and the social in nuanced and holistic ways?
- At the level of human development, we cannot claim knowledge of how the outcomes we are evaluating and measuring at early childhood will make a direct positive impact on peaceful lives as well as communal and global peace.
- With respect to sensitive periods and timing, we do not know enough about the reversibility and irreversibility of harm. This suggests great ethical issues of resource allocation, because if damage cannot be reversed, then intervention during the sensitive periods of development becomes an even more urgent priority.
- Have we assessed the new knowledge on early childhood development and peace sufficiently? When can we say that we have synthesized the knowledge well enough to communicate it for policy?

- A rigorous research agenda is needed to link the biology of human development and group and intergroup behavior.
- Mapping the field of existing best practices and effective methodology and knowledge accumulated in the field of peacebuilding by early childhood peace agencies can enhance the various capacities to develop intervention programs.

For Policy

Global Level

- Existing opportunities and spaces at the United Nations should be explored and utilized, such as the World Program for Human Rights Education and the work of the Special Representative of the Secretary General on Violence against Children. The first phase of the World Program (2005–2009) focused on school education, and the second phase (2010–2014) is addressing higher education. We recommend that a third phase focus on early childhood and peace education. (Note: peace education is one of the key elements of human rights education in general and in particular for children; see Article 29 (1) (d) of the Convention on the Rights of the Child.)
- We also recommend that the Special Representative of the Secretary General on Violence against Children take up the issue of early childhood intervention as her thematic report to the General Assembly, if this has not already been done. This should be done as soon as possible because (a) 2014 marks the 25th anniversary of the Convention on the Rights of the Child and (b) the third phase of the World Program begins in 2015.
- New knowledge about child development and peace needs to be translated into concrete policies, such as a UN Convention on early childhood and peace. Internationally accepted existing human rights instruments and UN documents should be used as backup references, including the Convention on the Rights of the Child, Declaration and Program of Action on a Culture of Peace, UN Secretary General's Study on Violence against Children, etc.

Local Level

Mayors for Peace originated in Hiroshima, Japan in 1992, at the initiative of Mayor Akiba and his colleague from Nagasaki. Since then, it has grown exponentially from two cities to 5,700 cities in 158 countries. Though the focus of the organization is "total abolition of all nuclear weapons by 2020," this initiative could be a good vehicle to advance peace education in which cities as urban administrative units take the political lead. For this, an initial 25 cities could be chosen as pilot cities for introducing peace education. UNICEF country offices could help to identify these cities. Another proactive organization, *Peace Messenger Cities*, also works with mayors and city administrations, and could become a good partner to advance the peace education agenda. *City of Sanctuary Movement*, which originated in Sheffield in 2005, is another example that is taking root in different places of intercultural, interreligious conflict, most recently in Belfast. A City of Sanctuary is a place of safety and welcome for people whose lives are in danger in their own countries.

For Practitioners

Education

Reduction of violence could be an important part of goals for peace education. Given the fact violence exists in one form or another, it is equally important for children to develop the capacities and skills to be able to respond to violence, including learning skills on how to prevent it. Education for peace should be an integral part of the early childhood formal education (from Kindergarten through grade 3). Such programs are in dire need for development and dissemination. Peer mediation programs have been run successfully in primary schools from Boston to Belfast. At the university level, courses in International Peace Studies and in Ecumenics are attracting young researchers and practitioners keen to learn alongside others of different cultural and faith traditions. Dialog and mutual understanding based on shared knowledge of one another's traditions provide an educational key to peace, justice, and reconciliation.

New technology can be a huge asset for both formal and informal education, but it cannot simply be left alone to fulfill its function in education. If educators leave it alone it will not disappear or necessarily be used benignly; instead its effect will be negatively felt.

Health

- It would be wise to convene leadership of hospitals, especially those with children's facilities, to explore how the newly discovered science of early childhood and its links to long-term peace outcomes would offer an opportunity for them to fulfill part of their founding vision and mission.
- It is important to incorporate institutional peace education through socioeconomic development agencies programs, especially for those who work in providing basic health services in conflict areas and underdeveloped settings.

Media

- Instant learning responses, connectedness, offers great access to a huge diversity of opinion.
- Integrate social media and media use in formal institutional teacher training (ministry of education). Teachers are behind their students in using technology, especially in privileged communities.
- Regulating the exposure to violence by media and social media in formative childhood, via extensive work with communities, families, and media outlets—especially in societies that have strong media industries which globally export children's programs.
- Reach out to fathers and men and engage them in a pathway between early childhood and peace.

For Families and Communities

- Listening: the first sign of respect is to listen. The first step of participation and reciprocity is to be heard.
- Ensure that children, from an early age, benefit from education on the values, attitudes, modes of behavior, and ways of life so as to enable them to resolve any dispute peacefully with nondiscrimination and tolerance, in a spirit of reciprocity, and with respect for human dignity and social justice.
- Involve children in activities designed to instill in them the values and goals of a culture of peace and empower them to become agents of change.
- Ensure equality of access to education for women, especially girls, and enhance the social capital of mothers.

Conclusion

The innovative approach taken by the Ernst Strüngmann Forum has revealed both the potential and challenges of sharing of expertise across experiences and disciplines. As we end our work, we find that we still do not have a conclusion. We are left pondering whether formative childhoods can provide a pathway to peace.

Nonetheless, our understanding and belief in the importance of early childhood and the long-term impacts of early intervention on individual and social developmental processes has been reconfirmed. While early childhood development is potentially vital, peacefulness in children's environment is also key to positive development. Multiple types of interventions are needed to promote and sustain children in the earliest years and throughout childhood. There is a lack of systematic communication and coordination between scientists, practitioners, and policy makers that needs to be redressed. We see the need to treat the relationship with caution because peace is a huge construct and can be viewed in various modes: inner and outer, direct and indirect, personal and structural. Thus, we cannot attribute a causally direct relationship between early childhood development and all manifestations of peace. Interdisciplinary conversation and in-depth study have increased the realization that this is a far more complex issue.

The well-being of children is fundamental to peace. Early childhood as a pathway to peace is populated with areas of evidence and also knowledge gaps that need to be addressed. For example, safety can also be understood and measured across the spectrum of sciences from biological to social. However the properties of safety, when conceptualized at the level of biology and the individual person, might be characterized by different properties when compared to the societal level (e.g., rule of law and human security). In sum, there is a traceable thread, of safety, that connects the individual person to society and social contexts that has the potential for making linkages between security in early childhood and security and peace at a social level. However, the nature and characteristics of safety change when the unit of analyses changes from one to many.

Because the worlds of early childhood and peace are seemingly disparate, there is a need to strengthen the interconnectedness, coordination of partnerships, and collaboration at many levels and among researchers from different disciplines and policy and practice community. For example, media and education are powerful channels to promote peace. We need to create or strengthen mechanisms and processes between these organizations and civil society that work on early childhood, peace, and peacebuilding. One such example is the Early Childhood Peace Consortium,[2] which brings together sectors engaged in either peacebuilding or early childhood to pursue jointly an agenda for promoting peace through the transformative power of the formative years of life.

Roles of family members, community leaders, educators, practitioners, policy makers, and scientists are not static. Depending on the context and situation, they can be knowledge generators, knowledge translators, or knowledge consumers. For example, when teaching children, educators are knowledge consumers; when observing their students, educators are knowledge generators; and when communicating this information to parents, educators are knowledge translators. The roles are dependent on the function and context, not on the affiliation to a particular sector. This conclusion has implications for the fluidity of knowledge. Thus, peacebuilders, policy makers, and practitioners need to take into account the realities and needs of early childhood when understanding this knowledge.

The promotion of secure childhood and sustainable peace benefits from applying the following principles to knowledge generation, use, and translation.

---

[2] http://www.unicef.org/earlychildhood/index_70959.html (accessed June 6, 2014).

Programs need to be sensitive, inclusive, participatory, and adaptable to the particular cultural contexts. A capabilities-based approach to practice, policy, and programs should be promoted that encourages human capabilities, cultural and community assets, and the emancipatory vision and practices. Coordination across social, cultural, economic, and ecological conditions/systemic structures should be rooted in the promotion of human security and human rights.

In closing, we are living in a world that is increasingly marked by violence: across nations as well as within countries, communities, and families. As a world community, we must put an end to this violence and find the "moral equivalent of war" (James 1995). War (or violence) provides human beings with opportunities to express their spiritual inclusions toward self-sacrifice and personal honor. We must find a way to give expression to these profoundly human values through peaceful engagement, beginning with the earliest years of life.

Future Research

Early childhood and peace knowledge is inclusive of, but not limited to, a range of scientific disciplines: anthropology (cultural, social, religious), economics, education, theology, developmental psychology, peace studies, gender studies, biobehavioral sciences, together with those pertaining to more applied fields of inquiry such as communications, group dynamics/organizational behavior, conflict resolution, peacebuilding, and the creation of a culture of peace. Thus, we need to expand our knowledge fields in the exploration of the association between early childhood and peace:

- Research and scholarship needs to generate evidence and knowledge that will facilitate the reconceptualization of the individual life course, from childhood through adolescence, with the aspiration of global citizenship and the reconceptualization of groups and societies with the aspiration of a culture of peace.
- New research is needed to examine the association between the traditional layers of influence that emphasized proximal to distal environments using an ecological nested systems model with the emerging associations of networks that cut across the levels, not just in concentric circles but through the interplay of network connections.
- Research should focus on the effectiveness and relevance of peace across a range of strategies (e.g., formal and informal education, parenting and community strategies, and the media).
- What is the most effective way to translate knowledge on early childhood for communities engaged in building peace? Where are the entry points and what are the resonant disciplinary paradigms that can be established to promote the uptake of this knowledge for policies and programs?

Bibliography

Note: Numbers in square brackets denote the chapter in which an entry is cited.

Aber, L., L. Biersteker, A. Dawes, and L. Rawlings. 2013. Social Protection and Welfare Systems: Implications for Early Childhood Development. In: Handbook of Early Childhood Development Research and Its Impact on Global Policy, ed. P. R. Britto et al., pp. 260–274. New York: Oxford Univ. Press. [13]

Abrams, D. A., S. Ryali, T. Chen, et al. 2013. Inter-Subject Synchronization of Brain Responses During Natural Music Listening. *Eur. J. Neurosci.* **37**:1458–1469. [7]

Abu-Nimer, M. 1999. Dialogue, Conflict Resolution and Change: Arab-Jewish Encounters in Israel. Albany: SUNY Press. [17, 19]

Abu-Nimer, M., and I. Nasser. 2013. Forgiveness in the Arab and Islamic Contexts: Between Theology and Practice. *J. Relig. Ethics* **41**:474–494. [15]

Acheson, D., D. Feifel, S. deWilde, et al. 2013. The Effect of Intranasal Oxytocin Treatment on Conditioned Fear Extinction and Recall in a Healthy Human Sample. *Psychopharmacology* **229**:199–208. [4]

Acheson, D., J. E. Gresack, and V. B. Risbrough. 2012. Hippocampal Dysfunction Effects on Context Memory: Possible Etiology for Posttraumatic Stress Disorder. *Neuropharmacology* **62**:674–685. [12]

Adolphs, R. 2009. The Social Brain: Neural Basis of Social Knowledge. *Annu. Rev. Psychol.* **60**:693–716. [4]

Adolphs, R., and M. L. Spezio. 2006. Role of the Amygdala in Processing Visual Social Stimuli. *Prog. Brain Res.* **156**:363–378. [9]

Ahmed, S. H., and M. N. Siddiqi. 2006. Healing through Art Therapy in Disaster Settings. *Lancet* **368**:S28–S29. [15]

Ainsworth, M. D. S. 1967. Infancy in Uganda: Infant Care and the Growth of Love. Baltimore: Johns Hopkins Univ. Press. [2]

―――. 1977. Infant Development and Mother-Infant Interaction among Ganda and American Families. In: Culture and Infancy: Variations in the Human Experience, ed. P. H. Leiderman et al., pp. 119–149. New York: Academic Press. [2]

Ainsworth, M. D. S., M. C. Blehar, E. Waters, and S. Wall. 1978. Patterns of Attachment. Hillsdale, NJ: Erlbaum. [2]

Ainsworth, M. D. S., and J. Bowlby. 1991. An Ethological Approach to Personality Development. *Am. Psychol.* **46**:331–341. [18]

Alderman, H., J. Hoddinott, and B. Kinsey. 2006. Long-Term Consequences of Early Childhood Malnutrition. *Oxford Econ. Papers* **58**:450–474. [13]

Al-Hassan, S. M., and J. E. Lansford. 2010. Evaluation of the Better Parenting Programme in Jordan. *Early Child Dev. Care* **180**:1203–1213. [3, 16]

Al-Krenawi, A., J. R. Graham, and M. A. Sehwail. 2007. Tomorrow's Players under Occupation: An Analysis of the Association of Political Violent with Psychological Functioning and Domestic Violence, among Palestinian Youth. *Am. J. Orthopsychiatry* **77**:427–433. [12]

Allport, G. W. 1954. The Nature of Prejudice. Reading: Addison-Wesley. [15]

Almas, A. N., K. A. Degnan, A. Radulescu, et al. 2012. Effects of Early Intervention and the Moderating Effects of Brain Activity on Institutionalized Children's Social Skills at Age 8. *PNAS* **109**:17228–17231. [7]

Alvares, G. A., I. B. Hickie, and A. J. Guastella. 2010. Acute Effects of Intranasal Oxytocin on Subjective and Behavioral Responses to Social Rejection. *Exp. Clin. Psychopharmacol.* **18**:316–321. [10]

Amstutz, L. S., and J. H. Mullet. 2005. The Little Book of Restorative Discipline for Schools: Teaching Responsibility; Creating Caring Climates. Intercourse, PA: Good Books. [17]

Anacker, A. M. J., and A. K. Beery. 2013. Life in Groups: The Roles of Oxytocin in Mammalian Sociality. *Front. Behav. Neurosci.* **7**:185. [7]

Anastasi, A. 1958. Heredity, Environment and the Question "How"? *Psychol. Rev.* **65**:197–208. [13]

Anda, R. F., V. J. Felitti, J. D. Bremner, et al. 2006. The Enduring Effects of Abuse and Related Adverse Experiences in Childhood: A Convergence of Evidence from Neurobiology and Epidemiology. *Eur. Arch. Psychiatry Clin. Neurosci.* **256**:174–186. [11]

Apicella, C., F. Marlowe, J. Fowler, and N. Christakis. 2012. Social Networks and Cooperation in Hunter-Gatherers. *Nature* **481**:497–502. [6]

Appiah, K. A. 2010. The Honor Code. New York: Norton. [2]

Appleyard, K., C. Yang, and D. K. Runyan. 2010. Delineating the Maladaptive Pathways of Child Maltreatment: A Mediated Moderation Analysis of the Roles of Self-Perception and Social Support. *Dev. Psychopathol.* **22**:337–352. [12]

Arnsten, A. F., and B. M. Li. 2005. Neurobiology of Executive Functions: Catecholamine Influences on Prefrontal Cortical Functions. *Biol. Psychiatry* **57**:1377–1384. [7]

Aronson, E., N. Blaney, C. Stephan, J. Sikes, and M. Snapp. 1978. The Jigsaw Classroom. Beverly Hills: Sage Publications. [6]

Ashby, N., and C. Neilsen-Hewett. 2012. Approaches to Conflict and Conflict Resolution in Toddler Relationships. *J. Early Child Res.* **10**:145–161. [17]

Assor, A., G. Roth, and E. L. Deci. 2004. The Emotional Costs of Parents' Conditional Regard: A Self-Determination Theory Analysis. *J. Pers.* **72**:47–88. [10]

Astuto, J., and M. D. Ruck. 2010. Early Childhood as a Foundation for Civic Engagement. In: Handbook of Research of Civic Engagement in Youth, ed. L. Sherrod et al., pp. 249–275. Hoboken, NJ: Wiley. [3, 19]

Attanayake, V., R. McKay, M. Joffres, et al. 2009. Prevalence of Mental Disorders among Children Exposed to War: A Systematic Review of 7,920 Children. *Med. Confl. Surviv.* **25**:4–19. [1, 12]

Avruch, K. 1998. Culture and Conflict Resolution. Washington, D.C.: U.S. Institute of Peace. [17]

Avruch, K., and P. W. Black. 1987. A Generic Theory of Conflict Resolution: A Critique. *J. Negotiation* **3**:87–96. [17]

———. 1991. The Culture Question and Conflict Resolution. *Peace & Change* **16**:22–45. [17]

Babiloni, C., G. Albertini, P. Onorati, et al. 2010. Cortical Sources of EEG Rhythms Are Abnormal in Down Syndrome. *Clin. Neurophysiol.* **121**:1205–1212. [9]

Baker, A., and N. Shalhoub-Kevorkian. 1999. Effects of Political and Military Traumas on Children: The Palestinian Case. *Clin. Psychol. Rev.* **19**:935–950. [12]

Bakermans-Kranenburg, M. J., and M. H. van IJzendoorn. 2006. Gene-Environment Interaction of the Dopamine D4 Receptor (DRD4) and Observed Maternal Insensitivity Predicting Externalizing Behavior in Preschoolers. *Dev. Psychobiol.* **48**:406–409. [10]

———. 2007. Genetic Vulnerability or Differential Susceptibility in Child Development: The Case of Attachment. *J. Child Psychol. Psychiatry* **48**:1160–1173. [10]

———. 2008. Oxytocin Receptor (OXTR) and Serotonin Transporter (5-HTT) Genes Associated with Observed Parenting. *Soc. Cogn. Affect. Neurosci.* **3**:128–134. [10]

———. 2011. Differential Susceptibility to Rearing Environment Depending on Dopamine-Related Genes: New Evidence and a Meta-Analysis. *Dev. Psychopathol.* **23**:39–52. [10]

———. 2013. Sniffing around Oxytocin: Review and Meta-Analyses of Trials in Healthy and Clinical Groups with Implications for Pharmacotherapy. *Transl. Psychiatry* **3**:e258. [10]

———. 2015. The Hidden Efficacy of Interventions: Gene x Environment Experiments from a Differential Susceptibility Perspective. *Annu. Rev. Psychol.*, in press.[10]

Bakermans-Kranenburg, M. J., M. H. van IJzendoorn, and F. Juffer. 2003. Less Is More: Meta-Analyses of Sensitivity and Attachment Interventions in Early Childhood. *Psychol. Bull.* **129**:195–215. [2, 11]

Bakermans-Kranenburg, M. J., M. H. van IJzendoorn, J. Mesman, L. R. Alink, and F. Juffer. 2008. Effects of an Attachment-Based Intervention on Daily Cortisol Moderatored by Dopamine Receptor D4: A Randomized Control Trial on 1- to 3-Year-Olds Screened for Externalizing Behavior. *Dev. Psychopathol.* **20**:805–820. [11]

Bakermans-Kranenburg, M. J., M. H. van IJzendoorn, M. M. E. Riem, M. Tops, and L. R. A. Alink. 2012. Oxytocin Decreases Handgrip Force in Reaction to Infant Crying in Females without Harsh Parenting Experiences. *Soc. Cogn. Affect. Neurosci.* **7**:951–957. [10]

Bandura, A. 2000. Exercise of Human Agency through Collective Efficacy. *Curr. Dir. Psychol. Sci.* **9**:75–78. [15]

Banks, J. A. 2010. Multicultural Education: Characteristics and Goals. In: Multicultural Education: Issues and Perspectives (7th edition), ed. J. A. Banks and C. A. M. Banks, pp. 3–30. Hoboken, NJ: Wiley. [17]

Barath, A. 2000. Treating War Trauma in Children and Youth from the Former Yugoslavia. In: Managing Multiethnic Local Communities in the Countries of the Former Yugoslavia, ed. N. Dimitrijevic, pp. 355–368. Budapest: Local Government and Public Service Reform Initiative. Open Society Institute. [12]

Barber, B. K. 2001. Political Violence, Social Integration, and Youth Functioning: Palestinian Youth from the Intifada. *J. Community Psychol.* **29**:259–280. [12]

———, ed. 2009a. Adolescents and War: How Youth Deal with Political Violence. New York: Oxford Univ. Press. [14]

———. 2009b. Making Sense and No Sense of War: Issues of Identity and Meaning in Adolescents' Experience with Political Conflict. In: Adolescents and War: How Youth Deal with Political Violence, ed. B. K. Barber, pp. 281–311. New York: Oxford Univ. Press. [14]

———. 2013. Annual Research Review: The Experience of Youth with Political Conflict: Challenging Notions of Resilience and Encouraging Research Refinement. *J. Child Psychol. Psychiatry* **54**:461–473. [12, 14]

Barber, B. K., and J. M. Schluterman. 2008. Connectedness in the Lives of Children and Adolescents: A Call for Greater Conceptual Clarity. *J. Adolesc. Health* **43**:209–216. [12]

Bar-Haim, Y., T. Ziv, D. Lamy, and R. M. Hodes. 2006. Nature and Nurture in Own-Race Face Processing. *Psychol. Sci.* **17**:159–163. [15]

Barhight, L. R., J. Hubbard, and C. T. Hyde. 2012. Children's Physiological and Emotional Reactions to Witnessing Bullying Predict Bystander Intervention. *Child Dev.* **84**:375–390. [11]

Barnard, A. 1983. Contemporary Hunter-Gatherers: Current Theoretical Issues in Ecology and Social Organization. *Annu. Rev. Anthropol.* **12**:193–214. [6]

Bar-On, D. 1999. The Indescribable and the Undiscussable: Reconstructing Human Discourse after Trauma. Budapest: Central European Univ. Press. [12]

Barouki, R., P. D. Gluckman, P. Grandjean, M. Hanson, and J. J. Heindel. 2012. Developmental Origins of Non-Communicable Disease: Implications for Research and Public Health. *Environ. Health* **11**:42. [1]

Barry, R. J., A. R. Clarke, and S. J. Johnstone. 2003. A Review of Electrophysiology in Attention-Deficit/Hyperactivity Disorder. I: Qualitative and Quantitative Electroencephalography. *Clin. Neurophysiol.* **114**:171–183. [9]

Bar-Tal, D. 1996. Development of Social Categories and Stereotypes in Early Childhood: The Case of "the Arab" Concept Formation, Stereotype and Attitudes of Jewish Children in Israel. *Intl. J. Intercult. Relat.* **20**:341–370. [18]

———. 2007. Sociopsychological Foundations of Intractable Conflicts. *Am. Behav. Sci.* **50**:1430–1453. [15]

———. 2013. Intractable Conflicts: Socio-Psychological Foundations and Dynamics. New York: Cambridge Univ. Press. [16]

Bartz, J. A., J. Zaki, N. Bolger, et al. 2010a. Effects of Oxytocin on Recollections of Maternal Care and Closeness. *PNAS* **107**:21371–21375. [10]

———. 2010b. Oxytocin Selectively Improves Empathic Accuracy. *Psychol. Sci.* **21**:1426–1428. [3, 10]

Bartz, J. A., J. Zaki, N. K. Bolger, and K. N. Ochsner. 2011. Social Effects of Oxytocin in Humans: Context and Person Matter. *Trends Cogn. Sci.* **15**:301–309. [4]

Batson, C. D. 1998. Prosocial Behavior and Altruism. In: The Handbook of Social Psychology (4th edition), ed. D. Gilbert et al., vol. 4, pp. 282–316. New York: McGraw-Hill. [15]

Bauer, P. M., J. L. Hanson, R. K. Pierson, R. J. Davidson, and S. D. Pollak. 2009. Cerebellar Volume and Cognitive Functioning in Children Who Experienced Early Deprivation. *Biol. Psychiatry* **66**:1100–1106. [9]

Baumgartner, T., M. Heinrichs, A. Vonlanthen, U. Fischbacher, and E. Fehr. 2008. Oxytocin Shapes the Neural Circuitry of Trust and Trust Adaptation in Humans. *Neuron* **58**:639–650. [10]

Bayer, J. K., H. Hiscock, O. C. Ukoumunne, K. Scalzo, and M. Wake. 2010. Three-Year-Old Outcomes of a Brief Universal Parenting Intervention to Prevent Behaviour Problems: Randomised Controlled Trial. *Arch. Dis. Child.* **95**:187–192. [16]

Beckes, L., J. A. Coan, and K. Hasselmo. 2013. Familiarity Promotes the Blurring of Self and Other in the Neural Representation of Threat. *Cogn. Affect. Behav. Neurosci.* **8**:670–677. [10]

Behrman, J. R. 2010. The International Food Policy Research Institute (IFPRI) and the Mexican Progresa Anti-Poverty and Human Resource Investment Conditional Cash. *World Dev.* **38**:1473–1485. [15]

Behrman, J. R., M. C. Calderon, S. H. Preston, et al. 2009. Nutritional Supplementation of Girls' Influences the Growth of Their Children: Prospective Study in Guatemala. *Am. J. Clin. Nutr.* **90**:1372–1379. [15]

Behrman, J. R., and H.-P. Kohler. 2014. Population Quantity, Quality and Mobility. In: Towards a Better Global Economy: Policy Implications for Global Citizens in the 21st Century, ed. J. R. Behrman and S. Fardoust. Oxford: Oxford Univ. Press. [15]

Bekerman, Z., and M. Zembylas. 2011. Teaching Contested Narratives: Identity, Memory and Reconciliation in Peace Education and Beyond. Cambridge: Cambridge Univ. Press. [16]

Bellier, I., and T. Wilson. 2000. Building, Imagining, and Experiencing Europe: Institutions and Identities in the European Union. In: An Anthropology of the European Union, ed. I. Bellier and T. Wilson, pp. 1–27. Oxford: Berg. [6]

Belsky, J. 1997. Variation in Susceptibility to Rearing Influences: An Evolutionary Argument. *Psychol. Inq.* **8**:182–186. [8]

———. 2008. War, Trauma and Children's Development: Observations from a Modern Evolutionary Perspective. *Intl. J. Behav. Dev.* **32**:260–271. [12]

Belsky, J., M. J. Bakermans-Kranenburg, and M. H. van IJzendoorn. 2007. For Better and for Worse: Differential Susceptibility to Environmental Influences. *Curr. Dir. Psychol. Sci.* **16**.300–304. [8, 10, 14]

Belsky, J., and M. Pluess. 2013. Beyond Risk, Resilience, and Dysregulation: Phenotypic Plasticity and Human Development. *Dev. Psychopathol.* **25**:1243–1261. [7]

Belsky, J., G. L. Schlomer, and B. J. Ellis. 2012. Beyond Cumulative Risk: Distinguishing Harshness and Unpredictability as Determinants of Parenting and Early Life History Strategy. *Dev. Psychol.* **48**:662–673. [7]

Belsky, J., L. Steinberg, and P. Draper. 1991. Childhood Experience, Interpersonal Development, and Reproductive Strategy: An Evolutionary Theory of Socialization. *Child Dev.* **62**:647–670. [7, 8]

Benatar, S., and R. Kirsch. 1987. Baragwanath: A Hospital in Despair. *S. Afr. Med. J.* **72**:307. [13]

Bercovitch, J., ed. 1996. Resolving International Conflicts: The Theory and Practice of Mediation. Boulder: Lynne Rienne Publishers. [17]

Berdasco, M., and M. Esteller. 2013. Genetic Syndromes Caused My Mutations in Epigenetic Genes. *Hum. Genet.* **132**:359–383. [5]

Bergman, K., P. Sarkar, T. G. O'Connor, N. Modi, and V. Glover. 2007. Maternal Stress During Pregnancy Predicts Cognitive Ability and Fearfulness in Infancy. *J. Am. Acad. Child Adolesc. Psychiatry* **46**:1454–1463. [11]

Bernard, K., M. Dozier, J. Bick, et al. 2012. Enhancing Attachment Organization among Maltreated Children: Results of a Randomized Clinical Trial. *Child Dev.* **83**:623–636. [11]

Bernard van Leer Foundation Program Staff. 2007. Early Childhood Programs in Two Divided Societies: Northern Ireland and Israel. *Early Childhood Matters* **108**:43–46. [18]

Berndt, R. 1972. The Walmadjeri and Gugardja. In: Hunters and Gatherers Today, ed. M. G. Bicchieri, pp. 177–212. New York: Holt, Rinehart & Winston. [6]

Bernhard, H., U. Fischbacher, and E. Fehr. 2006. Parochial Altruism in Humans (Letter). *Nature* **442**:912–915. [7]

Berrueta-Clement, J. R., L. J. Schweinhart, W. S. Barnett, A. Epstein, and D. P. Weikart. 1984. Changed Lives: The Effects of the Perry Preschool Program on Youths through Age 19. Ypsilanti: High/Scope Press. [16]

Berry, L., L. Biersteker, A. Dawes, L. Lake, and C. Smith, eds. 2013. South African Child Gauge 2013. Cape Town: Children's Institute, Univ. of Cape Town. [13]

Betancourt, T. S., I. Borisova, T. P. Williams, et al. 2013a. Psychosocial Adjustment and Mental Health in Former Child Soldiers: Systematic Review of the Literature and Recommendations for Future Research. *J. Child Psychol. Psychiatry* **54**:17–36. [12, 14, 15]

Betancourt, T. S., R. McBain, E. A. Newnham, and R. T. Brennan. 2013b. Trajectories of Internalizing Problems in War-Affected Sierra Leonean Youth: Examining Conflict and Postconflict Factors. *Child Dev.* **84**:455–470. [14]

Betancourt, T. S., S. E. Meyers-Ohki, A. P. Charrow, and W. A. Tol. 2013c. Interventions for Children Affected by War: An Ecological Perspective on Psychosocial Support and Mental Health Care. *Harv. Rev. Psychiatry* **21**:70–91. [12]

Bethlehem, R. A., S. Baron-Cohen, B. A. J. van Honk, and P. A. Bos. 2014. The Oxytocin Paradox. *Front. Behav. Neurosci* **8**:48. [4]

Bick, J., O. Naumova, S. Hunter, et al. 2012. Childhood Adversity and DNA Methylation of Genes Involved in the Hypothalamus-Pituitary-Adrenal Axis and Immune System: Whole-Genome and Candidate-Gene Associations. *Dev. Psychopathol.* **24**:1417–1425. [1]

Biglan, A., B. R. Flay, D. D. Embry, and I. N. Sandler. 2012. The Critical Role of Nurturing Environments for Promoting Human Well-Being. *Am. Psychol.* **67**:257–271. [14]

Blair, C., D. Berry, R. Mills-Koonce, et al. 2013. Cumulative Effects of Early Poverty on Cortisol in Young Children: Moderation by Autonomic Nervous System Activity. *Psychoneuroendocrinology* **38**:2666–2675. [7]

Blair, C., and C. C. Raver. 2012a. Child Development in the Context of Adversity: Experiential Canalization of Brain and Behavior. *Am. Psychol.* **67**:309–318. [7]

———. 2012b. Individual Development and Evolution: Experiential Canalization of Self-Regulation. *Dev. Psychol.* **48**:647–657. [7]

Blok, H., R. G. Fukkink, E. C. Gebhardt, and P. M. Leseman. 2005. The Relevance of Delivery Mode and Other Program Characteristics for the Effectiveness of Early Childhood Intervention. *Intl. J. Behav. Dev.* **29**:35–47. [16]

Blumenshine, P., S. Egerter, C. J. Barclay, C. Cubbin, and P. A. Braverman. 2010. Socioeconomic Disparities in Adverse Birth Outcomes: A Systematic Review. *Am. J. Prev. Med.* **39**:263–272. [11]

Boehm, C. 1999. Hierarchy in the Forest: The Evolution of Egalitarian Behavior. Cambridge, MA: Harvard Univ. Press. [11]

———. 2012. Moral Origins: The Evolution of Virtue, Altruism, and Shame: Basic Books. [7]

Bohm, D. 1996. On Dialogue. London: Routledge. [17]

Bonnin, A., N. Goeden, K. Chen, et al. 2011. A Transient Placental Source of Serotonin for the Fetal Forebrain. *Nature* **472**:347–350. [5]

Boothby, N., J. Crawford, and J. Halperin. 2006. Mozambique Child Soldier Life Outcome Study: Lessons Learned in Rehabilitation and Reintegration Efforts. *Glob. Public Health* **1**:87–107. [14]

Bornstein, M. H., and D. L. Putnick. 2012. Cognitive and Socioemotional Caregiving in Developing Countries. *Child Dev.* **831**:46–61. [3]

Bowlby, J. 1952. Maternal Care and Mental Health: A Report Prepared on Behalf of the World Heatlh Organization as a Contribution to the United Nations Programme for the Welfare of Homeless Children. Geneva: World Health Organization. [9, 11]

———. 1969. Attachment and Loss, vol. I: Attachment. London: Hogarth Press. [2]

———. 1982. Attachment and Loss: Retrospect and Prospect. *Am. J. Orthopsychiatry* **52**:664–678. [12]

————. 1991. Postscript. In: Attachment across the Life Cycle, ed. C. M. Parkes et al., pp. 293–297. London: Routledge. [2]

Bowman, B. T., M. S. Donovan, and M. S. Burns, eds. 2001. Eager to Learn: Educating Our Preschoolers. Washington, D.C.: National Research Council. [3]

Boxer, P., L. Rowell Huesmann, E. F. Dubow, et al. 2013. Exposure to Violence across the Social Ecosystem and the Development of Aggression: A Test of Ecological Theory in the Israeli-Palestinian Conflict. *Child Dev.* **84**:163–177. [12, 14, 15]

Boyce, W. T. 2007. A Biology of Misfortune: Stress Reactivity, Social Context, and the Ontogeny of Psychopathology in Early Life. In: Multilevel Dynamics in Developmental Psychopathology: Pathways to the Future. The Minnesota Symposia on Child Psychology, ed. A. S. Masten, pp. 45–82. Mahwah, NJ: Erlbaum. [14]

Boyce, W. T., P. K. Den Besten, J. Stamperdahl, et al. 2010. Social Inequalities in Childhood Dental Caries: The Convergent Roles of Stress, Bacteria and Disadvantage. *Soc. Sci. Med.* **71**:1644–1652. [11]

Boyce, W. T., and B. J. Ellis. 2005. Biological Sensitivity to Context: I. An Evolutionary–Developmental Theory of the Origins and Functions of Stress Reactivity. *Dev. Psychopathol.* **17**:271–301. [8]

Boyce, W. T., J. Obradovic, N. R. Bush, et al. 2012a. Social Stratification, Classroom Climate, and Behavioral Adaptation of Kindergarten Children. *PNAS* **109(Suppl 2)**:17168–17173. [3, 7, 11]

Boyce, W. T., M. B. Sokolowski, and G. E. Robinson. 2012b. Toward a New Biology of Social Adversity. *PNAS* **109**:17143–17148. [7]

Bradley, R. H., and R. F. Corwyn. 2005. Caring for Children around the World: A View from Home. *Intl. J. Behav. Dev.* **296**:468–478. [3]

Bradley, S. J., D. A. Jadaa, J. Brody, et al. 2003. Brief Psychoeducational Parenting Program: An Evaluation and 1-Year Follow-Up. *J. Am. Acad. Child Adolesc. Psychiatry* **42**:1171–1178. [16]

Bratton, S. C., D. Ray, T. Rhine, and L. Jones. 2005. The Efficacy of Play Therapy with Children: A Meta-Analytic Review of Treatment Outcomes. *Prof. Psychol. Res. Pr.* **36**:376–390. [12]

Bray, R. 2003. Predicting the Social Consequences of Orphanhood in South Africa. *Afr. J. AIDS Res.* **2**:39–55. [11]

Brewer, M. B. 1999. The Psychology of Prejudice: Ingroup Love and Outgroup Hate? *J. Soc. Iss.* **55**:429–444. [15]

Brewin, C. R., J. D. Gregory, M. Lipton, and N. Burgess. 2010. Intrusive Images in Psychological Disorders: Characteristics, Neural Mechanisms, and Treatment Implications. *Psychol. Rev.* **117**:210–232. [12]

Britto, P. R., P. L. Engle, and C. M. Super, eds. 2013. Handbook of Early Childhood Development Research and Its Impact on Global Policy. New York: Oxford Univ. Press. [1, 3, 14, 16, 19]

Britto, P. R., and S. L. Kagan. 2010. Global Status of Early Learning and Development Standards. In: International Encyclopedia of Education, ed. P. Peterson et al., vol. 2, pp. 138–143. Oxford: Elsevier. [3, 17]

Britto, P. R., and N. Ulkuer. 2012. Child Development in Developing Countries: Child Rights and Policy Implications. *Child Dev.* **831**:92–103. [3]

Britto, P. R., H. Yoshikawa, and K. Boller. 2011. Quality of Early Childhood Development Programs in Global Contexts. *Soc. Policy Rep.* **25**:1–31. [16]

Broad, K. D., and E. B. Keverne. 2011. Placental Protection of the Fetal Brain During Short-Term Food Deprivation. *PNAS* **108**:15237–15241. [5, 7]

Broadhead, P. 2009. Conflict Resolution and Children's Behaviour: Observing and Understanding Social and Cooperative Play in Early Years Educational Settings. *Early Years* **29**:105–118. [17]

Bronfenbrenner, U. 1979. The Ecology of Human Development: Experiments by Nature and Design. Cambridge, MA: Harvard Univ. Press. [1, 10, 15, 17]

———. 2005. Ecological Systems Theory. In: Making Human Beings Human: Bioecological Perspectives on Human Development, pp. 106–173. Thousand Oaks, CA: Sage Publications. [12]

Bronfenbrenner, U., and P. A. Morris. 2006. The Bioecological Model of Human Development. In: The Handbook of Child Psychology: Theoretical Models of Human Development (6th edition), ed. R. M. Lerner and W. Damon, vol. 1, pp. 793–828. Hoboken, NJ: Wiley. [14]

Brooker, I., and D. Poulin-Dubois. 2013. Is Parental Emotional Reliability Predictive of Toddlers' Learning and Helping? *Infant Behav. Dev.* **36**:403–418. [10]

Broome, B. J. 1993. Managing Differences in Conflict Resolution: The Role of Relational Empathy. In: Conflict Resolution Theory and Practice: Integration and Application, ed. D. J. Sandole and H. van der Merwe, pp. 95–111. Manchester: Manchester Univ. Press. [17]

Brown, G. W., and S. Davidson. 1978. Social Class, Psychiatric Disorder of Mother, and Accidents to Children. *Lancet* **1**:378–381. [11]

Brown, R. 2011. Prejudice: Its Social Psychology. New York: John Wiley and Sons. [15]

Brownell, C. A., M. Svetlova, and S. Nichols. 2009. To Share or Not to Share: When Do Toddlers Respond to Another's Needs? *Infancy* **14**:117–130. [7]

Brunton, P. J., and J. A. Russell. 2011. Neuroendocrine Control of Maternal Stress Responses and Fetal Programming by Stress in Pregnancy. *Prog. Neuropsychopharmacol. Biol. Psychiatry* **35**:11278–11191. [5]

Bruton, M. N., ed. 1989. Alternative Life-History Styles of Animals. Dordrecht: Kluwer Academic. [7]

Bugental, D. B. 2012. Adaptive Calibration of Children's Physiological Responses to Family Stress: The Utility of Evolutionary Developmental Theory. Comment on Del Giudice et al. (2012) and Sturge-Apple et al. (2012). *Dev. Psychol.* **48**:806–809. [7]

Buisman-Pijlman, F., N. M. Sumracki, J. J. Gordon, et al. 2013. Individual Differences Underlying Susceptibility to Addiction: Role for the Endogenous Oxytocin System. *Biochem. Pharmacol. Behav.* **119**:22–38. [4]

Burchinal, M. R., F. A. Campbell, D. M. Bryant, B. A. Wasik, and C. T. Ramey. 1997. Early Intervention and Mediating Processes in Cognitive Performance of Children of Low-Income African-American Families. *Child Dev.* **68**:935–954. [16]

Burnstein, E., C. Crandall, and S. Kitayama. 1994. Some Neo-Darwinian Decision Rules for Altruism: Weighing Cues for Inclusive Fitness as a Function of the Biological Importance of the Decision. *J. Pers. Soc. Psychol.* **67**:773–789. [10]

Burton, J. W., and F. Dukes. 1990a. Conflict: Practices in Management, Settlement and Resolution. New York: St. Martin's Press. [17]

———, eds. 1990b. Conflict: Readings in Management and Resolution. New York: St. Martin's Press. [17]

Bush, R. A. B., and J. Folger. 1994. The Promise of Mediation: Responding to Conflict through Empowerment and Recognition. San Francisco: Jossey-Bass Publishers. [17]

Bushman, B. J., and K. Newman, eds. 2013. Youth Violence: What We Need to Know. Report of the Subcommittee on Youth Violence of the Advisory Committee to the Social, Behavioral and Economic Sciences Directorate. Arlington: National Science Foundation. [14]

Buttelmann, D., and R. Böhm. 2014. The Ontogeny of the Motivation That Underlies In-Group Bias. *Psychol. Sci.* **25**:921–927. [7]

Cacioppo, J. T., and G. G. Berntson. 1992. Social Psychological Contributions to the Decade of the Brain: Doctrine of Multilevel Analysis. *Am. Psychol.* **47**:1019–1028. [15]

Cacioppo, S., C. Frum, E. Asp, et al. 2013. A Quantitative Meta-Analysis of Functional Imaging Studies of Social Rejection. *Sci. Reports* **3**:2027. [11]

Cameron, L., A. R. Rutland, R. Brown, and R. Douch. 2006. Changing Children's Intergroup Attitudes toward Refugees: Testing Different Models of Extended Contact. *Child Dev.* **77**:1208–1219. [15]

Cameron, N. M. 2011. Maternal Programming of Reproductive Function and Behavior in the Female Rat. *Front. Evol. Neurosci.* **3**:10. [7]

Cameron, N. M., F. A. Champagne, C. Parent, et al. 2005. The Programming of Individual Differences in Defensive Responses and Reproductive Strategies in the Rat through Variations in Maternal Care. *Neurosci. Biobehav. Rev.* **29**:843–865. [7]

Cameron, N. M., E. Soehngen, and M. J. Meaney. 2011. Variation in Maternal Care Influences Ventromedial Hypothalamus Activation in the Rat. *J. Neuroendocrinol.* **23**:393–400. [7]

Campbell, E. A., and C. T. Ramey. 1994. Effects of Early Intervention on Intellectual and Academic Achievement: A Follow-up Study of Children from Low-Income Families. *Child Dev.* **65**:684–698. [16]

Campbell, F. A., G. Conti, J. J. Heckman, et al. 2014. Early Childhood Investments Substantially Boost Adult Health. *Science* **343**:1478–1485. [1]

Campbell, F. A., C. T. Ramey, E. P. Pungello, J. Sparling, and S. Miller-Johnson. 2002. Early Childhood Education: Young Adult Outcomes from the Abecedarian Project. *Appl. Dev. Sci.* **6**:42–57. [16]

Carnevale, P. J., and D. G. Pruitt. 1992. Negotiation and Mediation. *Annu. Rev. Psychol.* **43**:531–582. [15]

Carré, J. M., A. M. Iselin, K. M. Welker, A. R. Hariri, and K. A. Dodge. 2014. Testosterone Reactivity to Provocation Mediates the Effect of Early Intervention on Aggressive Behavior. *Psychol. Sci.* **25**:1140–1146. [7]

Carretero, M. 2011. Constructing Patriotism. Charlotte: InfoAge Publishing. [3, 19]

Carrion, V. G., S. S. Wong, and H. Kletter. 2013. Update on Neuroimaging and Cognitive Functioning in Maltreatment-Related Pediatric PTSD: Treatment Implications. *J. Fam. Violence* **28**:53–61. [12]

Carter, C. S. 1998. Neuroendocrine Perspectives on Social Attachment and Love. *Psychoneuroendocrinology* **23**:779–818. [4, 7]

———. 2005. The Chemistry of Child Neglect: Do Oxytocin and Vasopressin Mediate the Effects of Early Experience? *PNAS* **102**:18247–18248. [7]

———. 2007. Sex Differences in Oxytocin and Vasopressin: Implications for Autism Spectrum Disorders? *Behav. Brain Res.* **176**:170–186. [4]

———. 2014. Oxytocin Pathways and the Evolution of Human Behavior. *Annu. Rev. Psychol.* **65**:17–39. [3, 4, 7]

Carter, C. S., E. M. Boone, H. Pournajafi-Nazarloo, and K. L. Bales. 2009. The Consequences of Early Experiences and Exposure to Oxytocin and Vasopressin Are Sexually Dimorphic. *Dev. Neurosci.* **31**:332–341. [4, 7]

Carter, C. S., A. C. DeVries, and L. L. Getz. 1995. Physiological Substrates of Monogamy: The Prairie Vole Model. *Neurosci. Biobehav. Rev.* **19**:303–314. [4]

Carter, C. S., and S. W. Porges. 2013. The Biochemistry of Love: An Oxytocin Hypothesis. *EMBO Rep.* **14**:12–16. [3, 4, 7]

Caspi, A., J. McClay, T. E. Moffitt, et al. 2002. Role of Genotype in the Cycle of Violence in Maltreated Children. *Science* **297**:851–854. [11]

Cassidy, J. 2001. Truth, Lies, and Intimacy: An Attachment Perspective. *Attach. Hum. Dev.* **3**:121–155. [11]

———. 2008. The Nature of the Child's Ties. In: Handbook of Attachment: Theory, Research, and Clinical Applications, ed. J. Cassidy and P. Shaver, pp. 3–22. New York: Guilford Press. [2]

Catani, C., A. H. Gewirtz, E. Wieling, et al. 2010. Tsunami, War, and Cumulative Risk in the Lives of Sri Lankan School Children. *Child Dev.* **81**:1175–1190. [14]

Catani, C., E. Schauer, and F. Neuner. 2008. Beyond Individual War Trauma: Domestic Violence against Children in Afghanistan and Sri Lanka. *J. Marital Fam. Ther.* **34**:165–176. [7, 12]

Chaffin, M., J. F. Silovsky, B. Funderburk, et al. 2004. Parent-Child Interaction Therapy with Physically Abusive Parents: Efficacy for Reducing Future Abuse Reports. *J. Consult. Clin. Psychol.* **72**:500–510. [14]

Champagne, F. A. 2012. Interplay between Social Experiences and the Genome: Epigenetic Consequences for Behavior. *Adv. Genet.* **77**:33–57. [4]

Champagne, F. A., J. Diorio, S. Sharma, and M. J. Meaney. 2001. Naturally Occurring Variations in Maternal Behavior in the Rat Are Associated with Differences in Estrogen-Inducible Central Oxytocin Receptors. *PNAS* **98**:12736–127341. [7]

Champagne, F. A., and M. J. Meaney. 2006. Stress During Gestation Alters Postpartum Maternal Care and the Development of the Offspring in a Rodent Model. *Biol. Psychiatry* **59**:1227–1235. [7]

Chan, M. 2013. Linking Child Survival and Child Development for Health, Equity, and Sustainable Development. *Lancet* **381**:1415–1514. [13]

Chandy, L., and G. Gertz. 2011. The Changing State of Global Poverty. In: Child Poverty Inequality: New Perspectives, ed. I. Ortiz et al., pp. 42–47. New York: UNICEF. [15]

Chapman, A. 2007. Truth Commissions and Intergroup Forgiveness: The Case of the South African Truth and Reconciliation Commission. *Peace Confl.* **13**:51–69. [12]

Chemtob, C. M., O. G. Gudino, and D. Laraque. 2013. Maternal Posttraumatic Stress Disorder and Depression in Pediatric Primary Care: Association with Child Maltreatment and Frequency of Child Exposure to Traumatic Events. *JAMA Pediatr.* **167**:1011–1018. [7]

Chen, X., and K. H. Rubin, eds. 2011. Socioemotional Development in Cultural Context. New York: Guilford Press. [2]

Chisholm, J. S. 1993. Death, Hope, and Sex: Life-History Theory and the Development of Reproductive Strategies. *Curr. Anthropol.* **34**:1–24. [8]

Christie, D. J. 2006. What Is Peace Psychology the Psychology Of? *J. Soc. Iss.* **62**:1–17. [15]

Christie, D. J., and A. Dawes. 2001. Tolerance and Solidarity. *Peace Confl.* **7(2)**:131–142. [13]

Christie, D. J., and C. J. Montiel. 2013. Contributions of Psychology to War and Peace. *Am. Psychol.* **68**:502–513. [15]

Christie, D. J., B. S. Tint, R. V. Wagner, and D. D. Winter. 2008. Peace Psychology for a Peaceful World. *Am. Psychol.* **63**:540–552. [15]

Christie, D. J., R. V. Wagner, and D. A. Winter. 2001. Peace, Conflict, and Violence: Peace Psychology for the 21st Century. Englewood Cliffs: Prentice-Hall. [3]

Chugani, H. T., M. E. Behen, O. Musik, et al. 2001. Local Brain Functional Activity Following Early Deprivation: A Study of Postinstitutionalized Romanian Orphans. *NeuroImage* **14**:1290–1301. [9]

Cicchetti, D. 2010. Resilience under Conditions of Extreme Stress: A Multilevel Perspective. *World Psychiatry* **9**:145–154. [14]

———. 2013. Resilient Functioning in Maltreated Children: Past, Present and Future Perspectives. *J. Child Psychol. Psychiat.* **54**:402–422. [4, 11, 14]

Cicchetti, D., and F. A. Rogosch. 1996. Equifinality and Multifinality in Developmental Psychopathology. *Dev. Psychopathol.* **8**:597–600. [14]

Cicchetti, D., and K. Valentino. 2006. An Ecological Transactional Perspective on Child Maltreatment: Failure of the Average Expectable Environment and Its Influence Upon Child Development. In: Developmental Psychopathology: Risk, Disorder, and Adaptation, ed. D. Cicchetti and D. J. Cohen, vol. 3, pp. 129–201. New York: Wiley. [12]

Cicirelli, V. G., J. W. Evans, and J. S. Schiller. 1969. The Impact of Head-Start Curricula: An Evaluation of the Effects of Head-Start on Children's Cognitive and Affective Development. Washington, D.C.: Westinghouse Learning Corporation. [16]

Claessens, S. E. F., N. P. Daskalakis, R. van der Veen, et al. 2011. Development of Individual Differences in Stress Responsiveness: An Overview of Factors Mediating the Outcome of Early Life Experiences. *Psychopharmacology* **214**:141–154. [7]

Clarke, A. R., R. J. Barry, R. McCarthy, et al. 2005. Quantitative EEG in Low IQ Children with Attention-Deficit/Hyperactivity Disorder. *Clin. Neurophysiol.* **117**:1708–1714. [9]

Clemens, J. L. 2012. Peace and Conflict Studies Versus Peace Science. In: Encyclopedia of Peace Psychology, ed. D. J. Christie, pp. 767–771. New York: Wiley-Blackwell. [15]

Cochrane, J. R. 2012. Religion, Health and the Economy. In: The Wiley-Blackwell Companion to African Religions, ed. E. K. Bongmba, pp. 430–442. Oxford: Wiley-Blackwell. [19]

Cohen, R. 1991. Negotiating across Cultures: Communication Obstacles in International Diplomacy. Washington, D.C.: U.S. Institute of Peace Press. [17]

Cohen, S., D. Janicki-Deverts, E. Chen, and K. A. Matthews. 2010. Childhood Socioeconomic Status Adult Health. *Ann. NY Acad. Sci.* **1186**:37–55. [11]

Cole, C. 2008. Begin with the Children: What Research on Sesame Street's International Coproductions Reveals About Using Media to Promote a New More Peaceful World. *Intl. J. Behav. Dev.* **32**:359–365. [18]

Coleman, J. 1988. Social Capital in the Creation of Human Capital. *Am. J. Sociol.* **94**:S95–S120. [1, 3]

Coleman, P. T. 2003. Characteristics of Protracted, Intractable Conflict: Toward the Development of a Metaframework. *Peace Confl.* **9**:1–37. [15]

Conger, R. D., K. J. Conger, and M. J. Martin. 2010. Socioeconomic Status, Family Processes, and Individual Development. *J. Marriage Fam.* **72**:685–704. [14]

Connolly, P. 2011. Using Survey Data to Explore Preschool Children's Ethnic Awareness and Attitudes. *J. Early Child. Res.* **9**:175–187. [15]

Connolly, P., and J. Hayden. 2007. From Conflict to Peace Building: The Power of Early Childhood Initiatives. Lessons from around the World. Redmond, WA: World Forum Foundation. [3, 17–19]

Connolly, P., A. Smith, and B. Kelly. 2002. Too Young to Notice? The Cultural and Political Awareness of 3–6 Year Olds in Northern Ireland. Belfast: Community Relations Council. [3, 18, 19]

Connor, R. C. 2010. Cooperation Beyond the Dyad: On Simple Models and a Complex Society. *Philos. Trans. R. Soc. Lond. B* **365**:2687–2697. [7]

Convention on the Rights of the Child. 1989. United Nations Treaty Series 1577. [3, 11]

Cowan, P. A., C. P. Cowan, M. K. Pruett, K. Pruett, and J. J. Wong. 2009. Promoting Father Engagement with Children: Preventive Interventions for Low-Income Families. *J. Marriage Fam.* **71**:663–679. [1, 16]

Crawford, P. 2005. Primarily Peaceful: Nurturing Peace in the Primary Grades. *Early Childhood Educ. J.* **32**:321–328. [17]

Cremin, H. 2007. Peer Mediation: Citizenship and Social Inclusion Revisited. Buckingham: Open Univ. Press. [17]

Crick, N. R., J. M. Ostrov, and N. E. Werner. 2006. A Longitudinal Study of Relational Aggression, Physical Aggression and Children's Social-Psychological Adjustment. *J. Abnorm. Child Psychol.* **34**:131–142. [11]

Crookston, B. T., W. Schott, S. Cueto, et al. 2013. Postinfancy Growth, Schooling, and Cognitive Achievement: Young Lives. *Am. J. Clin. Nutr.* **98**:1555–1563. [15]

Cummings, E. M., M. El-Sheikh, C. D. Kouros, and J. A. Buckhalt. 2009. Children and Violence: The Role of Children's Regulation in the Marital Aggression-Child Adjustment Link. *Clin. Child Fam. Psychol. Rev.* **12**:3–15. [12]

Cummings, E. M., C. E. Merrilees, A. C. Schermerhorn, et al. 2012. Political Violence and Child Adjustment: Longitudinal Tests of Sectarian Antisocial Behavior, Family Conflict, and Insecurity as Explanatory Pathways. *Child Dev.* **83**:461–468. [14]

Cummins, D. 2005. Dominance, Status and Social Hierarchies. In: The Handbook of Evolutionary Psychology, ed. D. M. Buss, pp. 676–697. New York: Wiley. [7]

D'Ambruoso, L. 2013. Global Health Post-2015: The Case for Universal Health Equity. *Glob. Health Action* **6**:19661. [1]

Dadds, M. R., C. Moul, A. Cauchi, et al. 2014. Methylation of the Oxytocin Receptor Gene and Oxytocin Blood Levels in the Development of Psychopathy. *Dev. Psychopathol.* **26**:33–40. [4]

Dai, L., C. S. Carter, J.Ying, et al. 2012. Oxytocin and Vasopressin Are Dysregulated in Williams Syndrome, a Genetic Disorder Affecting Social Behavior. *PLoS One* **7**:e38513. [4]

Darwin, C. 1871/1998. The Descent of Man. New York: Prometheus. [6]

Davies, L. 2008. Educating against Extremism. Sterling, VA: Trentham Books. [3]

Dawes, A., L. Biersteker, and L. Hendricks. 2012. Ilifalabantwana Sobambisana Initiative Partner Evaluation Report: The Ntataise Trust Play Group, Parent Support and Teacher Enrichment Programmes Rammulotsi/Viljoenskroon, Northern Free State. http://72.249.167.103/~ilifalab/wp-content/uploads/2012/09/Ntataise-partner-report1.pdf. (accessed May 8, 2014). [13]

Dawes, A., R. Bray, and A. van der Merwe. 2007. Monitoring Child Wellbeing: A South African Rights-Based Approach. Cape Town: HSRC Press. [13]

Dawes, A., and D. Donald. 1994. Childhood and Adversity: Psychological Perspectives from South African Research. Cape Town: David Philip. [13]

Dawes, A., and C. Ward. 2008. Levels, Trends, and Determinants of Child Maltreatment in the Western Cape Province. In: The State of Population in the Western Cape Province, ed. C. G. R. Marindo and S. Gaisie, pp. 97–125. Cape Town: HSRC Press. [13]

Dawson, D. 1996. The Origins of War: Biological and Anthropological Theories. *Hist. Theory* **35**:1–28. [17]

De Abreu, G. 2000. Relationships between Macro and Micro Socio-Cultural Contexts: Implications for the Study of Interactions in the Mathematics Classroom. *Educational Stud. Math.* **41**:1–29. [17]

Deaton, A. M., and A. Bird. 2011. CpG Islands and the Regulation of Transcription. *Genes Dev.* **25**:1010–1022. [5]

De Bellis, M. D., E. R. Broussard, D. J. Herring, et al. 2001. Psychiatric Co-Morbidity in Caregivers and Children Involved in Maltreatment: A Pilot Research Study with Policy Implications. *Child Abuse Negl.* **25**:923–944. [7]

De Bellis, M. D., S. R. Hooper, D. P. Woolley, and C. E. Shenk. 2010. Demographic, Maltreatment, and Neurobiological Correlates of PTSD Symptoms in Children and Adolescents. *J. Pediatr. Psychol.* **35**:570–577. [12]

De Bellis, M. D., and L. A. Thomas. 2003. Biologic Findings of Post-Traumatic Stress Disorder and Child Maltreatment. *Curr. Psychiatry Rep.* **5**:108–117. [12]

Decety, J., and P. L. Jackson. 2004. The Functional Architecture of Human Empathy. *Behav. Cogn. Neurosci. Rev.* **3**:71–100. [15]

De Dreu, C. K. 2012. Oxytocin Modulates Cooperation within and Competition between Groups: An Integrative Review and Research Agenda. *Horm. Behav.* **61**:419–428. [4]

De Dreu, C. K., L. L. Greer, M. J. J. Handgraaf, et al. 2010. The Neuropeptide Oxytocin Regulates Parochial Altruism in Intergroup Conflict among Humans. *Science* **328**:1408–1411. [10]

De Dreu, C. K., L. L. Greer, G. A. Van Kleef, S. Shalvi, and M. J. Handgraaf. 2011. Oxytocin Promotes Human Ethnocentrism. *PNAS* **1084**:1262–1266. [3]

De Dreu, C. K., S. Shalvi, L. L. Greer, G. A. Van Kleef, and M. J. Handgraaf. 2012. Oxytocin Motivates Non-Cooperation in Intergroup Conflict to Protect Vulnerable In-Group Members. *PLoS One* **7**:e46751. [7]

Del Giudice, M. 2009. Sex, Attachment, and the Development of Reproductive Strategies. *Behav. Brain Sci.* **32**:1–67. [8]

———. 2014. An Evolutionary Life-History Framework for Psychopathology. *Psychol. Inq.*, in press. [8]

Del Giudice, M., B. J. Ellis, and E. A. Shirtcliff. 2011. The Adaptive Calibration Model of Stress Responsivity. *Neurosci. Biobehav. Rev.* **35**:1562–1592. [8]

de Quervain, D. J.-F., I.-T. Kolassa, S. Ackermann, et al. 2012. PKCα Is Genetically Linked to Memory Capacity in Healthy Subjects and to Risk for Posttraumatic Stress Disorder in Genocide Survivors. *PNAS* **109**:8746–8751. [7]

de Quervain, D. J.-F., I.-T. Kolassa, V. Ertl, et al. 2007. A Deletion Variant of the Alpha2b-Adrenoceptor Is Related to Emotional Memory in Europeans and Africans. *Nat. Neurosci.* **10**:137–139. [7]

de Waal, F. B. M. 1996. Good Natured: The Origins of Right and Wrong in Humans and Other Animals. Cambridge, MA: Harvard Univ. Press. [7]

———. 2008. Putting the Altruism Back into Altruism: The Evolution of Empathy. *Annu. Rev. Psychol.* **59**:279–300. [10]

———. 2009. The Age of Empathy. New York: Three Rivers Press. [7]

de Waal, F. B. M., and D. L. Johanowicz. 1993. Modification of Reconciliation Behavior through Social Experience: An Experiment with Two Macaque Species. *Child Dev.* **64**:897–908. [8]

De Wolff, M. S., and M. H. van IJzendoorn. 1997. Sensitivity and Attachment: A Meta-Analysis on Parental Antecedents of Infant Attachment. *Child Dev.* **68**:571–591. [2]

Demuth, C. 2008. Talking to Infants: How Culture Is Instantiated in Early Mother-Infant Interactions. The Case of Cameroonian Farming Nso and North German Middle-Class Families. Doctoral Thesis. Osnabrück University: School of Human Sciences, Department of Culture and Psychology. [11]

Deng, L.-F. 2012. Parenting About Peace: Exploring Taiwanese Parents and Children's Perceptions in a Shared Political and Sociocultural Context. *Fam. Relat.* **61**:115–128. [17]

Dennis, M. 1993. Cultivating a Landscape of Peace: Iroquois-European Encounters in Seventeenth-Century America. Ithaca: Cornell Univ. Press. [6]

Dept. of Social Development, SASSA, and UNICEF. 2012. South African Child Support Grant Impact Assessment. Pretoria: Dept. of Social Development. http://www.unicef.org/evaldatabase/files/CSG_QUANTITATIVE_STUDY_FULL_REPORT_2012.pdf. (accessed May 8, 2014). [13]

Deutsch, M. 1973. The Resolution of Conflict: Constructive and Destructive Processes. New Haven: Yale Univ. Press. [6]

———. 1977. The Resolution of Conflict: Constructive and Destructive Processes. New Haven: Yale Univ. Press. [15]

———. 2006a. Cooperation and Competition. In: The Handbook of Conflict Resolution, ed. M. Deutsch et al., pp. 23–42. San Francisco: Jossey-Bass. [6]

———. 2006b. Justice and Conflict. In: The Handbook of Conflict Resolution, ed. M. Deutsch et al., pp. 43–68. San Francisco: Jossey-Bass. [6]

Dewey, J. 1938. Experience and Education. Kappa Delta Pi Lecture Series. New York: Macmillan. [17]

Dewey, K., and K. Begum. 2011. Long-Term Consequences of Stunting in Early Life. *Matern. Child Nutr.* **7(Suppl. 3)**:5–18. [13]

Diab, M., R.-L. Punamäki, E. Palosaari, and S. R. Qouta. 2014. Can Psychosocial Intervention Improve Social Relations among War–Affected Children? Intervention Impact and Mediating Role of Peer and Sibling Relations in a Randomized Controlled Trial. *Soc. Dev.* **23**:215–231. [12]

Diab, S. Y. 2011. The Psychosocial Factors That Undermine Children's Academic Potentials: A Multi-Level Study of the Main Psychosocial Factors That Contribute to Palestinian Children's Academic Underachievement. Berlin: Lambert Academic Publishing. [12]

Dias, B. G., and K. J. Ressler. 2014. Parental Olfactory Experience Influences Behavior and Neural Structure in Subsequent Generations. *Nat. Neurosci.* **17**:89–96. [7]

Dimitry, L. 2012. A Systematic Review on the Mental Health of Children and Adolescents in Areas of Armed Conflict in the Middle East. *Child Care Health Dev.* **38**:153–161. [14]

Dishion, T. J., D. Shaw, A. Connell, et al. 2008. The Family Check-up with High-Risk Indigent Families: Preventing Problem Behavior by Increasing Parents' Positive Behavior Support in Early Childhood. *Child Dev.* **79**:1395–1414. [14]

Dishion, T. J., and J. M. Tipsord. 2011. Peer Contagion in Child and Adolescent Social and Emotional Development. *Annu. Rev. Psychol.* **62**:189–214. [14]

Doan, S. N., and G. W. Evans. 2011. Maternal Responsiveness Moderates the Relationship between Allostatic Load and Working Memory. *Dev. Psychopathol.* **23**:873–880. [7]

Dodge, K. A., J. E. Bates, and G. S. Pettit. 1990. Mechanisms in the Cycle of Violence. *Science* **250**:1678–1683. [11]

Dodge, K. A., M. T. Greenberg, P. S. Malone, and the Conduct Problems Prevention Research Group. 2008. Testing an Idealized Dynamic Cascade Model of the Development of Serious Violence in Adolescence. *Child Dev.* **79**:1907–1927. [14]

Dodge, K. A., and D. R. Somberg. 1987. Hostile Attributional Biases among Aggressive Boys Are Exacerbated under Conditions of Threats to the Self. *Child Dev.* **58**:213–224. [11]

Domes, G., M. Heinrichs, A. Michel, C. Berger, and S. C. Herpertz. 2007. Oxytocin Improves "Mind-Reading" in Humans. *Biol. Psychiatry* **61**:731–733. [3]

Domschke, K. 2012. Patho-Genetics of Postraumatic Stress Disorder. *Psychiatr. Danub.* **24**:267–273. [5]

Doris, J. M., and the Moral Psychology Research Group. 2010. The Moral Psychology Handbook. New York: Oxford Univ. Press. [10]

Dovidio, J., S. Gaertner, and G. Kafati. 2000. Group Identity and Intergroup Relations: The Common In-Group Identity Model. *Adv. Group Processes* **17**:1–35. [6]

Dovidio, J. F., S. Gaertner, and T. Saguy. 2009. Commonality and the Complexity of "We": Social Attitudes and Social Change. *Pers. Soc. Psychol. Rev.* **13**:3–20. [6, 15]

Dowd, J. B., A. Zajaova, and A. Aiello. 2009. Early Origins of Health Disparities: Burden of Infection, Health, and Socioeconomic Status in U.S. Children. *Soc. Sci. Med.* **68**:699–707. [11]

Dozier, M., K. C. Stoval, K. E. Albus, and B. Bates. 2001. Attachment for Infants in Foster Care: The Role of Caregiver State of Mind. *Child Dev.* **72**:1467–1477. [11]

Dube, S. R., R. F. Anda, V. J. Felitti, et al. 2001a. Childhood Abuse, Household Dysfunction, and the Risk of Attempted Suicide Throughout the Life Span. *JAMA* **286**:3089–3096. [11]

———. 2001b. Growing up with Parental Alcohol Abuse: Exposure to Childhood Abuse, Neglect and Household Dysfunction. *Child Abuse Negl.* **25**:1627–1640. [7]

Dubow, E. F., P. Boxer, L. R. Huesmann, et al. 2012. Cumulative Effects of Exposure to Violence on Posttraumatic Stress in Palestinian and Israeli Youth. *J. Clin. Child Adolesc. Psychol.* **41**:837–844. [12]

Dugan, E. M., M. S. Snow, and S. R. Crowe. 2010. Working with Children Affected by Hurricane Katrina: Two Case Studies in Play Therapy. *Child Adolesc. Ment. Health* **15**:52–55. [15]

Dunbar, R. 2008. Cognitive Constraints on the Structure and Dynamics of Social Networks. *Group Dyn.* **12**:7–16. [7]

Duncan, G. J., J. Brooks-Gunn, W. J. Yeung, and J. R. Smith. 1998. How Much Does Childhood Poverty Affect the Life Chances of Children? *Am. Sociol. Rev.* **63**:406–423. [3]

Dunfield, K. A., and V. A. Kuhlmeier. 2013. Classifying Prosocial Behavior: Children's Responses to Instrumental Need, Emotional Distress, and Material Desire. *Child Dev.* **84**:1766–1776. [7]

Dunfield, K. A., V. A. Kuhlmeier, L. O'Connell, and E. Kelley. 2011. Examining the Diversity of Prosocial Behavior: Helping, Sharing, and Comforting in Infancy. *Infancy* **16**:227–247. [7]

Dunn, J. 2006. Moral Development in Early Childhood and Social Interaction in the Family. In: Handbook of Moral Development, ed. M. Killen and J. Smetana, pp. 331–350. New York: Psychology Press. [15]

Durakovic-Belko, E., A. Kulenovic, and R. Dapic. 2003. Determinants of Posttraumatic Adjustment in Adolescents from Sarajevo Who Experienced War. *J. Clin. Psychol.* **59**:27–40. [12]

Durston, S., K. M. Thomas, Y. Yang, et al. 2002. A Neural Basis for the Development of Inhibitory Control. *Dev. Sci.* **5**:9–16. [10]

Eagleton, T. 1991. Ideology: An Introduction. London: Verso. [13]

Eagly, A. H., and L. L. Carli. 2007. Through the Labyrinth: The Truth About How Women Become Leaders. Cambridge, MA: Harvard Business Review Press. [11]

Eagly, A. H., and M. Crowley. 1986. Gender and Helping-Behavior: A Meta-Analytic Review of the Social Psychological Literature. *Psychol. Bull.* **100**:283–308. [10]

Ebstein, R. P., A. Knafo, D. Mankuta, S. H. Chew, and P. S. Lai. 2012. The Contributions of Oxytocin and Vasopressin Pathway Genes to Human Behavior. *Horm. Behav.* **61**:359–379. [4]

Ecker, J. R., W. A. Bickmore, I. Barroso, et al. 2012. Genomics, Encode Explained. *Nature* **489**:57–74. [5]

Edward, V. J., G. W. Holden, V. J. Felitti, and R. F. Anda. 2003. Relationship between Multiple Forms of Childhood Maltreatment and Adult Mental Health in Community Respondents: Results from the Adverse Childhood Experiences Study. *Am. J. Psychiatry* **160**:1453–1460. [11]

Eggerman, M., and C. Panter-Brick. 2010. Suffering, Hope, and Entrapment: Resilience and Cultural Values in Afghanistan. *Soc. Sci. Med.* **71**:71–83. [12, 15]

———. 2014. Life Feeds on Hope: Family Mental Health, Culture and Resilience. In: Children of Afganistan, ed. J. Heath and A. Zahedi. Austin: Univ. of Texas Press. [12]

Ehlers, A., and D. M. Clark. 2000. A Cognitive Model of Posttraumatic Stress Disorder. *Behav. Res. Ther.* **38**:319–345. [12]

Ehrenreich, B. 1997. Blood Rites: Origins and History of the Passions of War. New York: Metropolitan Books. [17]

Ein-Dor, T., G. Doron, Z. Solomon, M. Mikulincer, and P. R. Shaver. 2010. Together in Pain: Attachment-Related Dyadic Processes and Posttraumatic Stress Disorder. *J. Counsel. Psychol.* **57**:317–327. [12]

Eisenberg, N. 2002. Empathy-Related Emotional Responses, Altruism, and Their Socialization. Oxford: Oxford Univ. Press. [15]

Eisenberg, N., and R. A. Fabes. 1998. Prosocial Development. In: Handbook of Child Psychology (5th edition), vol. 3: Social, Emotional, and Personality Development, ed. N. Eisenberg, pp. 701–778, W. Damon, series ed. New York: Wiley. [10]

Eisenberg, N., R. A. Fabes, and T. L. Spinrad. 1998. Prosocial Development. New York: Wiley and Sons. [15]

Eisenberg, N., and P. A. Miller. 1987. The Relation of Empathy to Prosocial and Related Behaviors. *Psychol. Bull.* **101**:91–119. [15]

Eisenberger, N. I., J. M. Jarcho, M. D. Lieberman, and B. D. Naliboff. 2006. An Experimental Study of Shared Sensitivity to Physical Pain and Social Rejection. *Pain* **126**:132–138. [10]

Eisenberger, N. I., and M. D. Lieberman. 2004. Why Rejection Hurts: A Common Neuralalarm System for Physical and Social Pain. *Trends. Cogn. Sci.* **8**:294–300. [10, 11]

Eisenberger, N. I., M. D. Lieberman, and K. D. Williams. 2003. Does Rejection Hurt? An fMRI Study of Social Exclusion. *Science* **302**:290–292. [7]

Elder, G. H., Jr. 1974/1999. Children of the Great Depression: Social Change in Life Experience. Boulder: Westview Press. [14]

Elias, N. 1939/2000. The Civilizing Process: Sociogenetic and Psychogenetic Investigations (revised edition). Cambridge, MA: Blackwell. [7]

Ellis, B. J. 2004. Timing of Pubertal Maturation in Girls: An Integrated Life History Approach. *Psychol. Bull.* **130**:920–958. [8]

Ellis, B. J., and D. F. Bjorklund. 2012. Beyond Mental Health: An Evolutionary Analysis of Development under Risky and Supportive Environmental Conditions: An Introduction to the Special Section. *Dev. Psychol.* **48**:591–597. [7]

Ellis, B. J., W. T. Boyce, J. Belsky, M. J. Bakermans-Kranenburg, and M. H. van Ijzendoorn. 2011. Differential Susceptibility to the Environment: An Evolutionary-Neurodevelopmental Theory. *Dev. Psychopathol.* **23**:7–28. [4, 7, 10]

Ellis, B. J., and M. Del Giudice. 2014. Beyond Allostatic Load: Rethinking the Role of Stress in Regulating Human Development. *Dev. Psychopathol.* **26**:1–20. [7, 14]

Ellis, B. J., M. Del Giudice, T. J. Dishion, et al. 2012. The Evolutionary Basis of Risky Adolescent Behavior: Implications for Science, Policy, and Practice. *Dev. Psychol.* **48**:598–623. [7]

Ellis, B. J., A. J. Figueredo, B. H. Brumbach, and G. L. Schlomer. 2009. Fundamental Dimensions of Environmental Risk. Human Nature: The Impact of Harsh Versus Unpredictable Environments on the Evolution and Development of Life History Strategies. *Hum. Nat.* **20**:204–268. [7]

Eluvathingal, T. J., H. T. Chugani, M. E. Behen, et al. 2006. Abnormal Brain Connectivity in Children after Early Severe Socioemotional Deprivation: A Diffusion Tensor Imaging Study. *Pediatrics* **117**:2093–2100. [5, 9]

Engle, P. L., M. M. Black, J. Behrman, et al. 2007. Strategies to Avoid the Loss of Developmental Potential in More Than 200 Million Children in the Developing World. *Lancet* **369**:229–242. [13–15, 19]

Engle, P. L., L. C. H. Fernald, H. Alderman, et al. 2011. Strategies for Reducing Inequalities and Improving Developmental Outcomes for Young Children in Low-Income and Middle-Income Countries. *Lancet* **378**:1339–1353. [13–16]

Enright, R. D. 2001. Forgiveness Is a Choice: A Step-by-Step Process for Resolving Anger and Restoring Hope. Washington, D.C.: American Psychological Association. [15]

Evans, S. E., C. Davies, and D. DiLillo. 2008. Exposure to Domestic Violence: A Meta-Analysis of Child and Adolescent Outcomes. *Aggress. Violent Behav.* **13**:131–143. [12]

Evans, G. W., and P. Kim. 2012. Childhood Poverty, Chronic Stress, Self-Regulation, and Coping. *Child Dev. Perspect.* **7**:43–48. [14]

Farmer, P. E., B. Nizeye, S. Stulac, and S. Keshavjee. 2006. Stuctural Violence and Clinical Medicine. *PloS Med.* **3**:e449. [1]

Farrington, D. P., R. Loeber, and M. M. Ttofi. 2012. Risk and Protective Factors for Offending. In: The Oxford Handbook of Crime Prevention, ed. B. C. Welsh and D. P. Farrington, pp. 46–69. New York: Oxford Univ. Press. [14]

Fearon, R. P., M. J. Bakermans-Kranenburg, M. H. van IJzendoorn, A. Lapsley, and G. I. Roisman. 2010. The Significance of Insecure Attachment and Disorganization in the Development of Children's Externalizing Behavior: A Meta-Analytic Study. *Child Dev.* **81**:435–456. [11]

Feddes, A. R., P. Noack, and A. Rutland. 2009. Direct and Extended Friendship Effects on Minority and Majority Children's Interethnic Attitudes: A Longitudinal Study. *Child Dev.* **80**:377–390. [15]

Fehr, E., H. Bernhard, and B. Rockenbach. 2008. Egalitarianism in Young Children. *Nature* **454**:1079–1083. [7]

Feinberg, A., and R. Irizarry. 2010. Stochastic Epigenetic Variation as a Driving Force of Development, Evolutionary Adaptation, and Disease. *PNAS* **107**:1757–1065. [8]

Feinberg, M. E., D. E. Jones, M. L. Kan, and M. C. Goslin. 2010. Effects of Family Foundations on Parents and Children: 3.5 Years after Baseline. *J. Fam. Psychol.* **24**:534–542. [3, 16]

Feldman, R. 2012. Oxytocin and Social Affiliation in Humans. *Horm. Behav.* **61**:380–391. [4]

Feldman, R., I. Gordon, M. Influs, T. Gutbir, and R. P. Ebstein. 2013. Parental Oxytocin and Early Caregiving Jointly Shape Children's Oxytocin Response and Social Reciprocity. *Neuropsychopharmacology* **38**:1154–1162. [1]

Feldman, R., S. Masalha, and R. Derdikman-Eiron. 2010. Conflict Resolution in the Parent–Child, Marital, and Peer Contexts and Children's Aggression in the Peer Group: A Process-Oriented Cultural Perspective. *Dev. Psychol.* **46**:310–325. [18]

Feldman, R., A. Vengrober, and R. P. Ebstein. 2014. Affiliation Buffers Stress: Cumulative Genetic Risk in Oxytocin-Vasopressin Genes Combines with Early Caregiving to Predict PTSD in War-Exposed Young Children. *Transl. Psychiatry* **4**:e370. [4]

Feldman, R., A. Weller, O. Zagoory-Sharon, and A. Levine. 2007. Evidence for a Neuroendocrinological Foundation of Human Affiliation Plasma Oxytocin Levels across Pregnancy and the Postpartum Period Predict Mother-Infant Bonding. *Psychol. Sci.* **18**:965–970. [11]

Feldman, R., O. Zagoory-Sharon, O. Weisman, et al. 2012. Sensitive Parenting Is Associated with Plasma Oxytocin and Polymorphisms in the OXTR and CD38 Genes. *Biol. Psychiatry* **72**:175–181. [7]

Felitti, M. D., J. Vincent, M. D. Anda, et al. 1998. Relationship of Childhood Abuse and Household Dysfunction to Many of the Leading Causes of Death in Adults: The Adverse Childhood Experiences (ACE) Study. *Am. J. Prev. Med.* **14**:245–258. [11]

Ferguson, R. B. 2013. Pinker's List: Exaggerating Prehistoric War Mortality. In: War, Peace, and Human Nature: Convergence of Evolutionary and Cultural Views, ed. D. P. Fry, pp. 112–131. New York: Oxford Univ. Press. [6]

Ferris, C. F. 2008. Functional Magnetic Resonance Imaging and the Neurobiology of Vasopressin and Oxytocin. *Prog. Brain Res.* **170**:305–320. [4]

Festinger, L. 1954. A Theory of Social Comparison Processes. *Hum. Relat.* **7**:117–140. [7]

Finn, A., and M. Leibbrandt. 2013. Mobility and Inequality in the First Three Waves of NIDS. Saldru Working Paper Number 120, NIDS Discussion Paper 2013/2. Cape Town: SALDRU, Univ. of Cape Town. [13]

Fisch, S. M., and R. T. Truglio. 2000. G Is for Growing: Thirty Years of Research on Children and Sesame Street. London: Lawrence Erlbaum Associates. [18]

Fisher, J., M. C. de Mello, V. Patel, et al. 2012. Prevalence and Determinants of Common Perinatal Mental Disorders in Women in Low-and Lower-Middle-Income Countries: A Systematic Review. *Bull. WHO* **9**:139–149. [15]

Fisher, R., and W. L. Ury. 1983. Getting to Yes: Negotiating Agreement without Giving In. New York: Penguin Books. [15, 17]

Fisher, R. J. 1990. The Social Psychology of Intergroup and International Conflict Resolution. New York: Springer. [15]

———. 1997. Interactive Conflict Resolution. Syracuse: Syracuse Univ. Press. [17]

———. 2005. Paving the Way: Contributions of Interactive Conflict Resolution to Peacemaking. Lanham, MD: Lexington Books. [17]

Fiske, A. P. 1992. The Four Elementary Forms of Sociality: Framework for a Unified Theory of Social Relations. *Psychol. Rev.* **99**:689–723. [7]

———. 2004. Four Modes of Constituting Relationships: Consubstantial Assimilation; Space, Magnitude, Time, and Force; Concrete Procedures; Abstract Symbolism. In: Relational Models Theory: A Contemporary Overview, ed. N. Haslam, pp. 61–146. Mahwah, NJ: Erlbaum. [7]

Flores, E., D. Cicchetti, and F. A. Rogosch. 2005. Predictors of Resilience in Maltreated and Nonmaltreated Latino Children. *Dev. Psychol.* **41**:338–351. [12]

Fonagy, P., M. Steele, G. Moran, H. Steele, and A. Higgitt. 1993. Measuring the Ghost in the Nursery: An Empirical Study of the Relation between Parents' Mental Representations of Childhood Experiences and Their Infants' Security of Attachment. *J. Am. Psychoanal. Assoc.* **41**:957–989. [11]

Fox, S. E., P. Levitt, and C. A. Nelson. 2010. How the Timing and Quality of Early Experiences Influence the Development of Brain Architecture. *Child Dev.* **81**:28–40. [9]

Fraiberg, S., E. Adelson, and V. Shapiro. 1975. Ghosts in the Nursery: A Psychoanalytic Approach to the Problems of Impaired Infant-Mother Relationships. *J. Am. Acad. Child Adolesc. Psychiatry* **14**:387–421. [11]

Freeman, D., K. Aquino, and B. McFerran. 2009. Overcoming Beneficiary Race as an Impediment to Charitable Donations: Social Dominance Orientation, the Experience of Moral Elevation, and Donation Behavior. *Pers. Soc. Psychol. Bull.* **35**:72–84. [10]

Freire, P. 1985. The Politics of Education: Culture, Power, and Liberation. Westport, CT: Greenwood Publishing Group. [11]

Fries, A. B., T. E. Ziegler, J. R. Kurian, S. Jacoris, and S. D. Pollak. 2005. Early Experience in Humans Is Associated with Changes in Neuropeptides Critical for Regulating Social Behavior. *PNAS* **102**:17237–17240. [10]

Fry, D. P. 2006. The Human Potential for Peace: An Anthropological Challenge to Assumptions About War and Violence. New York: Oxford Univ. Press. [6, 11]

———. 2009. Anthropological Insights for Creating Non-Warring Social Systems. *J. Aggr. Confl. Peace Res.* **1**:4–15. [6]

———. 2012. Life without War. *Science* **336**:879–884. [6]

Fry, D. P., and M. Miklikowska. 2012. Cultures of Peace. In: Psychological Components of Sustainable Peace, ed. P. T. Coleman and M. Deutsch, pp. 227–243. New York: Springer. [6]

Fry, D. P., and P. Söderberg. 2013. Lethal Aggression in Mobile Forager Bands and Implications for the Origins of War. *Science* **341**:270–273. [4, 6]

Fry, D. P., and G. Souillac. 2013. The Relevance of Nomadic Forager Studies to Moral Foundations Theory: Moral Education and Global Ethics in the Twenty-First Century. *J. Moral Educ.* **42**:346–359. [6]

Fry, D. P., and A. Szala. 2013. The Evolution of Agonism: The Triumph of Restraint in Nonhuman and Human Primates. In: War, Peace, and Human Nature: The Convergence of Evolutionary and Cultural Views, ed. D. P. Fry, pp. 451–474. New York: Oxford Univ. Press. [7]

Galler, J. R., C. P. Bryce, D. P. Waber, et al. 2012. Infant Malnutrition Predicts Conduct Problems in Adolescents. *Nutr. Neurosci.* **15**:186–192. [13, 15]

Galobardes, B., J. W. Lynch, and G. Davey Smith. 2004. Childhood Socioeconomic Circumstances and Cause-Specific Mortality in Adulthood: Systematic Review and Interpretation. *Epidemiol. Rev.* **26**:5–21. [11]

Galtung, J. 1969. Violence, Peace, and Peace Research. *J. Peace Res.* **63**:167–191. [3, 13, 15, 17]

———. 1994. Human Rights in Another Key. Cambridge: Polity Press. [13]

———. 1996. Peace by Peaceful Means: Peace and Conflict, Development and Civilization. Thousand Oaks, CA: Sage Publications. [1, 15, 17]

———. 2008. 50 Years: 100 Peace and Conflict Perspectives. Porto: Transend Univ. Press. [19]

Gandhi, M. 1948. Autobiography: The Story of My Experiments with Truth. New York: Courier Dover Publications. [15]

Gapp, K., A. Jawaid, P. Sarkies, et al. 2014. Implication of Sperm RNAs in Transgenerational Inheritance of the Effects of Early Trauma in Mice. *Nat. Neurosci.* **17**:667–669. [7]

Gardner, H. 1983. Frames of Mind: The Theory of Multiple Intelligences Theory. New York: Basic Books. [17]

Garmezy, N. 1983. Stressors of Childhood. In: Stress, Coping, and Development, ed. N. Garmezy and M. Rutter, pp. 43–84. New York: McGraw Hill. [14]

Garner, A. S., and J. P. Shonkoff. 2012. Early Childhood Adversity, Toxic Stress, and the Role of the Pediatrician: Translating Developmental Science into Lifelong Health. *Pediatrics* **129**:e224–231.662. [7]

Garon, N., S. E. Bryson, and I. M. Smith. 2008. Executive Function in Preschoolers: A Review Using an Integrative Framework. *Psychol. Bull.* **134**:31–60. [16]

Garrison, J. L., E. Z. Macosko, S. Bernstein, et al. 2012. Oxytocin/Vasopressin-Related Peptides Have an Ancient Role in Reproductive Behavior. *Science* **338**:540–543. [3]

Gartrell, D. 2012. Education for a Civil Society: How Guidance Teaches Young Children Democratic Life Skills. Washington, D.C.: Natl. Association for the Education of Young Children. [17]

Gasparini, L., and N. Lustig. 2011. The rise and fall of income inequality in Latin America. The Oxford Handbook of Latin American Economics, pp. 691–714. Oxford: Oxford Univ. Press. [15]

Gautvik, K. M., L. d. Lecea, V. T. Gautvik, et al. 1996. Overview of the Most Prevalent Hypothalamus-Specific mRNAs, as Identified by Directional Tag PCR Subtraction. *PNAS* **93**:8733–8738. [4]

Gehlert, S., D. Sohmer, T. Sacks, et al. 2008. Targeting Health Disparities: A Model Linking Upstream Determinants to Downstream Interventions. *Health Aff.* **27**:339–349. [15]

Georgiev, A., A. C. E. Klimczuk, D. M. Traficonte, and D. Maestripieri. 2013. When Violence Pays: A Cost-Benefit Analysis of Aggressive Behavior in Animals and Humans. *Evol. Psychol.* **11**:678–699. [8]

Geraci, A., and L. Surian. 2011. The Developmental Roots of Fairness: Infants' Reactions to Equal and Unequal Distributions of Resources. *Dev. Sci.* **14**:1012–1020. [7]

Gerstein, M. B., A. Kundaje, M. Hariharan, et al. 2012. Architecture of the Human Gene Regulatory Network Derived from Encode Data. *Nature* **489**:91–100. [5]

Gertler, P., A. Zanolini, R. Pinto, et al. 2013. Labor Market Returns to Early Childhood Stimulation: A 20-Year Follow-up to the Jamaica Study. Policy Research Working Paper 6529. Washington, D.C.: World Bank. [16]

Gilissen, R., M. J. Bakermans-Kranenburg, M. H. van IJzendoorn, and M. Linting. 2008. Electrodermal Reactivity During the Trier Social Stress Test for Children: Interaction between the Serotonin Transporter Polymorphism and Children's Attachment Representation. *Dev. Psychobiol.* **50**:615–625. [10]

Gilligan, J. 1997. Violence: Reflections on a National Epidemic. New York: Vintage Books. [15]

Gluckman, P. D., M. A. Hanson, P. Bateson, et al. 2009. Towards a New Developmental Synthesis: Adaptive Developmental Plasticity and Human Disease. *Lancet* **373**:1654–1657. [11]

Gluckman, P. D., M. A. Hanson, and C. Pinal. 2005. The Developmental Origins of Adult Disease. *Matern. Child Nutr.* **1**:130–141. [11]

Goldenberg, H., and I. Goldenberg, I. 2013. Family Therapy: An Overview (8th edition). Belmont, CA: Brooks/Cole. [14]

Goldfarb, W. 1945. Effects of Psychological Deprivation in Infancy and Subsequent Stimulation. *Am. J. Psychiatry* **102**:18–33. [9]

Gonzalez, A., J. M. Jenkins, M. Steiner, and A. S. Fleming. 2012. Maternal Early Life Experiences and Parenting: The Mediating Role of Cortisol and Executive Function. *J. Am. Acad. Child Adolesc. Psychiatry* **51**:673–682. [7]

Goodman, R. 1997. The Strengths and Difficulties Questionnaire: A Research Note. *J. Child Psychol. Psychiatry* **38**:581–586. [10]

Gordon, I., J. F. Leckman, and D. N. Berg. 2014. From Attachment to Groups: Tapping into the Neurobiology of Our Interconnectedness. *J. Am. Acad. Child Adolesc. Psychiatry* **53**:130–132. [1, 7]

Gordon, I., C. Martin, R. Feldman, and J. F. Leckman. 2011. Oxytocin and Social Motivation. *Dev. Cogn. Neurosci.* **14**:471–493. [3, 7]

Gottlieb, A. 2004. The Afterlife Is Where We Come From: The Culture of Infancy in West Africa. Chicago: Univ. of Chicago Press. [11]

Govindan, R. M., M. E. Behren, E. Helder, M. I. Makki, and H. T. Chugani. 2010. Altered Water Diffusivity in Cortical Association Tracts in Children with Early Deprivation Identified with Tract-Based Spatial Statistics (TBSS). *Cereb. Cortex* **20**:561–569. [9]

Graignic-Philippe, R., J. Dayan, S. Chokron, A.-Y. Jacquet, and S. Tordjman. 2014. Effects of Prenatal Stress on Fetal and Child Development: A Critical Literature Review. *Neurosci. Biobehav. Rev.* **43C**:137–162. [7]

Granger, B., F. Tekaia, A. M. Le Sourd, P. Rakic, and J. P. Bourgeois. 1995. Tempo of Neurogenesis and Synaptogenesis in the Primate Cingulate Mesocortex: Comparison with the Neocortex. *J. Comp. Neurol.* **360**:363–376. [9]

Grantham-McGregor, S., Y. B. Cheung, S. Cueto, et al. 2007. Developmental Potential in the First 5 Years for Children in Developing Countries. *Lancet* **369**:60–70. [16]

Grantham-McGregor, S. M., C. A. Powell, S. P. Walker, and J. H. Himes. 1991a. Nutritional Supplementation, Psychosocial Stimulation, and Mental Development of Stunted Children: The Jamaican Study. *Lancet* **338**:1–5. [13, 16]

Grantham-McGregor, S. M., S. P. Walker, S. M. Powell, and J. H. Himes. 1991b. Effects of Early Childhood Supplementation with and without Stimulation on Later Development in Stunted Jamaican Children. *Lancet* **6**:1–5. [1]

Greenberg, M. T., R. P. Weissberg, M. U. O'Brien, et al. 2003. Enhancing School-Based Prevention and Youth Development through Coordinated Social, Emotional, and Academic Learning. *Am. Psychol.* **58**:466–474. [15]

Greenough, W. T., J. E. Black, and C. S. Wallace. 1987. Experience and Brain Development. *Child Dev.* **58**:539–559. [9]

Gregor, T., and C. Robarchek. 1996. Two Paths to Peace: Semai and Mehinaku Nonviolence. In: A Natural History of Peace, ed. T. Gregor, pp. 159–188. Nashville: Vanderbilt Univ. Press. [6]

Gregory, S. G., J. J. Connelly, A. J. Towers, et al. 2009. Genomic and Epigenetic Evidence for Oxytocin Receptor Deficiency in Autism. *BMC Med.* **7**:62. [4]

Grice, H. P. 1975. Logic and Conversation. In: Syntax and Semantics: Speech Acts, ed. P. Cole and J. L. Moran, vol. 3, pp. 41–58. New York: Academic Press. [11]

————. 1989. Studies in the Way of Words. Cambridge, MA: Harvard Univ. Press. [11]

Groh, A. M., R. P. Fearon, M. J. Bakermans-Kranenburg, et al. 2014. The Significance of Attachment Security for Children's Social Competence with Peers: A Meta-Analytic Study. *Attach. Hum. Dev.* **16**:103–136. [2]

Grossmann, K. E., I. Bretherton, E. Waters, and K. Grossmann, eds. 2013. Maternal Sensitivity: Observational Studies Honouring Mary Ainsworth's 100th Year. *Attach. Hum. Dev.* **15**:443–681. [2]

Gruenewald, T., and A. Karlamangla. 2012. History of Socioeconomic Disadvantage and Allostatic Load in Later Life. *Soc. Sci. Med.* **74**:75–83. [7]

Grunberg, N. E., V. A. Maycock, and B. J. Anthony. 1985. Material Altruism in Children. *Basic Appl. Soc. Psych.* **6**:1–11. [10]

Guastella, A. J., S. L. Einfeld, K. M. Gray, et al. 2009. Intranasal Oxytocin Improves Emotion Recognition for Youth with Autism Spectrum Disorders. *Biol. Psychiatry* **67**:692–694. [3]

Gudsnuk, K., and F. A. Champagne. 2012. Epigenetic Influence of Stress and the Social Environment. *ILAR J.* **53**:279–288. [7]

Guillemin, C., N. Provencal, Sunderman, M. et al. 2014. DNA Methylation Signature of Childhood Chronic Physical Aggression in T Cells of Both Men and Women. *PLoS One* **9**:e86822 [5]

Gump, B. B., J. Reihman, P. Stewart, et al. 2007. Blood Lead (Pb) Levels: A Potential Environmental Mechanism Explaining the Relation between Socioeconomic Status and Cardiovascular Reactivity in Children. *Health Psychol.* **26**:296–304. [11]

Gunderson, G. G., and J. R. Cochrane. 2012. Religion and the Health of the Public: Shifting the Paradigm. New York: Palgrave MacMillan. [19]

Gunnar, M., and A. M. Herrera. 2013. The Development of Stress Reactivity: A Neurobiological Perspective. In: The Oxford Handbook of Developmental Psychology, ed. P. D. Zelazo, vol. 2: Self and Other, pp. 45–80. New York: Oxford Univ. Press. [14, 15]

Gunnar, M., and K. Quevedo. 2007. The Neurobiology of Stress and Development. *Annu. Rev. Psychol.* **58**:145–173. [7]

Gutkowska, J., and M. Jankowski. 2012. Oxytocin Revisited: Its Role in Cardiovascular Regulation. *J. Neuroendocrinol.* **24**:599–608. [4]

Guzman, Y. F., N. C. Tronson, V. Jovesevic, et al. 2013. Fear-Enhancing Effects of Septal Oxytocin Receptors. *Nat. Neurosci.* **16**:1185–1187. [4]

Haas, J. 1996. War. In: Encyclopedia of Cultural Anthropology, ed. D. Levinson and M. Ember, vol. 4, pp. 1357–1361. New York: Henry Holt and Company. [6]

———. 2001. Warfare and the Evolution of Culture. In: Archaeology at the Millennium: A Sourcebook, ed. G. Feinman and T. D. Price, pp. 329–350. New York: Kluwer Academic/Plenum. [6]

Haas, J., and M. Piscitelli. 2013. The Prehistory of Warfare: Misled by Ethnography. In: War, Peace, and Human Nature: Convergence of Evolutionary and Cultural Views, ed. D. P. Fry, pp. 168–190. New York: Oxford Univ. Press. [6]

Hackett, J. A., R. Sengupta, J. J. Zylic, et al. 2013. Germline DNA Demethylation Dynamics and Imprint Erasure through 5-Hydroxymethylcytosine. *Science* **339**:448–452. [5]

Hackman, D. A., M. J. Farah, and M. J. Meaney. 2010. Socioeconomic Status and the Brain: Mechanistic Insights from Human and Animal Research. *Nat. Rev. Neurosci.* **11**:651–659. [7]

Haidt, J. 2007. The New Synthesis in Moral Psychology. *Science* **316**:998–1002. [10]

———. 2012. The Righteous Mind: Why Good People Are Divided by Religion and Politics. New York: Pantheon. [6]

Hamber, B. 2009. Transforming Societies after Political Violence: Truth, Reconciliation, and Mental Health. New York: Springer. [15]

Hamilton, W. D. 1964. The Genetical Evolution of Social Behavior I–II. *J. Theor. Biol.* **7**:1–52. [7]

Hamlin, J. K., N. Mahajan, Z. Liberman, and K. Wynn. 2013. Not Like Me = Bad: Infants Prefer Those Who Harm Dissimilar Others. *Psychol. Sci.* **24**:589–594. [10]

Hamlin, J. K., K. Wynn, and P. Bloom. 2007. Social Evaluation by Preverbal Infants. *Nature* **450**:557–559. [7, 10]

Hammack, P. L. 2011. Narrative and the Politics of Identity: The Cultural Psychology of Israeli and Palestinian Youth. Oxford: Oxford Univ. Press. [17]

Hammock, E. A., and P. Levitt. 2006. The Discipline of Neurobehavioural Development: The Merging Interface of Processes That Build Circuits and Skills. *Hum. Dev.* **49**:294–309. [7]

Hammock, E. A., and L. J. Young. 2005. Microsatellite Instability Generates Diversity in Brain and Sociobehavioral Traits. *Science* **308**:1630–1634. [4]

Haque, F. N., I. I. Gottesman, and A. H. Wong. 2009. Not Really Identical: Epigenetic Differences in Monozygotic Twins and Implications for Twin Studies in Psychiatry. *Am. J. Med. Genet. C Semin. Med. Genet.* **151C**:136–141. [5]

Harkness, S., and C. M. Super. 2012. The Cultural Organization of Children's Environments. In: The Cambridge Handbook of Environment in Human Development, ed. L. C. Mayes and M. Lewis, pp. 498–516. New York: Cambridge Univ. Press. [15]

Harmon-Jones, E., P. A. Gable, and C. K. Peterson. 2010. The Role of Asymmetric Frontal Cortical Activity in Emotion-Related Phenomena: A Review and Update. *Biol. Psychol.* **84**:451–462. [10]

Harper, C., H. Alder, and P. Pereznieto. 2012. Escaping Poverty Traps: Children and Chronic Poverty. In: Child Poverty and Inequality: New Perspectives, ed. L. M. D. I. Ortiz and S. Engilbertsdottir, pp. 48–57. New York: UNICEF. [15]

Harris, A., and J. Seckl. 2011. Glucocorticoids, Prenatal Stress and the Programming of Disease. *Horm. Behav.* **59**:279–289. [5]

Hart, B., and T. R. Risley. 1995. Meaningful Differences in the Everyday Experiences of Young American Children. Baltimore: Brookes. [15]

Hart, H., and K. Rubia. 2012. Neuroimaging of Child Abuse: A Critical Review. *Front. Hum. Neurosci.* **6**:52. [12]

Hartshorne, H., and M. May. 1928. Studies in the Nature of Character. New York: Macmillian. [10]

Hasson, U., N. Yuval, I. Levy, G. Fuhrmann, and R. Malach. 2004. Intersubject Synchronization of Cortical Activity During Natural Vision. *Science* **303**:1634–1640. [7]

Hazan, C., and P. R. Shaver. 1987. Romantic Love Conceptualized as an Attachment Process. *J. Pers. Soc. Psychol.* **52**:511–524. [7]

Heard, E., and R. Martienssen. 2014. Transgenerational Epigenetic Inheritance: Myths and Mechanisms. *Cell* **157**:95–109. [7]

Heckman, J. J. 2006. Skill Formation and the Economics of Investing in Disadvantaged Children. *Science* **312**:1900–1902. [14, 15]

———. 2008. Schools, Skills and Synapses. *Econ. Inq.* **46**:289–324. [15]

———. 2009. The Case for Investing in Disadvantaged Young Children. In: Big Ideas for Children: Investing in Our Nations' Future. Washington, D.C.: First Focus. [3]

Heckman, J. J., and T. Kautz. 2013. Fostering and Measuring Skills: Interventions That Improve Character and Cognition. National Bureau of Economic Research, Working Paper 19656. http://www.nber.org/papers/w19656. (accessed April 26, 2014). [1, 3]

Heckman, J. J., and A. B. Krueger, eds. 2003. Inequality in America: What Role for Human Capital Policies? Cambridge, MA: MIT Press. [1, 3]

Heckman, J. J., and D. Masterov. 2007. The Productivity Argument for Investing in Young Children. *Rev. Agricult. Econ.* **29**:446–493. [3]

Heckman, J. J., S. H. Moon, R. Pinto, P. A. Savelyev, and A. Yavitz. 2009. The Rate of Return to the High/Scope Perry Preschool Program, IZA Discussion Paper 4533. Bonn: IZA. [15]

Heijmans, B. T., E. W. Tobi, A. D. Stein, et al. 2008. Persistent Epigenetic Differences Associated with Prenatal Exposure to Famine in Humans. *PNAS* **105**:17046–17049. [5]

Heim, C., L. J. Young, D. J. Newport, et al. 2009. Lower CSF Oxytocin Concentrations in Women with a History of Childhood Abuse. *Mol. Psychiatry* **14**:954–958. [10]

Hensch, T. K. 2005. Critical Period Plasticity in Local Cortical Circuits. *Nat. Rev. Neurosci.* **6**:877–888. [9]

Hewlett, B. S., and M. Lamb. 2005. Hunter-Gatherer Childhoods: Evolutionary, Developmental and Cultural Perspectives. New Brunswick: Aldine Transaction. [11]

Hewstone, M., and R. J. Brown. 1986. Contact Is Not Enough: An Intergroup Perspective on the Contact Hypothesis. In: Contact and Conflict in Intergroup Encounters, ed. M. Hewstone and R. Brown, pp. 1–44. Oxford: Basil Blackwell. [17]

Heydenberk, W., and R. Heydenberk. 2007. More Than Manners: Conflict Resolution in Primary Level Classrooms. *Early Child. Educ. J.* **35**:119–126. [15]

Hinde, R. A. 1987. Individuals, Relationships, and Culture. Cambridge: Cambridge Univ. Press. [2]

———. 1999. Why Gods Persist: A Scientific Approach to Religion. London: Routledge. [2]

———. 2011. Changing How We Live: Society from the Bottom Up. Nottingham: Spokesman. [1, 2, 18]

Hines, P., M. McCartney, J. Mervis, and B. Wible. 2011. Laying the Foundation for Lifetime Learning. Introduction to the Special Issue: Investing Early in Education. *Science* **333**:951. [16]

Hirst, J. J., H. K. Ralliser, D. M. Yates, T. Yawno, and D. W. Walker. 2008. Neurosteroids in the Fetus and Neonate: Potential Protective Role in Compromised Pregnancies. *Neurochem. Int.* **52**:602–610. [5]

Hiscock, H., J. K. Bayer, A. Price, et al. 2008. Universal Parenting Programme to Prevent Early Childhood Behavioural Problems: Cluster Randomised Trial. *BMJ* **336**:318–321. [16]

Ho, J. M., and J. E. Blevins. 2013. Coming Full Circle: Contributions of Central and Peripheral Oxytocin Actions to Energy Balance. *Endocrinology* **154**:589–596. [3]

Hoddinott, J. F., J. A. Maluccio, J. R. Behrman, R. Flores, and R. Martorell. 2008. Effect of a Nutrition Intervention During Early Childhood on Economic Productivity in Guatemalan Adults. *Lancet* **371**:411–416. [13, 15]

Hodgkin, R., and P. Newell. 2007. Implementation Handbook for the Convention on the Rights of the Child (3rd edition). Geneva: UNICEF. [3]

Hodgson, L. K., and E. H. Wertheim. 2007. Does Good Emotion Management Aid Forgiving? Multiple Dimensions of Empathy, Emotion Management and Forgiveness of Self and Others. *J. Soc. Pers. Relat.* **24**:931–949. [15]

Hoffman, M. L. 1975. Developmental Synthesis of Affect and Cognition and Its Implications for Altruistic Motivation. *Dev. Psychol.* **11**:607–622. [7, 15]

———. 1984. Interaction of Affect and Cognition in Empathy. In: Emotions, Cognitions and Behavior, ed. C. E. Izard et al., pp. 103–131. Cambridge: Cambridge Univ. Press. [10]

———. 2000. Empathy and Moral Development: Implications for Caring and Justice. Cambridge: Cambridge Univ. Press. [7, 10, 15]

Hong, J. S., M. J. Kral, D. L. Espelage, and P. Allen-Meares. 2012. The Social Ecology of Adolescent-Initiated Parent Abuse: A Review of the Literature. *Child Psychiatry Hum. Dev.* **43**:431–454. [12]

Honikman, S., T. S. van Heyningen, S. Field., E. Baron, and M. Tomlinson. 2012. Stepped Care for Maternal Mental Health: A Case Study of the Perinatal Mental Health Project in South Africa. *PloS Med.* **9**:e1001222. [13]

Honwana, A. M. 1997. Healing for Peace: Traditional Healers and Post-War Reconstruction in Southern Mozambique. *Peace Confl.* **3**:293–305. [15]

Horowitz, M. J. 1990. A Model of Mourning: Change in Schemas of Self and Other. *J. Am. Psychoanal. Assoc.* **38**:297–324. [12]

Hostinar, C. E., D. Cicchetti, and F. A. Rogosch. 2014. Oxytocin Receptor Gene Polymorphism, Perceived Social Support, and Psychological Symptoms in Male Treated Adolescents. *Dev. Psychopathol.* **26**:1–13. [4]

Hostinar, C. E., R. M. Sullivan, and M. R. Gunnar. 2013. Psychobiological Mechanism Underlying the Social Buffering of the Hypothalamic-Pituitary-Adrenocortical Axis: Review of Animal Models and Human Studies across Development. *Psychol. Bull.* **140**:256–282. [4]

Houweling, T. A., and A. E. Kunst. 2010. Socio-Economic Inequalities in Childhood Mortality in Low- and Middle-Income Countries: A Review of the International Evidence. *Br. Med. Bull.* **93**:7–26. [11]

Hoyt, W. T., F. D. Fincham, M. E. McCullough, G. Maio, and J. Davila. 2005. Responses to Interpersonal Transgressions in Families: Forgivingness, Forgivability, and Relationship-Specific Effects. *J. Pers. Soc. Psychol.* **89**:375–394. [12]

Hrdy, S. B. 2009. Mothers and Others: The Evolutionary Origins of Mutual Understanding. Cambridge, MA: Harvard Univ. Press. [4, 10, 11]

Huffmeijer, R., L. R. A. Alink, M. Tops, M. J. Bakermans-Kranenburg, and M. H. van IJzendoorn. 2012. Asymmetric Frontal Brain Activity and Parental Rejection Predict Altruistic Behavior: Moderation of Oxytocin Effects. *Cogn. Affect. Behav. Neurosci.* **12**:382–392. [10]

Huston, A. C. 1994. Children of Poverty: Designing Research to Affect Policy. *Soc. Policy Rep.* **8(2)**:1–12. [13]

Hutcherson, C. A., and J. J. Gross. 2011. The Moral Emotions: A Social Functionalist Account of Anger, Disgust, and Contempt. *J. Pers. Soc. Psychol.* **100**:719–737. [12]

Huttenlocher, P. R. 2009. Neural Plasticity. Cambridge, MA.: Harvard Univ. Press. [9]

Huttenlocher, P. R., and A. S. Dabholkar. 1997. Regional Differences in Synaptogenesis in Human Cerebral Cortex. *J. Comp. Neurol.* **387**:167–178. [9]

Irwin, L. G., A. Siddiqi, and C. Hertzman. 2007. Early Child Development: A Powerful Equalizer. Final Report. Geneva: World Health Organization. [13]

———. 2010. The Equalizing Power of Early Child Development: From the Commission on Social Determinants of Health to Action. *Child Health Educ.* **2**:3–18. [3]

Jacob, S., C. W. Brune, C. S. Carter, et al. 2007. Association of the Oxytocin Receptor Gene (OXTR) in Caucasian Children and Adolescents with Autism. *Neurosci. Lett.* **417**:6–9. [4]

Jaffe, J., B. Beebe, S. Feldstein, et al. 2001. Rhythms of Dialogue in Infancy: Coordinated Timing in Development. *Monogr. Soc. Res. Child Dev.* **66**:1–149. [11]

Jaffee, S. R., A. Caspi, T. E. Moffitt, et al. 2004. The Limits of Child Effects: Evidence for Genetically Mediated Child Effects on Corporal Punishment but Not on Physical Maltreatment. *Dev. Psychol.* **40**:1047–1058. [11]

James, W. 1995. The Moral Equivalent of War: Peace and Conflict (initially published in 1910). *Peace Confl.* **1**:17–26. [19]

Janoff-Bulman, R. 2006. Schema-Change Perspectives on Posttraumatic Growth. In: Handbook of Posttraumatic Growth, ed. L. G. Calhoun and R. G. Tedeschi, pp. 81–99. Mahwah, NJ: Laurence Erlbaum Associates. [12]

Jenkins Tucker, C., M. Holt, and D. Wiesen-Martin. 2013. Inter-Parental Conflict and Sibling Warmth During Adolescence: Associations with Female Depression in Emerging Adulthood. *Psychol. Reps.* **112**:243–251. [12]

Johnson, A., and T. Earle. 1987. The Evolution of Human Societies: From Foraging Group to Agrarian State. Stanford: Stanford Univ. Press. [6]

Johnson, D. W., and R. T. Johnson. 1990. Cooperative Learning. New York: Wiley-Blackwell Publishing. [15]

———. 1996. Conflict Resolution and Peer Mediation Programs in Elementary and Secondary Schools. *Rev. Educ. Res.* **66**:459–506. [17]

Johnson, S. B., A. W. Riley, D. A. Granger, and J. Riis. 2013. The Science of Early Life Toxic Stress for Pediatric Practice and Advocacy. *Pediatrics* **131**:319–327. [7]

Jolly, R. 2007. Early Childhood Development: The Global Challenge. *Lancet* **369**:8–9. [13]

Jordan, J. J., D. G. Rand, S. Arbesman, J. H. Fowler, and N. A. Christakis. 2013. Contagion of Cooperation in Static and Fluid Social Networks. *PLoS One* **8**:e66199. [1]

Jordans, M. J. D., W. A. Tol, I. H. Komproe, and J. V. T. M. de Jong. 2009. Systematic Review of Evidence and Treatment Approaches: Psychosocial and Mental Health Care for Children in War. *Child Adolesc. Ment. Health* **14**:2–14. [12]

Jost, J. T., B. W. Pelham, and M. R. Carvallo. 2002. Non-Conscious Forms of System Justification: Implicit and Behavioral Preferences for Higher Status Groups. *J. Exp. Soc. Psychol.* **38**:586–602. [15]

Judge, P. G. 2003. Conflict Resolution. In: Primate Psychology, ed. D. Maestripieri, pp. 41–68. Cambridge, MA: Harvard Univ. Press. [8]

Judt, T. 2010. Ill Fares the Land. London: Penguin Books and Allan Lane. [13]

Kabeer, N. 2010. Can the Mdgs Provide a Pathway to Social Justice? The Challenge of Intersecting Inequalities. New York: UNDP. [15]

Kagan, J., and S. Lamb. 1990. The Emergence of Morality in Young Children. Chicago: Univ. of Chicago Press. [10]

Kagan, S., and M. Madsen. 1971. Cooperation and Competition of Mexican, Mexican-American, and Anglo-American Children of Two Ages under Four Instruction Sets. *Dev. Psychol.* **5**:32–39. [6]

Kagitcibasi, C. 2007. Family, Self, and Human Development across Cultures. Mahwah, NJ: Erlbaum. [16]

Kagitcibasi, C., D. Sunar, and S. Bekman. 2001. Long-Term Effects of Early Intervention: Turkish Low-Income Mothers and Children. *J. Appl. Dev. Psychol.* **22**:333–361. [1, 3, 16]

Kagitcibasi, C., D. Sunar, S. Bekman, N. Baydar, and Z. Cemalcilar. 2009. Continuing Effects of Early Intervention in Adult Life: The Turkish Early Enrichment Project 22 Years Later. *J. Appl. Dev. Psychol.* **30**:764–779. [1, 13, 15, 16]

Kaldor, M. 2013. In Defence of New Wars. *Stability: Intl. J. Security Dev.* **2**:4. [18]

Kallgren, C. A., R. R. Reno, and R. B. Cialdini. 2000. A Focus Theory of Normative Conduct: When Norms Do and Do Not Affect Behavior. *Pers. Soc. Psychol. Bull.* **26**:1002–1012. [10]

Kaminski, J. W., L. A. Walle, J. H. Filene, and C. L. Boyle. 2008. A Meta-Analytic Review of Components Associated with Parent Training Program Effectiveness. *J. Abnorm. Child Psychol.* **364**:567–589. [3]

Kang, D. H., H. J. Jo, W. H. Jung, et al. 2013. The Effect of Meditation on Brain Structure: Cortical Thickness Mapping and Diffusion Tensor Imaging. *Soc. Cogn. Affect. Neurosci.* **8**:27–33. [10]

Kang, H. J., Y. I. Kawasawa, F. Cheng, et al. 2011. Spatio-Temporal Transcriptome of the Human Brain. *Nature* **478**:483–489. [1]

Kaplan, H. S., and S. W. Gangestad. 2005. Life History Theory and Evolutionary Psychology. In: Handbook of Evolutionary Psychology, ed. D. M. Buss, pp. 68–95. New York: Wiley. [8]

Karatsoreos, I. N., and B. S. McEwen. 2013. The Neurobiology and Physiology of Resilience and Adaptation across the Life Course. *J. Child Psychol. Psychiatry* **54**:337–347. [1, 14]

Kawachi, I., N. E. Adler, and W. H. Dow. 2010. Money, Schooling, and Health: Mechanisms and Causal Evidence. *Ann. NY Acad. Sci.* **1186**:56–68. [11]

Kazdin, A. 2014. Special Series Introduction: Reenvisioniong Clinical Science Training. *Clin. Psychol. Sci.* **2**:6–7. [11]

Keen, D. 2012. Useful Enemies: When Waging War Is More Important Than Winning Them. New Haven: Yale Univ. Press. [18]

Keller, H. 2003. Socialization for Competence: Cultural Models of Infancy. *Hum. Dev.* **46**:288–311. [11]

———. 2007. Cultures of Infancy. Mahwah, NJ: Erlbaum. [11]

Keller, H., H. Otto, B. Lamm, R. D. Yovsi, and J. Kaertner. 2008. The Timing of Verbal/Vocal Communications between Mothers and Their Infants: A Longitudinal Cross-Cultural Comparison. *Infant Behav. Dev.* **31**:217–226. [11]

Kellermann, N. P. F. 2001. The Long-Term Psychological Effects and Treatment of Holocaust Trauma. *J. Loss Trauma* **6**:197–218. [12]

Kelly, D. J., P. C. Quinn, A. M. Slater, et al. 2005. Three-Month-Olds, but Not Newborns, Prefer Own-Race Faces. *Dev. Sci.* **8**:F31–F36. [15]

Kelly, R. C. 2000. Warless Societies and the Origin of War. Ann Arbor: Univ. of Michigan Press. [6]

Kelly, R. L. 1995. The Foraging Spectrum: Diversity in Hunter-Gatherer Lifeways. Washington, D.C.: Smithsonian Institution Press. [6]

Kelman, H. C. 1981. Reflections on the History and Status of Peace Research. *Confl. Manag. Peace Sci.* **5**:95–110. [15]

———. 1999. The Interdependence of Israeli and Palestinian National Identities: The Role of the Other in Existential Conflicts. *J. Soc. Iss.* **55**:581–600. [15]

Kelman, H. C., and S. Cohen. 1976. The Problem-Solving Workshop: A Social Psychological Contribution to the Resolution of Conflict. *J. Peace Res.* **8**:79–90. [17]

Kelman, H. C., and R. J. Fisher. 2003. Conflict Analysis and Resolution. In: Oxford Handbook of Political Psychology, ed. D. O. Sears et al., pp. 315–353. Oxford: Oxford Univ. Press. [17]

Kenkel, W., J. Paredes, J. R. Yee, et al. 2012a. Exposure to an Infant Releases Oxytocin and Facilitates Pair-Bonding in Male Prairie Voles. *J. Neuroendocrinol.* **24**:874–886. [4]

———. 2012b. Neuroendocrine and Behavioural Responses to Exposure to an Infant in Male Prairie Voles. *J. Neuroendocrinol.* **24**:874–886. [7]

Kenkel, W. M., J. Paredes, G. F. Lewis, et al. 2013. Autonomic Substrates of the Response to Pups in Male Prairie Voles. *PLoS One* **8**:e69965. [4, 7]

Kenkel, W. M., J. R. Yee, and C. S. Carter. 2014. Is Oxytocin a Maternal-Fetal Signaling Molecule at Birth? Implications for Development. *J. Neuroendocrinol.*, in press. [4]

Kent, G. 2006. Children as Victims of Structural Violence. *Societies Without Borders* **1**:53–67. [13]

Kessler, R. C., K. A. McLaughlin, J. G. Green, et al. 2010. Childhood Adversities and Adult Psychopathology in the WHO World Mental Health Surveys. *Br. J. Psychiatry* **197**:378–385. [1]

Keverne, E. B. 2006. Trophoblast Regulation of Maternal Endocrine Function and Behaviour. In: Biology and Pathology of Trophoblast, ed. A. Moffett et al., pp. 148–163. New York: Cambridge Univ. Press. [5]

———. 2007. Genomic Imprinting and the Evolution of Sex Differences in Mammalian Reproductive Strategy. In: Genetics of Sexual Differentiation and Sexually Dimorphic Behaviors, ed. D. Yamamoto, pp. 217–243. New York: Academic Press. [5]

———. 2014. Significance of Epigenetics for Understanding Brain Development, Brain Evolution and Behaviour. *Neuroscience* **264**:207–217. [5, 7]

Khan, Y., and Z. A. Bhutta. 2010. Nutritional Deficiencies in the Developing World: Current Status and Opportunities for Intervention. *Pediatr. Clin. North Am.* **57**:1409–1441. [11]

Khazipov, R., R. Tyzio, and Y. Ben-Ari. 2008. Effects of Oxytocin on GABA Signalling in the Foetal Brain During Delivery. *Prog. Brain Res.* **170**:243–257. [4]

Killen, M., and A. Rutland. 2011. Children and Social Exclusion: Morality, Prejudice, and Group Identity. New York: Wiley-Blackwell. [15]

Killen, M., and E. Turiel. 1991. Conflict Resolution in Preschool Social Interactions. *Early Educ. Dev.* **2**:240–255. [7]

Kim, J. 2006. Emergence: Core Ideas and Issues. *Synthese* **151**:347–354. [3]

Kim, P., G. Evans, M. Angstadt, et al. 2013. Effects of Childhood Poverty and Chronic Stress on Emotion Regulatory Brain Function in Adulthood. *PNAS* **100**:18442–18447. [7]

Kim, P., R. Feldman, L. C. Mayes, et al. 2011. Breastfeeding, Brain Activation to Own Infant Cry, and Maternal Sensitivity. *J. Child Psychol. Psychiatry* **528**:907–915. [3]

Kirpal, S. 2002. Communities Can Make a Difference: Five Cases across Continents. In: From Early Child Development to Human Development: Investing in Our Children's Future, ed. M. E. Young, p. 293–362. Washington, D.C.: World Bank. [16]

Knafo, A., S. Israel, and R. P. Ebstein. 2011. Heritability of Children's Prosocial Behavior and Differential Susceptibility to Parenting by Variation in the Dopamine Receptor D4 Gene. *Dev. Psychopathol.* **23**:53–67. [10]

Knafo, A., C. Zahn-Waxler, M. Davidov, et al. 2009. Empathy in Early Childhood: Genetic, Environmental and Affective Contributions. Values, Empathy and Fairness across Social Borders. *Ann. NY Acad. Sci.* **1167**:103–114. [16]

Knafo, A., C. Zahn-Waxler, C. Van Hulle, J. L. Robinson, and S. H. Rhee. 2008. The Developmental Origins of a Disposition toward Empathy: Genetic and Environmental Contributions. *Emotion* **8**:737–752. [10]

Knauft, B. 1991. Violence and Sociality in Human Evolution. *Curr. Anthropol.* **32**:391–428. [6]

Knight, S. R., C. Davidson, A. M. Young, and C. L. Gibson. 2012. Allopregnanolone Protects against Dopamine-Induced Striatal Damage after *in Vitro* Ischaemia Via Interaction at GABA A Receptors. *J. Neuroendocrinol.* **24**:1135–1143. [5]

Knudsen, E. I. 2004. Sensitive Periods in the Development of the Brain and Behavior. *J. Cogn. Neurosci.* **16**:1412–1425. [9]

Knudsen, E. I., J. J. Heckman, J. L. Cameron, and J. P. Shonkoff. 2006. Economic, Neurobiological, and Behavioral Perspectives on Building America's Future Workforce. *PNAS* **103**:10155–10162. [7]

Koçak, A., and S. Bekman. 2004. Mothers Speaking: A Study on the Experience of Mothers within the Mother-Child Education Programme (MOCEP). *Eur. Early Childhood Educ. Res. J.* **12**:115–129. [3]

Koch, H., K. McCormack, M. M. Sanchez, and D. Maestripieri. 2014. The Development of the Hypothalamic-Pituitary-Adrenal Axis in Rhesus Monkeys: Effects of Age, Sex, and Early Experience. *Dev. Psychobiol.* **56**:86–95. [8]

Kochanska, G., N. Aksan, and M. E. Joy. 2007. Children's Fearfulness as a Moderator of Parenting in Early Socialization: Two Longitudinal Studies. *Dev. Psychol.* **43**:222–237. [10]

Kochanska, G., N. Aksan, and A. L. Koenig. 1995. A Longitudinal Study of the Roots of Preschoolers' Conscience: Committed Compliance and Emerging Internalization. *Child Dev.* **66**:1752–1769. [10]

Kochanska, G., K. Murray, and K. C. Coy. 1997. Inhibitory Control as a Contributor to Conscience in Childhood: From Toddler to Early School Age. *Child Dev.* **68**:263–277. [16]

Koenig, A. L., D. Cicchetti, and F. A. Rogosch. 2004. Moral Development: The Association between Maltreatment and Young Children's Prosocial Behaviors and Moral Transgressions. *Soc. Dev.* **13**:87–106. [10]

Kohlberg, L. 1984. The Psychology of Moral Development, vol. 2: Essays on Moral Development. San Franscisco: Harper and Row. [10]

———. 1985. Resolving Moral Conflicts within the Just Community. In: Moral Dilemmas, ed. C. Harding, pp. 71–98. Chicago: Precedent Publishing. [10]

Kohli, R. M., and Y. Zhang. 2013. TET Enzymes, TDG and the Dynamics of DNA Demethylation. *Nature* **502**:472–479. [7]

Kohn, A. 1986. No Contest: The Case against Competition. New York: Houghton Mifflin. [6]

Kolassa, I.-T., V. Ertl, C. Eckart, et al. 2010a. Association Study of Trauma Load and Slc6a4 Promoter Polymorphism in PTSD: Evidence from Survivors of the Rwandan Genocide. *J. Clin. Psychiatry* **71**:543–547. [7]

Kolassa, I.-T., S. Kolassa, V. Ertl, A. Papassotiropoulos, and D. J.-F. De Quervain. 2010b. The Risk of Posttraumatic Stress Disorder after Trauma Depends on Traumatic Load and the Catechol-O-Methyltransferase Val(158)Met Polymorphism. *Biol. Psychiatry* **67**:304–308. [7]

Konner, M. 2006. Human Nature, Ethnic Violence, and War. In: The Psychology of Resolving Global Conflicts: From War to Peace, Nature Versus Nurture, ed. M. Fitzduff and C. Stout, vol. 1, pp. 1–39. Westport, CT: Praeger Security Intl. [6]

Kordi-Tamandani, D. M., R. Sahranavard, and A. Torkamanzehi. 2013. Analysis of Association between Dopamine Receptor Genes' Methylation and Their Expression Profile with the Risk of Schizophrenia. *Psychiatr. Genet.* **23**:183–187. [5]

Kostelny, K., and J. Garbarino. 2001. The War Close to Home: Children and Violence in the United States. In: Peace, Conflict, and Violence: Peace Psychology in the 21st Century, ed. D. J. Christie et al., pp. 110–120. New York: Prentice-Hall. [13]

Kosterman, R., and S. Feshbach. 1989. Toward a Measure of Patriotic and Nationalistic Attitudes. *Polit. Psychol.* **10**:257–274. [15]

Kriesberg, L. 1998. Constructive Conflict: From Escalation to Resolution. Lanham, MD: Rowman and Littlefield. [17]

Kuczynski, L. 2003. Beyond Bidirectionality: Bilateral Conceptual Frameworks for Understanding Dynamics in Parent-Child Relations. In: Handbook of Dynamics in Parent-Child Relations, ed. L. Kuczynski, pp. 3–24. London: Sage Publications. [2]

Kuczynski, L., and J. De Mol. 2015. Dialectical Models of Socialization. In: Theory and Method, vol. 1 of the Handbook of Child Psychology and Developmental Science, (7th ed.), ed. W. F. Overton and P. C. M. Molenaar. Hoboken, NJ: Wiley, in press. [2]

Kumar, A., M. E. Behen, P. Singsoonsud, et al. 2014. Microstructural Abnormalities in Language and Limbic Pathways in Orphanage-Reared Children: A Diffusion Tensor Imagining Study. *J. Child Neurol.* **29**:318–325. [5]

Kumsta, R., E. Hummel, F. S. Chen, and M. Heinrichs. 2013. Epigenetic Regulation of the Oxytocin Receptor Gene: Implications for Behavioral Neuroscience. *Front. Neurosci.* **7**:Article 83. [3, 4, 7]

Labonté, B. 2012. Genome-Wide Epigenetic Regulation by Early-Life Trauma. *Arch. Gen. Psychiatry* **69**:722–731. [7]

Labonté, B., M. Suderman, G. Maussion, et al. 2012. Genome-Wide Epigenetic Regulation by Early-Life Trauma. *Arch. Gen. Psychiatry* **697**:722–731. [3]

———. 2013. Genome-Wide Methylation Changes in the Brains of Suicide Completers. *Am. J. Psychiatry* **170**:511–520. [1]

Lacroix, L., C. Rousseau, M.-F. Gauthier, et al. 2007. Immigrant and Refugee Preschoolers' Sandplay Representations of the Tsunami. *Arts in Psychotherapy* **34**:99–113. [15]

La Greca, A. M., W. K. Silverman, B. Lai, and J. Jaccard. 2010. Hurricane-Related Exposure Experiences and Stressors, Other Life Events, and Social Support: Concurrent and Prospective Impact on Children's Persistent Posttraumatic Stress Symptoms. *J. Consult. Clin. Psychol.* **78**:794–805. [14]

Lamb, S., and B. Zakhireh. 1997. Toddlers' Attention to the Distress of Peers in a Daycare Setting. *Early Educ. Dev.* **8**:105–118. [10]

Lamm, B. 2008. Children's Ideas About Infant Care: A Comparison of Rural Nso Children from Cameroon and German Middle Class Children. Doctoral Thesis. Osnabrück University: School of Human Sciences, Department of Culture and Psychology. [11]

Langer, A., F. Stewart, and R. Venugopal, eds. 2012. Horizontal Inequalities and Post-Conflict Development. London: Palgrave Macmillan. [1]

Lansford, J. E., L. Chang, K. A. Dodge, et al. 2005. Physical Discipline and Children's Adjustment: Cultural Normativeness as a Moderator. *Child Dev.* **76**:1234–1246. [11]

Lansford, J. E., and K. Deater-Deckard. 2012. Childrearing Discipline and Violence in Developing Countries. *Child Dev.* **83**:62–75. [3, 14]

Lawlor, D. A., J. A. Sterne, P. Tynelius, G. Davey Smith, and F. Rasmussen. 2006. Association of Childhood Socioeconomic Position with Cause-Specific Mortality in a Prospective Record Linkage Study of 1,839,384 Individuals. *Am. J. Epidemiol.* **164**:907–915. [11]

Lazar, I., and R. B. Darlington. 1982. Lasting Effects of Early Education. *Monogr. Soc. Res. Child Dev.* **47**:1–151. [16]

Leavitt, G. 1977. The Frequency of Warfare: An Evolutionary Perspective. *Sociological Inquiry* **47**:49–58. [6]

Leavitt, K. S., S. A. Gardner, M. M. Gallagher, and G. Schamess. 1998. Severly Traumatized Siblings: A Treatment Strategy. *Clin. Soc. Work J.* **26**:55–71. [12]

Lederach, J. P. 1995. Preparing for Peace: Conflict Transformation across Cultures. Syracuse: Syracuse Univ. Press. [17]

———. 1997. Building Peace: Sustainable Reconciliation in Divided Societies. Washington, D.C.: U.S. Institute of Peace. [17]

————. 1999. Justpeace: The Challenge of the 21st Century. In: People Building Peace. 35 Inspiring Stories from around the World. Utrecht: European Center for Conflict Prevention. [15]

Lee, J. H., and C. F. Cole. 2009. Creating Global Citizens: The Panwapa Project. *Comm. Res. Trends* **28**:25–30. [1, 18]

Lee, R., and I. DeVore. 1968. Problems in the Study of Hunters and Gatherers. In: Man the Hunter, ed. R. Lee and I. DeVore, pp. 3–12. Chicago: Aldine. [6]

Lee, R., C. Ferris, L. D. V. d. Kar, and E. F. Coccaro. 2009. Cerebrospinal Fluid Oxytocin, Life History of Aggression and Personality Diorder. *Psychoneuroendocrinology* **34**:1567–1573. [4]

Leeb, R. T., T. Lewis, and A. J. Zolotor. 2009. A Review of Physical and Mental Health Consequences of Child Abuse and Neglect and Implications for Practice. *Am. J. Lifestyle Med.* **5**:454–468. [12]

Lemish, D., and M. Götz, eds. 2007. Children and Media in Times of War and Conflict. Newark: Hampton Press. [18]

Lengua, L. J., A. C. Long, K. I. Smith, and A. N. Meltzoff. 2005. Pre-Attack Symptomatology and Temperament as Predictors of Children's Responses to the September 11 Terrorist Attacks. *J. Child Psychol. Psychiatry* **46**:631–645. [12]

Leon, D. A., and G. Walt. 2001. Poverty, Inequality, and Health: An International Perspective. Oxford: Oxford Univ. Press. [15]

Lerner, M. J., and D. T. Miller. 1977. Just World Research and the Attribution Process: Looking Back and Ahead. *Psychol. Bull.* **85**:1030–1051. [13]

LeRoux, I., M. Tomlinson, N. Mbewu, et al. 2013. Outcomes of Home Visits for Pregnant Township Mothers and Their Infants in South Africa: A Cluster Randomised Controlled Trial. *AIDS* **27**:1461–1471. [15]

Leung, K., P. T. Koch, and L. Lu. 2002. A Dualistic Model of Harmony and Its Implications for Conflict Management in Asia. *Asia Pacific J. Manag.* **19**:201–220. [15]

LeVine, R. 1990. Enculturation: A Biosocial Perspective on the Development of Self. In: The Self in Transition: Infancy to Early Childhood, ed. D. Chicchetti and M. Beeghly, pp. 97–113. Chicago: Univ. of Chicago Press. [15]

LeVine, R. A., S. Dixon, S. LeVine, et al. 1996. Child Care and Culture: Lessons from Africa. Cambridge: Cambridge Univ. Press. [11]

Levy, S. 2006. Progress against Poverty: Sustaining Mexico's Progresa-Oportunidades Program. Washington, D.C.: Brookings Institution. [15]

Lewin, K. 1943. Defining the "Field at a Given Time". *Psychol. Rev.* **50**:292–310. [3]

————. 1951. Field Theory in Social Science. New York: Harper. [7, 15]

Lewis, M., C. Stranger, and M. W. Sullivan. 1989. Deception in 3-Year-Olds. *Dev. Psychol.* **25**:439–443. [10]

Lieberman, A. F. 2007. Ghosts and Angels: Intergenerational Patterns in the Transmission and Treatment of the Traumatic Sequelae of Domestic Violence. *Infant Ment. Health J.* **28**:422–439. [11]

Lieberman, A. F., E. Padrón, P. Van Horn, and W. W. Harris. 2005. Angels in the Nursery: The Intergenerational Transmission of Benevolent Parental Influences. *Infant Ment. Health J.* **26**:504–520. [11]

Lieberman, A. F., and P. Van Horn. 2011a. Child-Parent Psychotherapy: A Developmental Approach to Mental Health Treatment in Infancy and Early Childhood. In: Handbook of Infant Mental Health (3rd edition), ed. C. H. Zeanah, pp. 439–449. New York: Guilford Press. [14]

————. 2011b. Psychotherapy with Infants and Young Children: Repairing the Effects of Stress and Trauma on Early Attachment. New York: Guilford Press. [11]

Liu, J. 2011. Early Health Risk Factors for Violence: Conceptualisation, Evidence, and Implications. *Aggress. Violent Behav.* **16**:63–73. [15]

Liu, J., A. Raine, P. Venables, and S. A. Mednick. 2004. Malnutrition at Age 3 Years Predisposes to Externalizing Behavior Problems at Ages 8, 11 and 17 Years. *Am. J. Psychiatry* **161**:2005–2013. [13, 15]

Liu, J. H., and D. Paez. 2012. National Political Cultures. Encyclopedia of Peace Psychology, ed. D. J. Christie, pp. 691–695. New York: Wiley-Blackwell. [15]

Loeber, R., and D. P. Farrington, eds. 1998. Serious and Violence Juvenile Offenders: Risk Factors and Successful Interventions. Thousand Oaks, CA: Sage Publications. [14]

———. 2012. From Juvenile Delinquency to Adult Crime: Criminal Careers, Justice Policy, and Prevention. New York: Oxford Univ. Press. [14]

Lorenz, K. 1966. On Aggression. New York: Harcourt, Brace and World. [8, 17]

Lösel, F., and D. P. Farrington. 2012. Direct Protective and Buffering Protective Factors in the Development of Youth Violence. *Am. J. Prev. Med.* **43**:S8–S23. [14]

Love, J., E. E. Kisker, C. Ross, et al. 2005. The Effectiveness of Early Head Start for 3-Year-Old Children and Their Parents: Lessons for Policy and Programs. *Dev. Psychol.* **41**:885–901. [3, 16]

Luby, J. L., D. M. Barch, A. Belden, et al. 2012. Maternal Support in Early Childhood Predicts Larger Hippocampal Volumes at School Age. *PNAS* **109**:2854–2859. [7]

Lundberg, M., and A. Wuermli, eds. 2012. Children and Youth in Crisis: Protecting and Promoting Human Development in Times of Economic Shocks. Washington, D.C.: The World Bank. [14]

Luthar, S. S., D. Cicchetti, and B. Becker. 2000. The construct of resilience: A critical evaluation and guidelines for future work: *Child Dev.* **71**:543–562. [14]

Maccani, M. A., and V. S. Knopik. 2012. Cigarette Smoke Exposure-Associated Alternations to Non-Coding RNA. *Front. Genet.* **3**:53. [5]

Maccio, A., C. Madeddu, P. Chessa, et al. 2010. Oxytocin Both Increases Proliferative Response of Peripheral Blood Lymphomonocytes to Phytohemagglutinin and Reverses Immunosuppressive Estrogen Activity. *In Vivo* **24**:157–163. [3]

MacDonald, K., and D. Feifel. 2013. Helping Oxytocin Deliver: Considerations in the Development of Oxytocin-Based Therapeutics for Brain Development. *Front. Neurosci.* **7**:35. [4]

MacNair, R. 2003. The Psychology of Peace: An Introduction. Westport, CT: Praeger. [3]

Maestripieri, D. 2005a. Early Experience Affects the Intergenerational Transmission of Infant Abuse in Rhesus Monkeys. *PNAS* **102**:9726–9729. [8, 11]

———. 2005b. Effects of Early Experience on Female Behavioural and Reproductive Development in Rhesus Macaques. *Proc. Roy. Soc. Lond. B* **272**:1243–1248. [8]

Maestripieri, D., and K. A. Carroll. 1998. Risk Factors for Infant Abuse and Neglect in Group-Living Rhesus Monkeys. *Psychol. Sci.* **9**:143–145. [8]

Maestripieri, D., J. D. Higley, S. G. Lindell, et al. 2006. Early Maternal Rejection Affects the Development of Monoaminergic Systems and Adult Abusive Parenting in Rhesus Macaques. *Behav. Neurosci.* **120**:1017–1024. [8]

Maestripieri, D., J. R. Roney, N. DeBias, K. M. Durante, and G. M. Spaepen. 2004. Father Absence, Menarche, and Interest in Infants among Adolescent Girls. *Dev. Sci.* **7**:560–566. [8]

Maestripieri, D., K. Wallen, and K. A. Carroll. 1997. Infant Abuse Runs in Families of Group-Living Pigtail Macaques. *Child Abuse Negl.* **21**:465–471. [8]

Maguire, E. A., D. G. Gadian, I. S. Johnsrude, et al. 2000. Navigation-Related Structural Change in the Hippocampi of Taxi Drivers. *PNAS* **97**:44398–44403. [10]

Mah, B. L., M. J. Bakermans-Kranenburg, M. H. Van IJzendoorn, and R. Smith. 2014. Oxytocin Promotes Protective Behavior in Depressed Mothers: A Pilot Study with the Enthusiastic Stranger Paradigm. *Depress. Anxiety* doi: 10.1002/da.22245 (Epub ahead of print). [7]

Main, M., E. Hesse, and R. Goldwyn. 2008. Studying Differences in Language Usage in Recounting Attachment History: An Introduction to the AAI. In: Clinical Applications of the Adult Attachment Interview, ed. H. Steele and M. Steele, pp. 31–68. New York: Guilford Press. [11]

Main, M., N. Kaplan, and J. Cassidy. 1985. Security in Infancy, Childhood, and Adulthood: A Move to the Level of Representation. *Monogr. Soc. Res. Child Dev.* **50**:66–104. [11]

Malinowski, B. 1941. An Anthropological Analysis of War. *Am. J. Sociol.* **46**:521–550. [6]

Maluccio, J. A., J. Hoddinott, J. R. Behrman, et al. 2009. The Impact of Improving Nutrition During Early Childhood on Education among Guatemalan Adults. *Econ. J.* **119**:734–763. [15]

Maoz, I. 2004. Coexistence Is in the Eye of the Beholder: Evaluating Intergroup Encounter Interventions between Jews and Arab in Israel. *J. Soc. Iss.* **60**:403–418. [17]

Marais, H. 2001. South Africa: Limits to Change: The Political Economy of Transition. New York: Palgrave Macmillan. [15]

Marlowe, F. 2010. The Hadza Hunter-Gatherers of Tanzania. Berkeley: Univ. of California Press. [6]

Marshall, P. J., Y. Bar-Haim, and N. A. Fox. 2002. Development of the EEG from 5 Months to 4 Years of Age. *Clin. Neurophysiol.* **113**:1199–1208. [9]

Marshall, P. J., N. A. Fox, and the Bucharest Early Intervention Project Core Group. 2004. A Comparison of the Electroencephalogram between Institutionalized and Community Children in Romania. *J. Cogn. Neurosci.* **16**:1327–1338. [9]

Marshall, P. J., B. J. Reeb, N. A. Fox, C. A. Nelson, and C. H. Zeanah. 2008. Effects of Early Intervention on EEG Power and Coherence in Previously Institutionalized Children in Romania. *Dev. Psychopathol.* **20**:861–880. [9, 10]

Martin, W. L., and C. S. Carter. 2013. Oxytocin and Vasopressin Are Sequestered in Plasma. In: 10th World Congress of Neurohypophyseal Hormones Abstracts. www.vasopressin.org. (accessed April 6, 2014). [4]

Mascaro, O., and G. Csibra. 2014. Human Infants' Learning of Social Structures: The Case of Dominance Hierarchy. *Psychol. Sci.* **25**:250–255. [7]

Masten, A. S. 2001. Ordinary magic: Resilience processes in development. *Am. Psychol.* **56**:227–238. [14]

———. 2007. Resilience in Developing Systems: Progress and Promise as the Fourth Wave Rises. *Dev. Psychopathol.* **19**: 921-930. [14]

———. 2011. Resilience in Children Threatened by Extreme Adversity: Frameworks for Research, Practice, and Translational Synergy. *Dev. Psychopathol.* **23**:493–506. [12, 14, 15]

———. 2013. Risk and Resilience in Development. In: The Oxford Handbook of Developmental Psychology, vol. 2, Self and Other, ed. P. D. Zelazo, pp. 579–608. New York: Oxford Univ. Press. [14]

———. 2014a. Global Perspectives on Resilience in Children and Youth. *Child Dev.* **85**:6–20. [14]

——— 2014b. Ordinary Magic: Resilience in Development. New York: Guilford Press. [14]

Masten, A. S., and D. Cicchetti. 2010. Developmental Cascades. *Dev. Psychopathol.* **22**:491–495. [14, 15]

Masten, A. S., J. D. Long, S. I.-C. Kuo, C. M. McCormick, and C. D. Desjardins. 2009. Developmental Models of Strategic Intervention. *Intl. J. Dev. Sci.* **3**:282–291. [14]

Masten, A. S., and A. R. Monn, A. R. 2014. Resilience in Children and Families: A Call for Integrating Science, Practice, and Training. *Fam. Relat.*, in press. [14]

Masten, A. S., and A. J. Narayan. 2012. Child Development in the Context of Disaster, War, and Terrorism: Pathways of Risk and Resilience. *Annu. Rev. Psychol.* **63**:227–257. [12, 14, 15]

Masten, A. S., A. J. Narayan, W. K. Silverman, and J. D. Osofsky. 2014. Children in War and Disaster. In: Handbook of Child Psychology and Developmental Science (7th edition), vol. 4, Ecological Settings and Processes in Developmental Systems, ed. R. M. Lerner et al., pp. 1288–1369. Hoboken, NJ: Wiley. [14]

Masten, A. S., and A. Tellegen, A. 2012. Resilience in Developmental Psychopathology: Contributions of the Project Competence Longitudinal Study. *Dev. Psychopathol.* **24**:345–361. [14]

Masten, C. L., N. I. Eisenberger, J. H. Pfeifer, and M. Dapretto. 2010. Witnessing Peer Rejection During Early Adolescence: Neural Correlates of Empathy for Experiences of Social Exclusion. *Soc. Neurosci.* **5**:496–507. [10]

Masten, C. L., A. E. Guyer, H. B. Hodgdon, et al. 2008. Recognition of Facial Emotions among Maltreated Children with High Rates of Post-Traumatic Stress Disorder. *Child Abuse Negl.* **32**:139–153. [12]

Masten, C. L., S. A. Morelli, and N. I. Eisenberger. 2011. An fMRI Investigation of Empathy for "Social Pain" and Subsequent Prosocial Behavior. *Neuroimage* **55**:381–388. [10]

Matthews, S. G., and D. I. Phillips. 2012. Transgenerational Inheritance of Stress Pathology. *Exp. Neurol.* **233**:95–101. [7]

Maughan, A., and D. Cicchetti. 2002. Impact on Child Maltreatment and Interadult Violence on Children's Emotion Regulation Abilities and Socioemotional Adjustment. *Child Dev.* **73**:1525–1542. [12]

Maurer, D., T. L. Lewis, H. P. Brent, and A. V. Levin. 1999. Rapid Improvement in the Acuity of Infants after Visual Input. *Science* **286**:108–110. [9]

Maxwell, J. 2007. Mediation in the Schools: Self-Regulation, Self-Esteem, and Self-Discipline. *Confl. Res. Q.* **7**:149–155. [17]

McCarthy, J. F., C. A. Scheraga, and D. E. Gibson. 2010. Culture, Cognition and Conflict: How Neuroscience Can Help to Explain Cultural Differences in Negotiation and Conflict Management. In: Neuroeconomics and the Firm, ed. A. A. Stanton et al., pp. 263–288. Cheltenham: Edward Elgar. [17]

McCartney, K., and D. A. Phillips, eds. 2006. Handbook of Early Childhood Development. Oxford: Blackwell Publishing. [3, 19]

McCormick, M. C., J. Brooks-Gunn, S. L. Buka, et al. 2006. Early Intervention in Low Birth Weight Premature Infants: Results at 18 Years of Age for the Infant Health and Development Program. *Pediatrics* **117**:771–780. [16]

McCormick, C. M., S. I-C. Kuo, and A. S. Masten. 2011. Developmental Tasks across the Lifespan. In: Handbook of Lifespan Development, ed. K. L. Fingerman, C. A. Berg, J. Smith, and T. C. Antonucci, pp. 117–140. New York: Springer. [14]

McCullough, M. E., E. J. Pedersen, J. M. Schroder, B. A. Tabak, and C. S. Carver. 2013. Harsh Childhood Environmental Characteristics Predict Exploitation and Retaliation in Humans. *Proc. Biol. Sci.* **280**:20122104. [11]

McCullough, M. E., K. C. Rachal, S. J. Sandage, et al. 1998. Interpersonal Forgiving in Close Relationships: II. Theoretical Elaboration and Measurement. *J. Pers. Soc. Psychol.* **75**:1586–1603. [15]

McEwen, B. S. 2012. Brain on Stress: How the Social Environment Gets under the Skin. *PNAS* **109**:17180–17185. [7, 13]

McGee, R. A., D. A. Wolfe, S. A. Yuen, S. K. Wilson, and J. Carnochan. 1995. The Measurement of Maltreatment: A Comparison of Approaches. *Child Abuse Negl.* **19**:233–249. [11]

McGowan, P. O., A. Sasaki, A. D'Alessio, et al. 2009. Epigenetic Regulation of the Glucocorticoid Receptor in Human Brain Associates with Childhood Abuse. *Nat. Neurosci.* **12**:342–348. [7, 10]

McGuinness, D., L. M. McGlynn, P. C. Johnson, et al. 2012. Socio-Economic Status Is Associated with Epigenetic Differences in the pSoBid Cohort. *Intl. J. Epidem.* **41**:151–160. [7]

McKown, C., and R. S. Weinstein. 2003. The Development and Consequences of Stereotype Consciousness in Middle Childhood. *Child Dev.* **74**:498–515. [7]

McLennan, D., and M. Pecaski. 2012. Using Sociodrama to Help Young Children Problem Solve. *Early Childhood Educ. J.* **39**:407–412. [17]

McLoyd, V. 1998. Socio-Economic Disadvantage and Child Development. *Am. Psychol.* **53**:185–204. [13]

Meaney, M. J. 2010. Epigenetics and the Biological Definition of Gene x Environment Interactions. *Child Dev.* **81**:41–79. [1]

Meaney, M. J., and M. Szyf. 2005. Maternal Care as a Model for Experience-Dependent Chromatin Plasticity? *Trends Neurosci.* **28**:456–463. [7]

Mee, S., B. G. Bunney, C. Reist, S. G. Potkin, and W. E. Bunney. 2006. Psychological Pain: A Review of Evidence. *J. Psychiatr. Res.* **40**:680–690. [11]

Meggitt, M. 1965. The Desert People: A Study of the Walbiri Aborigines of Central Australia. Chicago: Univ. of Chicago Press. [6]

Mehta, D., T. Klengel, K. N. Connelly, et al. 2013. Childhood Maltreatment Is Associated with Distinct Genomic and Epigenetic Profiles in Postraumatic Stress Disorder. *PNAS* **110**:8302–8307. [5]

Mehta, M. A., N. I. Golembo, C. Nosarti, et al. 2009. Amygdala, Hippocampal and Corpus Callosum Size Following Severe Early Institutional Deprivation: The English and Romanian Adoptees Study Pilot. *J. Child Psychol. Psychiatry* **50**:943–951. [9]

Meinlschmidt, G., and C. Heim. 2007. Sensitivity to Intranasal Oxytocin in Adult Men with Early Parental Separation. *Biol. Psychiatry* **61**:1109–1111. [10]

Meins, E., and C. Fernyhough. 1999. Linguistic Acquisitional Style and Mentalising Development: The Role of Maternal Mind-Mindedness. *Cogn. Dev.* **14**:363–380. [11]

Meiser-Stedman, R., T. Dalgleish, P. Smith, W. Yule, and E. Glucksman. 2007. Diagnostic, Demographic, Memory Quality, and Cognitive Variables Associated with Acute Stress Disorder in Children and Adolescents. *J. Abnorm. Psychol.* **116**:65–79. [12]

Menard, C. B., K. J. Bandeen-Roche, and H. D. Chilcoat. 2004. Epidemiology of Multiple Childhood Traumatic Events: Child Abuse, Parental Psychopathology, and Other Family-Level Stressors. *Soc. Psychiatry Psychiatr. Epidemiol.* **39**:857–865. [11]

Mendes, D. D., J. Mari, M. Singer, G. M. Barros, and A. F. Mello. 2009. Study Review of the Biological, Social and Environmental Factors Associated with Aggressive Behaviour. *Rev. Braz. Psychiatry* **31**:577–585. [15]

Menzies Lyth, I. 1959. The Functions of Social Systems as a Defence against Anxiety: A Report on a Study of the Nursing Service of a General Hospital. *Hum. Relat.* **13**:95–121. [18]

Meyer, M. L., C. L. Masten, Y. Ma, et al. 2013. Empathy for the Social Suffering of Friends and Strangers Recruits Distinct Patterns of Brain Activation. *Soc. Cogn. Affect. Neurosci.* **8**:446–454. [10]

Michalik, N. M., N. Eisenberg, T. L. Spinrad, et al. 2007. Longitudinal Relations among Parental Emotional Expressivity and Sympathy and Prosocial Behavior in Adolescence. *Soc. Dev.* **16**:286–309. [12]

Miklikowska, M., and D. P. Fry. 2010. Values for Peace: Ethnographic Lessons from the Semai of Malaysia and the Mardu of Australia. *Beliefs and Values* **2**:124–137. [6]

Mikton, C., and A. Butchart. 2009. Child Maltreatment Prevention: A Systematic Review of Reviews. *Bull. WHO* **875**:353–361. [3]

Mikulincer, M., and P. R. Shaver. 2008. Can't Buy Me Love: An Attachment Perspective on Social Support and Money as Psychological Buffers. *Psychol. Inq.* **19**:167–173. [10]

Mikulincer, M., P. R. Shaver, and N. Hores. 2006. Attachment Bases on Emotion Regulation and Posttraumatic Adjustment. In: Emotion Regulation in Families: Pathways to Dysfunction and Health, ed. D. K. Snyder et al., pp. 77–99. Washington, D.C.: American Psychological Association. [12]

Milgram, S. 1963. Behavioral Study of Obedience. *J. Abnorm. Psychol.* **67**:4. [10]

———. 1974. Obedience to Authority: An Experimental View. London: Tavistock Publications. [10]

Miller, F. G. 2009. The Randomized Controlled Trial as a Demonstration Project: An Ethical Perspective. *Am. J. Psychiatry* **166**:743–745. [9]

Miller, P. J., and J. J. Goodnow. 1995. Cultural Practices: Toward an Integration of Culture and Development. In: Cultural Practices as Contexts for Development, ed. J. J. Goodnow et al., pp. 5–16. San Francisco: Josey-Bass. [13]

Millum, J., and E. J. Emanuel. 2007. The Ethics of International Research with Abandoned Children. *Science* **318**:1874–1875. [9]

Minuchin, P. 1985. Families and Individual Development: Provocations from the Field of Family Therapy. *Child Dev.* **56**:289–302. [2]

Mitchell, C., J. Hobcraft, S. S. McLanahan, et al. 2014. Social Disadvantage, Genetic Sensitivity, and Children's Telomere Length. *PNAS* **111**:5944–5949. [1]

Miyake, K., C. Yang, Y. Minakuchi, et al. 2013. Comparison of Genomic and Epigenomic Expression in Monozygotic Twins Discordant for Rett Syndrome. *PLoS One* **8**:e66729. [5]

Moffitt, T. E., L. Arseneault, D. Belsky, et al. 2011. A Gradient of Childhood Self-Control Predicts Health, Wealth, and Public Safety. *PNAS* **108**:2693–2698. [7, 14]

Moll, J., F. Krueger, R. Zahn, et al. 2006. Human Fronto-Mesolimbic Networks Guide Decisions About Charitable Donation. *PNAS* **103**:15623–15628. [10]

Mollica, R. F., K. McInnes, C. Poole, and S. Tor. 1998. Dose-Effect Relationships of Trauma to Symptoms of Depression and Post-Traumatic Stress Disorder among Cambodian Survivors of Mass Violence. *Br. J. Psychiatry* **173**:482–488. [7]

Monk, C., J. Spicer, and F. Champagne. 2012. Linking Prenatal Maternal Adversity to Developmental Outcomes in Infants: The Role of Epigenetic Pathways. *Dev. Psychopathol.* **24**:1361–1376. [7]

Monks, C. P., P. K. Smith, and J. Swettenham. 2005. Psychological Correlates of Peer Victimization in Preschool: Social Cognitive Skills, Executive Function and Attachment Profiles. *Aggress. Behav.* **31**:571–588. [16]

Montero, M., and C. C. Sonn. 2009. Psychology of Liberation: Theory and Applications. New York: Springer. [15]

Montgomery, E. 2004. Tortured Families: A Coordinated Management of Meaning Analysis. *Fam. Proc.* **43**:349–371. [12]

———. 2010. Trauma and Resilience in Young Refugees: A 9-Year Follow-up Study. *Dev. Psychopathol.* **22**:477–489. [12]

Montiel, C. J. 2001. Toward a Psychology of Structural Peacebuilding. In: Peace, Conflict, and Violence: Peace Psychology for the 21st Century, ed. D. J. Christie et al., pp. 282–294. Englewood Cliffs: Prentice-Hall. [15]

Montiel, C. J., and N. M. Noor. 2009. Peace Psychology in Asia. New York: Springer. [15]

Moore, C. 2009. Fairness in Children's Resource Allocation Depends on the Recipient. *Psychol. Sci.* **20**:944–948. [15]

Moran, P., D. Ghate, and A. van der Merwe. 2004. What Works in Parenting Support? A Review of the International Evidence. UK Dept. of Education and Skills Research Report RR574. [3]

Morgan, D. K., and E. Whitelaw. 2008. The Case for Transgenerational Epigenetic Inheritance in Humans. *Mamm. Genome* **19**:394–397. [7]

Morgan, H. D., F. Santos, K. Green, W. Dean, and W. Reik. 2005. Epigenetic Reprogramming in Mammals. *Hum. Mol. Genet.* **14**:R47–R58. [5]

Morrill, C. 2013. A Brief Look at Sociological Perspectives on Peer Hierarchies, Organizational Conditions in Schools, and Youth Violence and Conflict. In: Youth Violence: What We Need to Know. Report of the Subcommittee on Youth Violence of the Advisory Committee to the Social, Behavioral and Economic Sciences Directorate, pp. 20–22. Washington, D.C.: National Science Foundation. [14]

Morrill, C., and M. Musheno. 2013. Youth Conflict: Culture and Control in an Urban Public School. Chicago: Univ. of Chicago Press. [14]

Morrow, R. W. 2006. Sesame Street and the Reform of Children's Television. Baltimore: The Johns Hopkins Univ. Press. [18]

Moser, J. S., S. P. Cahill, and E. B. Foa. 2010. Evidence for Poorer Outcome in Patients with Severe Negative Trauma-Related Cognitions Receiving Prolonged Exposure Plus Cognitive Restructuring: Implications for Treatment Matching in Posttraumatic Stress Disorder. *J. Nerv. Ment. Disorder* **198**:72–75. [12]

Motti-Stefanidi, F., J. Berry, X. Chryssochoou, D. L. Sam, and J. Phinney. 2012. Positive Immigrant Youth Adaptation in Context: Developmental, Acculturation, and Social-Psychological Perspectives. In: Realizing the Potential of Immigrant Youth, ed. A. S. Masten et al., pp. 116–158. New York: Cambridge Univ. Press. [14]

Msall, M., J. Bier, L. LaGasse, M. Tremont, and B. Lester. 1998. The Vulnerable Preschool Child: The Impact of Biomedical and Social Risks on Neurodevelopmental Function. *Semin. Pediatr. Neurol.* **5**:52–61. [11]

Murray, L., S. Halligan, and P. Cooper. 2010. Effects of Postnatal Depression on Mother–Infant Interactions and Child Development. In: The Wiley-Blackwell Handbook of Infant Development (2nd edition), vol. 2: Applied and Policy Issues, ed. J. G. Bremner and T. D. Wachs, pp. 192–220. Chichester: John Wiley. [7]

Mweru, M. 2010. Why Are Kenyan Teachers Still Using Corporal Punishment Eight Years after a Ban on Corporal Punishment? *Child Abuse Rev.* **19**:248–258. [11]

Myers, F. 1986. Pintupi Country, Pintupi Self: Sentiment, Place, and Politics among Western Desert Aborigines. Berkeley: Univ. of California Press. [6]

Näätänen, P., K. Kanninen, S. Qouta, and R.-L. Punamäki. 2002. Trauma-Related Emotional Patterns and Their Association with Post-Traumatic and Somatic Symptoms. *Anxiety Stress Coping* **15**:75–94. [12]

Naber, F. B. A., I. E. Poslawsky, M. H. van IJzendoorn, H. Van Engeland, and M. J. Bakermans-Kranenburg. 2012. Brief Report: Oxytocin Enhances Paternal Sensitivity to a Child with Autism: A Double-Blind Within-Subject Experiment with Intranasally Administered Oxytocin. *J. Autism Dev. Disord.* **43**:224–229. [10]

Nasser, I., and M. Abu-Nimer. 2007. Peace Education in a Bilingual and Bi-Ethnic School for Palestinians and Jews in Israel: Lessons and Challenges. In: Educational Response to Conflict: Systemic Issues, ed. Z. Bekerman and C. McGlynn. New York: Palgrave Macmillan. [19]

Nasser, I., M. Abu-Nimer, and O. Mahmouda. 2014. Contextual and Pedagogical Considerations in Teaching for Forgiveness in the Arab World. *Compare* **44**:32–52. [15]

National Research Council and Institute of Medicine. 2009. Preventing Mental, Emotional, and Behavioral Disorders among Young People: Progress and Possibilities. Washington, D.C.: National Academies Press. [14]

National Scientific Council on the Developing Child. 2008. Science Briefs: Focus and Planning Skills Can Be Improved before a Child Enters School. http://developing-child.harvard.edu/index.php/download_file/-/view/90/. (accessed June 5, 2014). [16]

Naumova, O. Y., M. Lee, R. Koposov, et al. 2012. Differential Patterns of Whole-Genome DNA Methylation in Institutionalized Children and Children Raised by Their Biological Parents. *Dev. Psychopathol.* **24**:143–155. [1]

Nelson, C. A., N. A. Fox, and C. H. Zeanah. 2014. Romania's Abandoned Children: Deprivation, Brain Development and Recovery. Cambridge, MA: Harvard Univ. Press. [9]

Nelson, C. A., C. H. Zeanah, N. A. Fox, et al. 2007. Cognitive Recovery in Socially Deprived Young Children: The Bucharest Early Intervention Project. *Science* **318**:1937–1940. [3]

Nesdale, D. 2008. Social Identity Development and Children's Ethnic Attitudes in Australia. Handbook of Race, Racism, and the Developing Child, ed. M. Bennett and F. Sani, pp. 313–338. New York: Psychology Press. [15]

Nestler, E. J. 2013. Epigenetic Mechanisms of Drug Addiction. *Neuropharmacology* **76(Pt B)**:259–268. [5]

Neugebauer, R., P. W. Fisher, J. B. Turner, et al. 2009. Post-Traumatic Stress Reactions among Rwandan Children and Adolescents in the Early Aftermath of Genocide. *Intl. J. Epidem.* **38**:1033–1045. [7]

Neumann, I. D., and R. Landgraf. 2012. Balance of Brain Oxytocin and Vasopressin: Implications for Anxiety, Depression and Social Behaviors. *Trends Neurosci.* **35**:649–659. [4]

Neuner, F., C. Catani, M. Ruf, et al. 2008. Narrative Exposure Therapy for the Treatment of Traumatized Children and Adolescents (KidNET): From Neurocognitive Theory to Field Intervention. *Child Adolesc. Psychiatr. Clin. N. Am.* **17**:641–664. [12]

Neuner, F., M. Schauer, U. Karunakara, et al. 2004. Psychological Trauma and Evidence for Enhanced Vulnerability for Posttraumatic Stress Disorder through Previous Trauma among West Nile Refugees. *BMC Psychiatry* **4**:34. [7]

Neville, H., and D. Bavellier. 1998. Neural Organization and Plasticity for Language. *Curr. Opin. Neurobiol.* **8**:254–258. [9]

Nevin, R. 2000. How Lead Exposure Relates to Temporal Changes in IQ, Violent Crime, and Unwed Pregnancy. *Environ. Res.* **83**:1–22. [11]

NICE. 2014. Post-Traumatic Stress Disorder (PTSD): The Management of PTSD in Adults and Children in Primary and Secondary Care. National Institute for Health and Clinical Excellence. http://www.nice.org.uk/CG26. (accessed Jan. 6, 2014). [12]

Noble, K. G., S. M. Houston, E. Kan, and E. R. Sowell. 2012. Neural Correlates of Socioeconomic Status in the Developing Human Brain. *Dev. Sci.* **15**:516–527. [7]

Noddings, N. 2012. Peace Education: How We Come to Love and Hate War. New York: Cambridge Univ. Press. [16]

Noor, N. M. 2009. The Future of Peace Psychology in Asia. In: Peace Psychology in Asia, ed. C. J. Montiel and N. M. Noor, pp. 307–321. New York: Springer. [15]

Nores, M., and S. W. Barnett. 2010. Benefits of Early Childhood Education Interventions across the World. *Econ. Ed. Rev.* **29**:271–282. [13, 15]

Norman, G. J., J. T. Cacioppo, J. S. Morris, et al. 2011. Oxytocin Increases Autonomic Cardiac Control: Moderation by Loneliness. *Biol. Psychol.* **86**:174–180. [4]

Norton, N. E. L., K. Smith, F. Kander, and K. Short. 2005. Permitanme Hablar: Allow Me to Speak. *Lang. Arts* **83**:118–127. [15]

Nunnally, J. C. 1970. Introduction to Psychological Measurement. New York: McGraw-Hill. [10]

Oberlander, T., J. Weinberg, M. Papsdorf, et al. 2008. Prenatal Exposure to Maternal Depression, Neonatal Methylation of Human Glucocorticoid Receptor Gene (NR3C1) and Infant Cortisol Stress Responses. *Epigenetics* **3**:97–106. [7]

Obradović, J., and W. T. Boyce. 2012. The Role of Stress Reactivity for Child Development: Indices, Correlates and Future Directions. In: The Cambridge Handbook of Environment in Human Development, ed. L. C. Mayes and M. Lewis, pp. 655–681. New York: Cambridge Univ. Press. (14)

O'Connell, M. E., T. Boat, and K. E. Warner, eds. 2009. Preventing Mental, Emotional, and Behavioral Disorders among Young People: Progress and Possibilities. Washington, D.C.: National Academies Press. [14]

O'Connell, M. J., N. B. Loughran, T. A. Walsh, et al. 2010. A Phylogenetic Approach to Test for Evidence of Parental Conflict or Gene Duplications Associated with Protein-Encoding Imprinted Orthologous Genes in Placental Mammals. *Mamm. Genome* **21**:486–498. [5]

O'Connor, M., and A. Elklit. 2008. Attachment Styles, Traumatic Events, and PTSD: A Cross-Sectional Investigation of Adult Attachment and Trauma. *Attach. Hum. Dev.* **10**:59–71. [12]

O'Connor, T. G., J. Heron, and V. Glover. 2002. Antenatal Anxiety Predicts Child Behavioral/Emotional Problems Independently of Postnatal Depression. *J. Am. Acad. Child Adolesc. Psychiatry* **41**:1470–1477. [11]

O'Connor, T. G., M. Rutter, C. Beckett, L. Keaveney, and J. M. Kreppner. 2000. The Effects of Global Severe Privation on Cognitive Competence: Extension and Longitudinal Follow-Up. English and Romanian Adoptees Study Team. *Child Dev.* **71**:376–390. [7]

Olds, D. L. 2006. The Nurse-Family Partnership: An Evidence-Based Preventive Intervention. *Infant Ment. Health J.* **27**:5–25. [11, 14]

Olff, M., J. L. Frijling, L. D. Kubzansky, et al. 2013. The Role of Oxytocin in Social Bonding, Stress Regulation and Mental Health: An Update on the Moderating Effects of Context and Interindividual Differences. *Psychoneuroendocrinology* **38**:1883–1894. [4]

Olson, K. R., and Spelke, E. S. 2008. Foundations of Cooperation in Young Children. *Cognition* **108**:222–231. [7]

Omidian, P. A., and N. J. Lawrence. 2007. A Community Based Approach to Focusing: The Islam and Focusing Project of Afghanistan. *Folio* **20**:152–162. [15]

Opotow, S. 2001. Social Injustice. In: Peace, Conflict, and Violence: Peace Psychology in the 21st Century, ed. D. J. Christie et al., pp. 102–110. New York: Prentice-Hall. [13]

Oser, F. K., W. Althof, and A. Higgins-D'Allessandro. 2008. The Just Community Approach to Moral Education: System Change or Individual Change? *J. Moral Educ.* **37**:395–415. [10]

Ostrov, J. M., K. E. Woods, E. A. Jansen, J. F. Casas, and N. R. Crick. 2004. An Observational Study of Delivered and Received Aggression, Gender and Social-Psychological Adjustment in Preschool: "This White Crayon Doesn't Work…" *Early Child Res. Q.* **19**:355–371. [16]

Otto, H. 2008. Culture-Specific Attachment Strategies in the Cameroonian Nso: Cultural Solutions to a Universal Developmental Task. Doctoral Thesis. Osnabrück University: School of Human Sciences, Department of Culture and Psychology. [11]

Otto, H., and H. Keller, eds. 2014. Different Faces of Attachment: Cultural Variation on a Universal Human Need. Cambridge: Cambridge Univ. Press. [11]

Ouyang, L., Fang, X., Mercy, J., Perou, R., and Grosse, S. D. 2008. Attention-Deficit/Hyperactivity Disorder Symptoms and Child Maltreatment: A Population-Based Study. *J. Pediatr.* **153(6)**:851–856. [12]

Overton, W. F. 2013. A New Paradigm for Developmental Science: Relationism and Relational-Developmental Systems. *Appl. Dev. Sci.* **17**:94–107. [14, 15]

Paardekooper, B., J. T. V. M. de Jong, and J. M. A. Hermanns. 1999. The Psychological Impact of War and the Refugee Situation on South Sudanese Children in Refugee Camps in Northern Uganda: An Exploratory Study. *J. Child Psychol. Psychiatry* **40**:529–536. [12]

Page, J. 2000. Reframing Early Childhood Curriculum: Educational Imperatives for the Future. London: Routledge Falmer. [17]

Pagotto, L., A. Voci, and V. Maculan. 2010. The Effectiveness of Intergroup Contact at Work: Mediators and Moderators of Hospital Workers' Prejudice Towards Immigrants. *J. Comm. Appl. Soc. Psychol.* **20**:317–330. [15]

Palosaari, E., R.-L. Punamäki, S. Qouta, and M. Diab. 2013. Intergenerational Effects of War Trauma among Palestinian Families Mediated Via Psychological Maltreatment. *Child Abuse Negl.* **37**:955–968. [12]

Pannebakker, F. D. 2007. Morality from Infancy to Middle Childhood. Leiden: Mostert and Onderen. [10]

Panter-Brick, C., A. Burgess, M. Eggerman, F. McAllister, K. Pruett, and J.F. Leckman. 2014a. Engaging Fathers: Recommendations for a Game Change in Parenting Interventions Based on a Systematic Review of the Global Evidence. *J. Child Psychol. Psychiatry* **55**, in press. [1, 3, 15, 16]

Panter-Brick, C., and M. Eggerman. 2012. Understanding Culture, Resilience, and Mental Health: The Production of Hope. In: The Social Ecology of Resilience: A Handbook of Theory and Practice, ed. M. Ungar. New York: Springer. [12]

Panter-Brick, C., M. Eggerman, V. Gonzalez, and S. Safdar. 2009. Ongoing Violence, Social Suffering and Mental Health: A School-Based Survey in Afghanistan. *Lancet* **374**:807–816. [7]

Panter-Brick, C., M. Eggerman, A. Mojadidi, and T. McDade. 2008. Social Stressors, Mental Health, and Physiological Stress in an Urban Elite of Young Afghans in Kabul. *Am. J. Hum Biol.* **20**:627–641. [1]

Panter-Brick, C., A. Goodman, W. Tol, and M. Eggerman. 2011. Mental Health and Childhood Adversities: A Longitudinal Study in Kabul, Afghanistan. *J. Am. Acad. Child Adolesc. Psychiatry* **50**:349–363. [7, 12, 15]

Panter-Brick, C., M. P. Grimon, and M. Eggerman. 2014b. Caregiver-Child Mental Health: A Prospective Study in Conflict and Refugee Settings. *J. Child Psychol. Psychiatry* **55**:313–327. [1, 12]

Panter-Brick, C., and J. F. Leckman. 2013. Resilience in Child Development: Interconnected Pathways to Well-Being. *J. Child Psychol. Psychiatry* **54**:333–336. [1, 3, 14, 15]

Parker, K. J., and D. Maestripieri. 2011. Identifying Key Features of Early Stressful Experiences That Produce Stress Vulnerability and Resilience in Primates. *Neurosci. Biobehav. Rev.* **35**:1466–1483. [8]

Parkes, C. M., J. Stevenson-Hinde, and P. Marris, eds. 1991. Attachment across the Life Cycle. London: Routledge. [2]

Patterson, G. R., M. S. Forgatch, and D. S. DeGarmo. 2010. Cascading Effects Following Intervention. *Dev. Psychopathol.* **22**:941–970. [14]

Paulus, M., N. Kühn-Popp, M. Licata, B. Sodian, and J. Meinhardt. 2013. Neural Correlates of Prosocial Behavior in Infancy: Different Neurophysiological Mechanisms Support the Emergence of Helping and Comforting. *NeuroImage* **66**:522–530. [10]

Pearce, E., C. Stringer, and R. I. Dunbar. 2013. New Insights into Differences in Brain Organization between Neanderthals and Anatomically Modern Humans. *Proc. Biol. Sci.* **280**:20130168. [4]

Pederson, D. R., and G. Moran. 1995. A Categorical Description of Mother–Infant Relationships in the Home and Its Relation to Q-Sort Measures of Infant-Mother Interaction. *Monogr. Soc. Res. Child Dev.* **60**:111–132. [10]

Peltonen, K., and E. Palosaari. 2013. Evidence-Based Resilience-Enhancing Intervention Methods for Children Affected by Armed Conflict. In: Handbook of Resilience in Children of War, ed. C. Fernando and M. Ferrari, pp. 267–284. New York: Springer. [12]

Peltonen, K., and R.-L. Punamäki. 2010. Preventative Interventions among Children Exposed to Trauma of Armed Conflict: A Literature Review. *Aggress. Behav.* **36**:95–116. [12, 14]

Peltonen, K., S. Qouta, E. El Sarraj, and R.-L. Punamäki. 2010. Military Trauma and Social Development: The Moderating and Mediating Roles of Peer and Sibling Relations in Mental Health. *Intl. J. Behav. Dev.* **34**:554–563. [12]

Peña, C. J., Y. D. Neugut, and F. A. Champagne. 2013. Developmental Timing of the Effects of Maternal Care on Gene Expression and Epigenetic Regulation of Hormone Receptor Levels in Female Rats. *Endocrinology* **154**11:4340–4351. [3]

Pennisi, E. 2012. Encode Project Writes Eulogy for Junk DNA. *Science* **337**:1159–1161. [1, 3]

Perroud, N., A. Paoloni-Giacobino, P. Prada, et al. 2011. Increased Methylation of Glucocorticoid Receptor Gene (NR3C1) in Adults with a History of Childhood Maltreatment: A Link with the Severity and Type of Trauma. *Trans. Psychiatry* **1**:e59. [7]

Pettigrew, T. F. 1998. Intergroup Contact Theory. *Annu. Rev. Psychol.* **49**:65–85. [15]

Pettigrew, T. F., and L. R. Tropp. 2006. A Meta-Analytic Test of Intergroup Contact Theory. *J. Pers. Soc. Psychol.* **90**:751–783. [15]

Piaget, J. 1932. The Moral Development of the Child. London: Kegan Paul. [15]

Pickett, K., and R. Wilkinson. 2010. The Spirit Level: Why Greater Equality Makes Societies Stronger. New York: Bloomsbury Publishing. [11]

Pinker, S. 2003. The Blank Slate: The Modern Denial of Human Nature. New York: Penguin Books. [7]

———. 2011. The Better Angels of Our Nature: Why Violence Has Declined. New York: Penguin Books. [7, 8]

Piquero, A. R., D. P. Farrington, B. C. Welsh, R. Tremblay, and W. G. Jennings. 2009. Effects of Early Family/Parent Training Programs on Antisocial Behavior and Delinquency. *J. Exp. Criminology* **5**:83–120. [14]

Plotsky, P. M., K. V. Thrivikraman, C. B. Nemeroff, et al. 2005. Long-Term Consequences of Neonatal Rearing on Central Corticotropin-Releasing Factor Systems in Adult Male Rat Offspring. *Neuropsychopharmacology* **30**:2192–2204. [7]

Pohlandt-Mccormick, H. 2000. I Saw a Nightmare: Violence and the Construction of Memory (Soweto, June 16, 1976). *Hist. Theory* **3**:23–44. [13]

Pollak, S. D., D. Cicchetti, K. Hornung, and A. Reed. 2000. Recognizing Emotion in Faces: Developmental Effects of Child Abuse and Neglect. *Dev. Psychol.* **36**:679–688. [11, 12]

Porges, S. W. 1998. Love: An Emergent Property of the Mammalian Autonomic Nervous System. *Psychoneuroendocrinology* **23**:837–861. [4]

Porges, S. W. 2011. The Polyvagal Theory: Neurophysiological Foundations of Emotions, Attachment, Communication and Self-Regulation. New York: W.W Norton. [4, 7]

Portmann-Lanz, C. B., A. Schoeberlein, R. Portmann, et al. 2010. Turning Placenta into Brain: Placental Mesenchymal Stem Cells Differentiate into Neurons and Oligodendrocytes. *Am. J. Obstet. Gynecol.* **202**:294.e291–294.e211. [5]

Posada, G., T. Lu, J. Trumbell, et al. 2013. Is the Secure Base Phenomenon Evident Here, There, and Anywhere: A Cross-Cultural Study of Child Behaviour and Experts' Definitions. *Child Dev.* **84**:1896–1905. [2]

Poutahidis, T., S. M. Kearney, T. Levkovich, et al. 2013. Microbial Symbionts Accelerate Wound Healing Via the Neuropeptide Hormone Oxytocin. *PLoS One* **8**10:e78898. [3]

Power, F. C. 1979. The Moral Atmosphere of a Just Community High School: A Four-Year Longitudinal Study. Doctoral Thesis. Harvard University: Graduate School of Education. [10]

Power, M., and T. Dalgleish. 2008. Cognition and Emotion: From Order to Disorder. Hove: Psychology Press. [12]

Preskill, H., N. Jones, and A. Tengue. 2013. Markers That Matter: Success Indicators in Early Learning and Education. Foundation Strategy Group. http://www.fsg.org/tabid/191/ArticleId/936/Default.aspx?srpush=true (accessed May 23, 2014). [17]

Preston, S. D., and F. de Waal. 2002. Empathy: Its Ultimate and Proximate Bases. *Behav. Brain Sci.* **25**:1–20. [15]

Provençal, N., M. J. Suderman, C. Guillemin, et al. 2012. The Signature of Maternal Rearing in the Methylome in Rhesus Macaque Prefrontal Cortex and T Cells. *J. Neurosci.* **32**:15626–15642. [1, 3, 5, 7, 8]

Provençal, N., M. J. Suderman, F. Vitaro, et al. 2013. Childhood Chronic Physical Aggression Associates with Adult Cytokine Levels in Plasma. *PloS One* **7**:69481. [5]

Pruett, M. K., C. P. Cowan, P. A. Cowan, and K. Pruett. 2009. Lessons Learned from Supporting Father Involvement Study: A Cross-Cultural Preventative Intervention for Low-Income Families with Young Children. *J. Soc. Serv. Res.* **352**:163–179. [3]

Punamäki, R.-L. 2002. The Uninvited Guest of War Enters Childhood: Developmental and Personality Aspects of War and Military Violence. *Traumatology* **8**:45–63. [12]

———. 2006. Resiliency in Conditions of War and Military Violence: Preconditions and Developmental Processes. In: Working with Children and Adolescents: An Evidence-Based Approach to Risk and Resilience, ed. M. E. Garralda and M. Flament, pp. 129–177. New York: Jason Aronson. [12]

————. 2007. Trauma and Dreaming: The Impact on Dream Recall, Content and Patterns, and the Mental Health Function of Dreaming. In: The New Science of Dreaming: Content, Recall, and Personality Correlates, ed. P. McNamara and D. Barret, vol. 2, pp. 211–252. Westport, CT: Praeger Publishing. [12]

Punamäki, R.-L., S. Qouta, M. El Masri, I. Komproe, and J. T. V. M. De Jong. 2005. The Deterioration and Mobilization Effects of Trauma on Social Support: Childhood Maltreatment and Adulthood Military Violence in a Palestinian Community Sample. *Child Abuse Negl.* **29**:351–373. [12]

Qouta, S., R.-L. Punamäki, and E. El Sarraj. 2008a. Child Development and Family Mental Health in War and Military Violence: The Palestinian Experience. *Intl. J. Behav. Dev.* **32**:310–324. [12, 14]

Qouta, S., R.-L. Punamäki, T. Miller, and E. El Sarraj. 2008b. Does War Beget Child Aggression? Military Violence, Gender, Age and Aggressive Behavior in Two Palestinian Samples. *Aggress. Behav.* **34**:231–244. [12]

Quinlan, R. J. 2007. Human Parental Effort and Environmental Risk. *Proc. R. Soc. B* **274**:121–125. [12]

Radtke, K. M., M. Ruf, H. M. Gunter, et al. 2011. Transgenerational Impact of Intimate Partner Violence on Methylation in the Promoter of the Glucocorticoid Receptor. *Trans. Psychiatry* **1**:e21. [7]

Rai, T. S., and A. P. Fiske. 2011. Moral Psychology Is Relationship Regulation: Moral Motives for Unity, Hierarchy, Equality, and Proportionality *Psychol. Rev.* **118**:57–75. [7]

Rakoczy, H., and M. F. H. Schmidt. 2013. The Early Ontogeny of Social Norms. *Child Dev. Perspect.* **7**:17–21. [7]

Ramey, C. T., and S. L. Ramey. 1998. Prevention of Intellectual Disabilities: Early Interventions to Improve Cognitive Development. *Prev. Med.* **27**:224–232. [16]

Ramirez, M., Y. Wu, S. Kataoka, et al. 2012. Youth Violence across Multiple Dimensions: A Study of Violence, Absenteeism, and Suspensions among Middle School Children. *J. Pediatr.* **161**:542–546. [11]

Rapee, R. M., S. Kennedy, M. Ingram, S. Edwards, and L. Sweeney. 2005. Prevention and Early Intervention of Anxiety Disorders in Inhibited Preschool Children. *J. Consult. Clin. Psychol.* **73**:488–497. [11]

Raver, C. C., C. Blair, and M. Willoughby. 2012. Poverty as a Predictor of 4-Year-Olds' Executive Function: New Perspectives on Models of Differential Susceptibility. *Dev. Psychol.* **49**:292–304. [7]

Rawls, J. 1971. A Theory of Justice. Cambridge MA: Harvard Univ. Press. [11]

Razin, A. 1998. CpG Methylation, Chromatin Structure and Gene Silencing–a Three-Way Connection. *EMBO J.* **1717**:4905–4908. [3]

Razin, A., and A. D. Riggs. 1980. DNA Methylation and Gene Function. *Science* **210**:604–610. [3]

Reed, R. V., M. Fazel, L. Jones, C. Panter-Brick, and A. Stein. 2012. Mental Health of Displaced Refugee Children Resettled in Low-Income and Middle-Income Countries: Risk and Protective Factors. *Lancet* **379**:250–265. [14]

Reichard, R. J., and S. J. Paik. 2012. Developing the Next Generation of Leaders: Research, Policy and Practice. In: Early Development and Leadership: Building the Next Generation of Leaders, ed. S. E. Murphy and R. J. Reichard, pp. 309–328. New York: Taylor and Francis. [18]

Reik, W., and J. Walter. 2001. Genomic Imprinting: Parental Influence on the Genome. *Nat. Rev. Genet.* **2**:21–32. [8]

Reitz, C., G. Tosto, R. Mayteaux, et al. 2012. Genetic Variants in the Fat and Obesity Associated (FTO) Gene and Risk of Alzheimer's Disease. *PLoS One* 7:e50354. [5]

Report of the Subcommittee on Youth Violence of the Advisory Committee to the SBE Sciences Directorate. 2013. Youth Violence: What We Need to Know. Arlington: National Science Foundation. [14]

Reyna, S. 1994. A Mode of Domination Approach to Organized Violence. In: Studying War: Anthropological Perspectives, ed. S. Reyna and R. Downs, pp. 29–65. Amsterdam: Gordon and Breach. [6]

Reynolds, A. J., H. Chang, and J. A. Temple. 1998. Early Childhood Intervention and Juvenile Delinquency: An Exploratory Analysis of the Chicago Child-Parent Centers. *Eval. Rev.* 22:341–372. [16]

Reynolds, A. J., and S.-R. Ou. 2004. Alterable Predictors of Child Well-Being in the Chicago Longitudinal Study. *Child. Youth Serv. Rev.* 26:1–14. [16]

Reynolds, A. J., A. J. Rolnick, M. M. Englund, and J. A. Temple, eds. 2010. Childhood Programs and Practices in the First Decade of Life: A Human Capital Integration. New York: Cambridge Univ. Press. [14]

Reynolds, A. J., J. A. Temple, B. A. B. White, S.-R. Ou, and D. L. Robertson. 2011. Age 26 Cost-Benefit Analysis of the Child-Parent Center Early Education Program. *Child Dev.* 82:379–404. [14]

Reynolds, P., and A. Dawes. 1999. Truth and Youth: Blame and Pain. *ISSBD Newsletter* 2:10–11. [13]

Richter, L. 2004. The Importance of Caregiver-Child Interactions for the Survival and Healthy Development of Young Children: A Review. Geneva: World Health Organization. [3]

———. 2013. Foreword. In: South African Child Gauge, ed. B. L. L. Biersteker et al., p. 7. Cape Town: Children's Institute: Univ. of Cape Town. [15]

Richter, L., J. Biersteker, C. Burns, et al. 2012. Diagnostic Review of Early Childhood Development, Pretoria: Department of Performance, Monitoring and Evaluation and Inter-Departmental Steering Committee on ECD. http://www.gov.za/documents/download.php?f=170644 (accessed June 6, 2014). [13]

Richter, L., and A. Dawes. 2008. Child Abuse in South Africa: Rights and Wrongs. *Child Abuse Rev.* 17:79–93. [13]

Richter, L., A. Dawes, and J. de Kadt. 2010. Early Childhood. In: Promoting Mental Health in Scarce-Resource Contexts, ed. I. Petersen et al., pp. 99–123. Cape Town: Human Science Research Council. [3]

Rid, A. 2012. When Is Research Socially Valuable? Lessons from the Bucharest Early Intervention Project. Commentary on a Case Study in the Ethics of Mental Health Research. *J. Nerv. Ment. Dis.* 200:248–249. [9]

Riem, M. M. E., M. J. Bakermans-Kranenburg, R. Huffmeijer, and M. H. van IJzendoorn. 2013a. Does Intranasal Oxytocin Promote Prosocial Behavior to an Excluded Fellow Player? A Randomized Controlled Trial with Cyberball. *Psychoneuroendocrinology* 38:1418–1425. [10]

Riem, M. M. E., M. J. Bakermans-Kranenburg, M. H. van IJzendoorn, D. Out, and S. A. Rombouts. 2012. Attachment in the Brain: Adult Attachment Representations Predict Amygdala and Behavioral Responses to Infant Crying. *Attach. Hum. Dev.* 14:533–551. [11]

Riem, M. M. E., M. H. van IJzendoorn, M. Tops, et al. 2013b. Oxytocin Effects on Complex Brain Networks Are Moderated by Experiences of Maternal Love Withdrawal. *Eur. Neuropsychopharmacol.* 23:1288–1295. [4, 10]

Rinaman, L., L. Banihashemi, and T. J. Koehnle. 2011. Early Life Experience Shapes the Functional Organization of Stress-Responsive Visceral Circuits. *Physiol. Behav.* **104**:632–640. [7]

Robjant, K., and M. Fazel. 2010. The Emerging Evidence for Narrative Exposure Therapy: A Review. *Clin. Psychol. Rev.* **30**:1030–1039. [12]

Rodrik, D. 2014. The Past, Present, and Future of Economic Growth. In: Towards a Better Global Economy: Policy Implications for Global Citizens in the 21st Century, ed. J. R. Behrman and S. Fardoust. Oxford: Oxford Univ. Press. [15]

Rogers, C. E., P. J. Anderson, D. K. Thompson, et al. 2012. Regional Cerebral Development at Term Relates to School-Age Social–Emotional Development in Very Preterm Children. *J. Am. Acad. Child Adolesc. Psychiatry* **51**:181–191. [10]

Rogoff, B. 2003. The Cultural Nature of Human Development. Oxford: Oxford Univ. Press. [15]

Ronsaville, B. J., K. M. Carroll, and L. S. Onken. 2001. A Stage Model of Behavioral Therapies Research: Getting Started and Moving on from Stage 1. *Clin. Psychol.* **8**:133–142. [11]

Roseboom, T., S. de Rooij, and R. Painter. 2006. The Dutch Famine and Its Long-Term Consequences to Adult Health. *Early Hum. Dev* **82**:485–491. [5]

Rosenberg, M., and L. M. Knox. 2005. The Matrix Comes to Youth Violence Prevention: A Strengths-Based, Ecologic, and Developmental Framework. *Am. J. Prev. Med.* **29**:185–190. [15]

Ross, D., and L. Brown, eds. 2009. The Nicomachean Ethics, by Aristotle (translated by D. Ross). Oxford: Oxford Univ. Press. [10]

Rotheram-Borus, M. J., I. M. le Roux, M. Tomlinson, et al. 2011. Philani Plus (+): A Mentor Mother Community Health Worker Home Visiting Program to Improve Maternal and Infants' Outcomes. *Prev. Sci.* **12**:372–388. [13, 15]

Rousseau, J. J. 1762. Emile, or on Education (translated by Allan Bloom). New York: Basic Books. [10]

Rubin, D. C., D. Berntsen, and M. Bohni, K. 2008. A Memory-Based Model of Posttraumatic Stress Disorder: Evaluating Basic Assumptions Underlying the PTSD Diagnosis. *Psychol. Rev.* **115**:985–1011. [12]

Rubin, D. C., M. F. Dennis, and J. C. Beckham. 2011. Autobiographical Memory for Stressful Events: The Role of Autobiographical Memory in Posttraumatic Stress Disorder. *Conscious Cogn.* **20**:840–856. [12]

Rubin, J., D. Pruitt, and S. Kim. 1994. Social Conflict: Escalation, Stalemate, and Settlement. New York: McGraw-Hill. [6]

Rubin, J. Z., and G. Levinger. 1995. Levels of Analysis: In Search of Generalizable Knowledge. In: Conflict, Cooperation, and Justice: Essays Inspired by the Work of Morton Deutsch, ed. B. B. Bunker and J. Z. Rubin, pp. 13–38. San Francisco: Jossey-Bass. [15]

Rubin, L. H., C. S. Carter, J. R. Bishop, et al. 2013. Peripheral Vasopressin but Not Oxytocin Relates to Severity of Acute Psychosis in Women with Acutely-Ill Untreated First-Episode Psychosis. *Schizophr. Res.* **146**:138–143. [4]

———. 2014. Reduced Levels of Vasopressin and Reduced Behavioral Modulation of Oxytocin in Psychotic Disorders. *Schizophr. Bull.* March 11 (Epub ahead of print). [4]

Ruble, D. N., J. Alvarez, M. Bachman, et al. 2004. The Development of a Sense of "We": The Emergence and Implications of Children's Collective Identity. In: The Development of Social Self, ed. M. Bennett and F. Sani, pp. 29–76. New York: Psychology Press. [19]

Rushton, J. P., C. H. Littlefield, and C. J. Lumsden. 1986. Gene Culture Coevolution of Complex Social Behavior: Human Altruism and Mate Choice. *PNAS* **83**:7340–7343. [10]

Rutter, M. 2012. Resilience as a Dynamic Concept. *Dev. Psychopathol.* **24**:335–344. [14]

Rutter, M., C. Beckett, J. Castle, et al. 2009. Effects of Profound Early Institutional Deprivation: An Overview of Findings from a UK Longitudinal Study of Romanian Adoptees. In: International Advances in Adoption Research for Practice, ed. G. M. Wrobel and E. Neil, pp. 332–350. Chichester: Wiley-Blackwell. [9]

Sachs, J. 2008. Common Wealth: Economics for a Crowded Planet. New York: Penguin Press. [6]

Sadeh, A., S. Hen-Gal, and L. Tikotzky. 2008. Young Children's Reactions to War-Related Stress: A Survey and Assessment of an Innovative Intervention. *Pediatrics* **121**:46–53. [15, 16]

Sagi, A., and M. L. Hoffman. 1976. Empathic Distress in the Newborn. *Dev. Psychol.* **12**:175–176. [10]

Saigh, P. A., A. E. Yasik, R. A. Oberfield, P. V. Halamandaris, and J. D. Bremner. 2006. The Intellectual Performance of Traumatized Children and Adolescents with or without Posttraumatic Stress Disorder. *J. Abnorm. Psychol.* **115**:332–340. [12]

Salamon, J. 2002. Israeli-Palestinian Battles Intrude on Sesame Street. *New York Times*, July 30, 2002. [18]

Salo, J., R.-L. Punamäki, and S. Qouta. 2004. Associations between Self and Other Representations and Posttraumatic Adjustment among Political Prisoners. *Anxiety Stress Coping* **17**:421–439. [12]

Saloojee, G., and G. Schneider. 2007. Monitoring Childhood Disability. In: Monitoring Child Well-Being. A South African Rights-Based Approach, ed. A. Dawes et al., pp. 191–121. Cape Town: HSRC Press. [13]

Saloojee, H. 2007. Monitoring Child Health. In: Monitoring Child Well-Being. A South African Rights-Based Approach, ed. A. Dawes et al., pp. 93–110. Cape Town: HSRC Press. [13]

Sameroff, A. 2009. How to Become a Developmental Scientist. SRCD Devel. **52(3)**. [2]

Sanchez, M. M., K. McCormack, A. P. Grand, et al. 2010. Effects of Sex and Early Maternal Abuse on Adrenocorticotropin Hormone and Cortisol Responses to the Corticotropin-Releasing Hormone Challenge During the First 3 Years of Life in Group-Living Rhesus Monkeys. *Dev. Psychopathol.* **22**:45–53. [8]

Sanders, M. 2003. Triple P – Positive Parenting Program: A Population Approach to Promoting Competent Parenting. *Adv. Mental Health* **2**:1–17. [13]

———. 2008. The Triple P: Positive Parenting Program as a Public Health Approach to Strengthening Parenting. *J. Fam. Psychol.* **22**:506–517. [12]

Sandler, I., E. Schoenfelder, S. Wolchik, and D. MacKinnon. 2011. Long-Term Impact of Prevention Programs to Promote Effective Parenting: Lasting Effects but Uncertain Processes. *Annu. Rev. Psychol.* **62**:299–329. [14]

Sandy, S., and S. Boardman. 2000. The Peaceful Kids Conflict Resolution Program. *Intl. J. Conflict Manag.* **11**:337–357. [17]

Sapienza, J. K., and A. S. Masten. 2011. Understanding and Promoting Resilience in Children and Youth. *Curr. Opin. Psychiatry* **24**:267–273. [14]

Sapolsky, R. M. 2013. Rousseau with a Tail: Maintaining a Tradition of Peace among Baboons. In: War, Peace, and Human Nature: The Convergence of Evolutionary and Cultural Views, ed. D. P. Fry, pp. 421–438. New York: Oxford Univ. Press. [7]

Sapolsky, R. M., and L. J. Share. 2004. A Pacific Culture among Wild Baboons: Its Emergence and Transmission. *PloS Biol.* **2**:E106. [11]

Saraceno, B., M. V. Ommeren, R. Batniji, et al. 2007. Barriers to Improvement of Mental Health Services in Low-Income and Middle-Income Countries. *Lancet* **370**:1164–1174. [15]

Saunders, D., D. Bradshaw, and N. Ngongo. 2010. The Status of Child Health in South Africa. In: South African Child Gauge 2009/2010, ed. M. Kibel et al., pp. 29–40. Cape Town: Children's Institute, Univ. of Cape Town. [13]

Schiff, M., R. Pat-Horenczyk, R. Benbenishty, et al. 2012. High School Students' Posttraumatic Symptoms, Substance Abuse and Involvement in Violence in the Aftermath of War. *Soc. Sci. Med.* **75**:1321–1328. [14]

Schmidt, M. F. H., and J. A. Sommerville. 2011. Fairness Expectations and Altruistic Sharing in 15-Month-Old Human Infants. *PLoS One* **6**:e23223. [7]

Schorr, E. A., N. A. Fox, V. van Wassenhove, and E. I. Knudsen. 2005. Auditory-Visual Fusion in Speech Perception in Children with Cochlear Implants. *PNAS* **102**:18748–18750. [9]

Schott, W. B., B. T. Crookston, F. A. Lundeen, et al. 2013. Child Growth from Ages 1 to 8 Years in Ethiopia, India, Peru and Vietnam: Key Distal Household and Community Factors. *Soc. Sci. Med.* **97**:278–287. [15]

Schrumpf, F., D. K. Crawford, and R. J. Bodine. 1997. Peer Mediation: Conflict Resolution in Schools. Champaign: Research Press. [17]

Schwebel, M., and D. J. Christie. 2001. Children and Structural Violence. In: Peace, Conflict, and Violence: Peace Psychology in the 21st Century, ed. D. J. Christie et al., pp. 120–130. New York: Prentice-Hall. [13]

Schweinhart, L. J., J. Montie, Z. Xiang, et al. 2005. Lifetime Effects: The High/Scope Perry Preschool Study through Age 40. Ypsilanti: High/Scope Educational Research Foundation. [16]

Scrimin, S., U. Moscardino, F. Capello, G. Altoè, and G. Axia. 2009. Recognition of Facial Expressions of Mixed Emotions in School-Age Children Exposed to Terrorism. *Dev. Psychol.* **45**:1341–1352. [12]

Seltzer, L. J., T. Ziegler, M. J. Connolly, A. R. Prososki, and S. D. Pollak. 2014. Stress-Induced Elevation of Oxytocin in Maltreated Children: Evolution, Neurodevelopment and Social Behavior. *Child Dev.* **85**:501–512. [4]

Sen, A. 1999. Development as Freedom. Oxford: Oxford Univ. Press. [13]

Seng, J., J. Miller, M. Sperlich, et al. 2013. Exploring Dissociation and Oxytocin as Pathways between Trauma Exposure and Trauma-Related Hyperemesis Gravidarum: A Test-of-Concept Pilot. *J. Trauma Dissociation* **14**:40–55. [4]

Service, E. 1962. Primitive Social Organization: An Evolutionary Perspective. New York: Random House. [6]

Seung, S. 2012. Connectome: How the Brain's Wiring Makes Us Who We Are. New York: Houghton Mifflin Harcourt. [1]

Sferruzzi-Perri, A. N., O. R. Vaughan, P. M. Coan, et al. 2011. Placental-Specific Igf2 Deficiency Alters Developmental Adaptations to Undernutrition in Mice. *Endocrinology* **152**:3202–3212. [5]

Shah, A. A., and R. H. Beinecke. 2009. Global Mental Health Needs, Services, Barriers, and Challenges. *Intl. J. Ment. Health* **38**:14–29. [15]

Shalev, I., T. E. Moffitt, K. Sugden, et al. 2013. Exposure to Violence During Childhood Is Associated with Telomere Erosion from 5 to 10 Years of Age: A Longitudinal Study. *Mol. Psychiatry* **18**:576–581. [11]

Shanab, M. E., and K. A. Yahya. 1977. Behavioral Study of Obedience in Children. *J. Pers. Soc. Psychol.* **35**:530–536. [10]

Sharp, S., and P. Smith. 2002. School Bullying: Insights and Perspectives. New York: Routledge. [17]

Shaver, P. R., and M. Mikulincer. 2002. Dialogue on Adult Attachment: Diversity and Integration. *Attach. Hum. Dev.* **4**:243–257. [12]

Shaw, D. S., T. J. Dishion, L. Supplee, F. Gardner, and K. Arnds. 2006. Randomized Trial of a Family-Centered Approach to the Prevention of Early Conduct Problems: 2-Year Effects of the Family Check-up in Early Childhood. *J. Consult. Clin. Psychol.* **74**:1–9. [14]

Shaw, D. S., and H. E. Gross. 2008. What We Have Learned About Early Childhood and the Development of Delinquency. In: The Long View of Crime: A Synthesis of the Longitudinal Research, ed. A. M. Liberman, pp. 79–127. New York: Springer. [14]

Shen, Y.-J. 2002. Short-Term Group Play Therapy with Chinese Earthquake Victims: Effects on Anxiety, Depression and Adjustment. *Intl. J. Play Therapy* **11**:43–63. [15]

Sheppes, G., S. Scheibe, G. Suri, et al. 2014. Emotion Regulation Choice: A Conceptual Framework and Supporting Evidence. *J. Exp. Psychol. Gen.* **143**:163–181. [12]

Sheridan, M., J. Howard, and D. Alderson. 2011. Play in Early Childhood: From Birth to Six Years (3rd edition). Oxon: Routledge. [7]

Sheridan, M., K. Sarsour, D. Jutte, M. D'Esposito, and W. T. Boyce. 2012a. The Impact of Social Disparity on Prefrontal Function in Childhood. *PLoS One* **7**:e35744. [7]

Sheridan, M., N. A. Fox, C. H. Zeanah, K. McLaughlin, and C. A. Nelson. 2012b. Variation in Neural Development as a Result of Exposure to Institutionalization Early in Childhood. *PNAS* **109**:12927–12932. [9]

Sherif, M. 1936. The Psychology of Social Norms. New York: Harper Collins. [7]

————. 1966. In Common Predicament: Social Psychology of Intergroup Conflict and Cooperation. Boston: Houghton Mifflin Company. [19]

Sherif, M., O. J. Harvey, B. J. White, W. R. Hood, and C. W. Sherif. 1954/1961. Intergroup Conflict and Cooperation: The Robber's Cave Experiment. Norman: Univ. of Oklahoma Press. [6, 7, 14]

Sherif, M., and C. W. Sherif. 1953. Groups in Harmony and Tension: An Integration of Studies on Intergroup Relations. New York: Harper. [17]

Shonkoff, J. P. 2010. Building a New Biodevelopmental Framework to Guide the Future of Early Childhood Policy. *Child Dev.* **81**:357–367. [7]

Shonkoff, J. P., and P. A. Fisher. 2013. Rethinking Evidence-Based Practice and Two-Generation Programs to Create the Future of Early Childhood Policy. *Dev. Psychopathol.* **25**:1635–1653. [7]

Shonkoff, J. P., A. S. Garner, B. S. Siegel, et al. 2012. The Lifelong Effects of Early Childhood Adversity and Toxic Stress. *Pediatrics* **129**:e232–e246. [14, 15]

Shonkoff, J. P., and P. Levitt. 2010. Neuroscience and the Future of Early Childhood Policy: Moving from Why to What and How. *Neuron* **67**:689–691. [7]

Shonkoff, J. P., and D. A. Phillips, eds. 2000. From Neurons to Neighborhoods: The Science of Early Childhood Development. Washington, D.C.: National Academies Press. [3, 17, 19]

Shulruf, B., C. O'Loughlin, and H. Tolley. 2009. Parenting Education and Support Policies and Their Consequences in Selected OECD Countries. *Child Youth Serv. Rev.* **31**:525–532. [3]

Siddiqui, A., and H. Ross. 2004. Mediation as a Method of Parent Intervention in Children's Disputes. *J. Fam. Psychol.* **18**:147–159. [16]

Siegel, D. J. 2012. The Developing Mind (2nd edition): How Relationships and the Brain Interact to Shape Who We Are. New York: Guilford Press. [7]

Simic, O., Z. Volcic, and C. R. Philpot. 2012. Peace Psychology in the Balkans: In Times Past, Present and Future. New York: Springer. [15]

Simon, L. 2010. Working to Change the World: An Examination of One Child's Social Activism. *Urban Rev.* **42**:296–315. [15]

Simpson, J. A., V. Griskevicius, S. I.-C. Kuo, S. Sung, and W. A. Collins. 2012. Evolution, Stress, and Sensitive Periods: The Influence of Unpredictability in Early Versus Late Childhood on Sex and Risky Behavior. *Dev. Psychol.* **48**:674–686. [7]

Singer, I. 2012. Beyond Violence: A Film and Workshop. http://movingbeyondviolence.org/index.html. (accessed June 6, 2014). [18]

Skoufias, E. 2001. Progresa and Its Impacts on the Welfare and Human Capital of Adults and Children in Rural Mexico: A Synthesis of the Results of an Evaluation by the International Food Policy Research Institute (IFPRI). Washington, D.C.: IFPRI, Food Consumption and Nutrition Division. [15]

Slade, A., L. Sadler, C. D. Dios-Kenn, et al. 2005. Minding the Baby: A Reflective Parenting Program. *Psychoanal. Study Child* **60**:74–100. [3]

Smallwood, S. A., and G. Kelsey. 2012. *De Novo* DNA Methylation: A Germ Cell Perspective. *Trends Genet.* **28**:33–42. [5]

Smilansky, M., and D. Nevo. 1979. The Gifted Disadvantaged. London: Gordon and Breach. [16]

Smith, H. J., T. F. Pettigrew, G. M. Pippin, and S. Bialosiewicz. 2012. Relative Deprivation: A Theoretical and Meta-Analytic Review. *Pers. Soc. Psychol. Rev.* **16**:203–232. [15]

Smith, K. E., E. C. Porges, G. J. Norman, J. J. Connelly, and J. Decety. 2014. Oxytocin Receptor Gene Variation Predicts Empathic Concern and Autonomic Arousal While Perceiving Harm to Others. *Soc. Neurosci.* **9**:1–9. [4]

Smith, P. K., and K. J. Connolly. 1980. The Ecology of Preschool Behavior. Cambridge: Cambridge Univ. Press. [7]

Snyder, M., R. Snyder, and R. Snyder, Jr. 1980. The Young Child as Person: Toward the Development of Healthy Conscience. New York: Human Sciences Press. [3]

Sommerville, J. A., M. F. H. Schmidt, J. Yun, and M. Burns. 2013. The Development of Fairness Expectations and Prosocial Behavior in the Second Year of Life. *Infancy* **18**:40–66. [7]

Soubry, A., C. Hoyo, R. L. Jirtle, and S. K. Murphy. 2014. A Paternal Environmental Legacy: Evidence for Epigenetic Inheritance through the Male Germ Line. *Bioessays* **36**:359–371. [1]

Souillac, G. 2011. The Burden of Democracy: The Claims of Cultures, Public Cultures, and Democratic Memory. Lanham, MD: Lexington Books. [6]

———. 2012. A Study in Transborder Ethics: Justice, Citizenship, Civility. Brussels: Peter Lang. [6]

Sowell, E. R., P. M. Thompson, K. D. Tessner, and A. W. Toga. 2001. Mapping Continued Brain Growth and Gray Matter Density Reduction in Dorsal Frontal Cortex: Inverse Relationships During Postadolescent Brain Maturation. *J. Neurosci.* **21**:8819–8829. [5]

Spiecker, B. 1991. Emoties En Morele Opvoeding (Emotions and Moral Education). Amsterdam: Boom. [10]

Spiel, C., and D. Strohmeier. 2012. Peer Relations in Multicultural Schools. In: Realizing the Potential of Immigrant Youth, ed. A. S. Masten et al., pp. 376–396. New York: Cambridge Univ. Press. [14]

Sroufe, L. A. 1996. Emotional Development: The Organization of Emotional Life in the Early Years. New York: Cambridge Univ. Press. [7]

Sroufe, L. A., B. Egeland, E. Carlson, and W. A. Collins. 2005. Placing Early Attachment Experiences in Developmental Context. In: Attachment from Infancy to Adulthood: The Major Longitudinal Studies, ed. K. E. Grossmann et al., pp. 48–70. New York: Guilford Press. [11]

Sroufe, L. A., and M. C. Sampson. 2000. Attachment Theory and Systems Concepts. *Hum. Dev.* **43**:321–326. [12]

Srour, W. A. 2005. Children Living under a Multi-Traumatic Environment: The Palestinian Case. *Isr. J. Psychiatry Relat. Sci.* **42**:88–95. [18]

Staff, R. T., A. D. Murray, T. S. Ahearn, et al. 2012. Childhood Socioeconomic Status and Adult Brain Size: Childhood Socioeconomic Status Influences Adult Hippocampal Size. *Ann. Neurol.* **71**:653–660. [7]

Staub, E. 1989. The Roots of Evil: The Origins of Genocide and Other Group Violence. New York: Cambridge Univ. Press. [6]

Staub, E., L. A. Pearlman, A. Gubin, and A. Hagengimana. 2005. Healing, Reconciliation, Forgiving and the Prevention of Violence after Genocide or Mass Killing: An Intervention and Its Experimental Evaluation in Rwanda. *J. Soc. Clin. Psychol.* **24**:297–334. [15]

Steele, H., and M. Steele. 2005. Understanding and Resolving Emotional Conflict: The View from 12 Years of Attachment Research across Generations and across Childhood. In: Attachment from Infancy to Adulthood: The Major Longitudinal Studies, ed. K. E. Grossmann et al., pp. 137–164. New York: Guilford Press. [11]

Steele, M., J. Hodges, J. Kaniuk, S. Hillman, and K. Henderson. 2003. Attachment Representations and Adoption: Associations between Maternal States of Mind and Emotion Narratives in Previously Maltreated Children. *J. Child Psychother.* **29**:187–205. [11]

Steele, M., J. Hodges, J. Kaniuk, et al. 2008. Forecasting Outcomes in Previously Maltreated Children: The Use of the AAI in a Longitudinal Adoption Study. In: Clinical Applications of the Adult Attachment Interview, ed. H. Steele and M. Steele, pp. 427–451. New York: Guilford Press. [11]

Stephan, W. G., and K. Finlay. 1999. The Role of Empathy in Improving Intergroup Relations. *J. Soc. Iss.* **55**:729–743. [15]

Steutel, J., and B. Spiecker. 2004. Cultivating Sentimental Dispositions through Aristotelian Habituation. *J. Philos. Educ.* **38**:531–549. [10]

Stewart, R. C., E. Umar, F. Kauye, et al. 2008. Maternal Common Mental Disorder and Infant Growth: A Cross-Sectional Study from Malawi. *Matern. Child Nutr.* **4**:209–219. [15]

Stoltenborgh, M., M. J. Bakermans-Kranenburg, L. R. Alink, and M. H. van IJzendoorn. 2012. The Universality of Childhood Emotional Abuse: A Meta-Analysis of Worldwide Prevalence. *J. Aggress. Maltreat. Trauma* **21**:870–890. [11]

Stoltenborgh, M., M. J. Bakermans-Kranenburg, and M. H. van IJzendoorn. 2013a. The Neglect of Child Neglect: A Meta-Analytic Review of the Prevalence of Neglect. *Soc. Psychiatry Psychiatr. Epidemiol.* **48**:345–355. [11]

Stoltenborgh, M., M. J. Bakermans-Kranenburg, M. H. van IJzendoorn, and L. R. Alink. 2013b. Cultural–Geographical Differences in the Occurrence of Child Physical Abuse? A Meta-Analysis of Global Prevalence. *Intl. J. Psychol.* **48**:81–94. [11]

Stoop, R. 2012. Neuromodulation by Osytocin and Vasopressin. *Neuron* **76**:142–159. [4]

Strathearn, L., P. Fonagy, J. Amico, and P. R. Montague. 2009. Adult Attachment Predicts Maternal Brain and Oxytocin Response to Infant Cues. *Neuropsychopharmacology* **3413**:2655–2666. [3]

Stratton, K. R., C. J. Howe, and F. C. Battaglia. 1996. Fetal Alcohol Syndrome Diagnosis, Epidemiology, Prevention, and Treatment. Institute of Medicine, Division of Biobehavioral Sciences and Mental Disorders, Committee to Study Fetal Alcohol Syndrome and National Institute on Alcohol Abuse and Alcoholism. Washington, D.C.: National Academy. [13]

Stribley, J. M., and C. S. Carter. 1999. Developmental Exposure to Vasopressin Increases Aggression in Adult Prairie Voles. *PNAS* **96**:12601–12604. [4]

Stuebe, A. M., K. Grewen, and S. Meltzer-Brody. 2013. Association between Maternal Mood and Oxytocin Response to Breastfeeding. *J. Womens Health* **22**:352–361. [4]

Stürmer, S., M. Snyder, and A. M. Omoto. 2005. Prosocial Emotions and Helping: The Moderating Role of Group Membership. *J. Pers. Soc. Psychol.* **88**:532. [15]

Suderman, M., P. O. McGowan, A. Sasaki, et al. 2012. Conserved Epigenetic Sensitivity to Early Life Experience in the Rat and Human Hippocampus. *PNAS* **109**:17266–17272. [5, 7]

Suedfeld, P., R. W. Cross, and M. Stewart. 2012. Levels of Analysis Problem. In: Encyclopedia of Peace Psychology, ed. D. J. Christie, pp. 595–599. New York: Wiley-Blackwell. [15]

Suess, G. J., K. Grossmann, and L. A. Sroufe. 1992. Effects of Infant Attachment to Mother and Father on Quality of Adaptation in Preschool: From Dyadic to Individual Organisation of Self. *Intl. J. Behav. Dev.* **15**:43–65. [11]

Sunar, D. 2009. Suggestions for a New Integration in the Psychology of Morality. *Soc. Personal. Psychol. Compass* **3**:447–474. [7]

Sunar, D., C. Kagitcibasi, J. F. Leckman, et al. 2013. Is Early Childhood Relevant for Peace-Building? *J. Peacebuilding Devel.* **8**:81–85. [1, 3]

Super, C. M., and S. Harkness. 1986. The Developmental Niche: A Conceptualization at the Interface of Child and Culture. *Intl. J. Behav. Dev.* **9**:545–569. [2]

Super, C. M., S. Harkness, and C. J. Mavridis. 2011. Parental Ethnotheories About Children's Socioemotional Development. In: Socioemotional Development in Cultural Context, ed. X. Chen and K. H. Rubin, pp. 73–98. New York: Guilford Press. [2]

Swart, H., and M. Hewstone. 2012. Intergroup Forgiveness. In: Encyclopedia of Peace Psychology, ed. D. J. Christie, pp. 445–449. New York: Wiley-Blackwell. [15]

Sweet, M. A., and M. I. Appelbaum. 2004. Is Home Visiting an Effective Strategy? A Meta-Analytic Review of Home Visiting Programs for Families with Young Children. *Child Dev.* **75**:1435–1456. [16]

Syme, S. L. 2008. Reducing Racial and Social-Class Inequalities in Health: The Need for a New Approach. *Health Aff.* **27**:456–459. [11]

Szyf, M. 2011. The Early Life Social Environment and DNA Methylation: DNA Methylation Mediating the Long-Term Impact of Social Environments Early in Life. *Epigenetics* **6**:971–978. [5]

———. 2013a. DNA Methylation, Behavior and Early Life Adversity. *J. Genet. Genomics* **40**:331–338. [7]

———. 2013b. How Do Environments Talk to Genes? *Nat. Neurosci.* **16**:2–4. [5]

Szyf, M., and J. Bick. 2013. DNA Methylation: A Mechanism for Embedding Early Life Experiences in the Genome. *Child Dev.* **84**:49–57. [1]

Tabibnia, G., and M. D. Lieberman. 2007. Fairness and Cooperation Are Rewarding: Evidence from Social Cognitive Neuroscience. *Ann. NY Acad. Sci.* **1118**:90–101. [7]

Tajfel, H. 1982. Social Identity and Intergroup Relations. Cambridge: Cambridge Univ. Press. [7]

Talwar, V., H. M. Gordon, and K. Lee. 2007. Lying in the Elementary School Years: Verbal Deception and Its Relation to Second-Order Belief Understanding. *Dev. Psychol.* **43**:804–810. [10]

Tam, T., M. Hewstone, J. B. Kenworthy, et al. 2008. Postconflict Reconciliation: Intergroup Forgiveness and Implicit Biases in Northern Ireland. *J. Soc. Iss.* **64**:303–320. [15]

Tedeschi, R. G., and L. G. Calhoun. 2004. A Clinical Approach to Posttraumatic Growth. In: Positive Psychology in Practice, ed. P. A. Linley and S. Joseph, pp. 405–419. Hoboken, NJ: Wiley. [12]

Telzer, E. H., C. Masten, L., E. T. Berkman, M. D. Lieberman, and A. J. Fuligni. 2011. Neural Regions Associated with Self-Control and Mentalizing Are Recruited During Prosocial Behaviors Towards the Family. *NeuroImage* **58**:242–249. [10]

Thabet, A. A., A. N. Ibraheem, R. Shivram, E. A. Winter, and P. Vostanis. 2009. Parenting Support and PTSD in Children of a War Zone. *Intl. J. Soc. Psychiatry* **55**:226–237. [12]

Thaler, R. H., and C. R. Sunstein. 2008. Nudge: Improving Decisions About Health, Wealth, and Happiness. New Haven: Yale Univ. Press. [10, 11]

Thayer, Z. M., and C. W. Kuzawa. 2014. Early Origins of Health Disparities: Material Deprivation Predicts Maternal Evening Cortisol in Pregnancy and Offspring Cortisol Reactivity in the First Few Weeks of Life. *Am. J. Hum. Biol.* doi: 10.1002/ajhb.22532 (Epub ahead of print). [7]

Themner, L., and P. Wallensteen. 2012. Armed Conflicts 1946–2011. *J. World Peace* **49**:565–575. [4]

Thomas, R., and M. J. Zimmer-Gembeck. 2011. Accumulating Evidence for Parent-Child Interaction Therapy in the Prevention of Child Maltreatment. *Child Dev.* **82**:177–192. [14]

Thompson, L. Y., C. R. Snyder, L. Hoffman, et al. 2005. Dispositional Forgiveness of Self, Others, and Situations. *J. Pers. Soc. Psychol.* **73**:313–360. [15]

Thompson, R. A. 2008. Early Attachment and Later Development: Familiar Questions, New Answers. In: Handbook of Attachment: Theory, Research, and Clinical Applications, ed. J. Cassidy and P. Shaver, pp. 348–365. New York: Guilford Press. [2]

Thompson, R. A., and E. K. Newton. 2013. Baby Altruists? Examining the Complexity of Prosocial Motivation in Young Children. *Infancy* **18**:120–133. [7]

Thomsen, L., W. E. Frankenhuis, M. Ingold-Smith, and S. Carey. 2011. Big and Mighty: Preverbal Infants Mentally Represent Social Dominance. *Science* **331**:477–480. [7, 11]

Tiemeier, H., F. P. Velders, E. Szekely, et al. 2012. The Generation R Study: A Review of Design, Findings to Date and a Study of the 5-HTTLPR by Environment Interaction from Fetal Life Onwards. *J. Am. Acad. Child Adolesc. Psychiatry* **51**:1119–1135. e1117. [10]

Tiffin, P. A., M. S. Pearce, and L. Parker. 2005. Social Mobility over the Lifecourse and Self Reported Mental Health at Age 50: A Prospective Cohort Study. *J. Epidemiol. Comm. Health* **59**:870–872. [7]

Tol, W., M. Jordans, B. Kohrt, T. Betancourt, and I. Komproe. 2014. Promoting Mental Health and Psychological Wellbeing in Children Affected by Political Violence: Current Evidence for an Ecological Resilience Approach. In: Children and War: A Handbook for Promoting Resilience, ed. C. Fernando and M. Ferrari, pp. 11–27. New York: Springer. [12]

Tol, W. A., V. Patel, M. Tomlinson, et al. 2011. Research Priorities for Mental Health and Psychosocial Support in Humanitarian Settings. *PLoS Med.* **8**:e1001096. [12]

Tol, W. A., S. Song, and M. J. D. Jordans. 2013. Resilience and Mental Health in Children and Adolescents Living in Areas of Armed Conflict: A Systematic Review of Findings in Low and Middle-Income Countries. *J. Child Psychol. Psychiat.* **54**:445–460. [4, 12]

Tomlinson, M. R., A. Dawes, and A. J. Flisher. 2012. Preventing the Development of Youth Violence in the Early Years: Implications for South African Practice. In: Youth Violence: Sources and Solutions in South Africa, ed. C. L. Ward et al., pp. 141–174. Cape Town: UCT Press. [13, 15]

Tomlinson, M., M. J. O'Connor, I. M. LeRoux, et al. 2014a. Multiple Risk Factors During Pregnancy in South Africa: The Need for a Horizontal Approach to Perinatal Care. *Prev. Sci.* **15**:277–282. [15]

Tomlinson, M., A. D. Rahman, J. Sanders, J. Maselko, and M. J. Rotheram-Borus. 2014b. Leveraging Paraprofessionals and Family Strengths to Improve Coverage and Penetration of Nutrition and Early Child Development Services. *Ann. NY Acad. Sci.* **1308**:162–171. [15]

Tomlinson, M., L. Swartz, and K. Daniels. 2011. No Health without Mental Health: The Global Effort to Improve Population Mental Health. In: Population Mental Health: Evidence, Policy, and Public Health Practice, ed. N. Cohen and S. Galea, pp. 174–191. London: Routledge. [15]

Tonkinson, R. 1974. The Jigalong Mob: Aboriginal Victors of the Desert Crusade. Menlo Park, CA: Cummings. [6]

———. 2004. Resolving Conflict within the Law: The Mardu Aborigines of Australia. In: Keeping the Peace: Conflict Resolution and Peaceful Societies around the World, ed. G. Kemp and D. P. Fry, pp. 89–104. New York: Routledge. [6]

Toth, S. L., and J. Gravener. 2012. Bridging Research and Practice: Relational Interventions for Maltreated Children. *Child Adolesc. Ment. Health* **17**:131–138. [14]

Toth, S. L., F. A. Rogosch, J. T. Manly, and D. Cicchetti. 2006. The Efficacy of Toddler-Parent Psychotherapy to Reorganize Attachment in the Young Offspring of Mothers with Major Depressive Disorder: A Randomized Preventive Trial. *J. Consult. Clin. Psychol.* **74**:1006–1016. [11]

Tottenham, N., T., A. Hare, A. Millner, et al. 2011. Elevated Amygdala Response to Faces Following Early Deprivation. *Dev. Sci.* **14**:190–204. [9]

Tottenham, N., T. A. Hare, B. T. Quinn, et al. 2010. Prolonged Institutional Rearing Is Associated with Atypically Large Amygdala Volume and Difficulties in Emotion Regulation. *Dev. Sci.* **13**:46–61. [9]

Tottenham, N., and M. A. Sheridan. 2009. A Review of Adversity, the Amygdala and the Hippocampus: A Consideration of Developmental Timing. *Front. Hum. Neurosci.* **3**:68. [9]

Toussint, L., and Webb, J. R. 2005. Theoretical and empirical connections between forgiveness, mental health, and well-being. In: Handbook of forgiveness, ed. E. L. Worthington, Jr., pp. 349–362. New York: Routledge.[12]

Trask, E. V., K. Walsh, and D. DiLillo. 2011. Treatment Effects for Common Outcomes of Child Sexual Abuse: A Current Meta-Analysis. *Aggress. Violent Behav.* **16**:6–19. [12]

Tremblay, R. E. 2010. Developmental Origins of Disruptive Behaviour Problems: The "Original Sin" Hypothesis, Epigenetics and Their Consequences for Prevention. *J. Child Psychol. Psychiatry* **51**:341–367. [10]

Trivers, R. L. 1971. The Evolution of Reciprocal Altruism. *Q. Rev. Biol.* **46**:35–57. [7]

Tronick, E. Z., and J. F. Cohn. 1989. Infant-Mother Face-to-Face Interaction: Age and Gender Differences in Coordination and the Occurrence of Miscoordination. *Child Dev.* **60**:85–92. [11]

Tronick, E. Z., G. A. Morelli, and S. Winn. 1987. Multiple Caretaking of Efe (Pygmy) Infants. *Am. Anthropol.* **89**:96–106. [11]

Troy, M., and L. A. Sroufe. 1987. Victimization among Preschoolers: Role of Attachment Relationship History. *J. Am. Acad. Child Adolesc. Psychiatry* **26**:166–172. [11]

Tung, Y. C., D. Ayuso, X. Shan, et al. 2010. Hypothalamic-Specific Manipulation of *Fto*, the Ortholog of Human Obesity Gene *FTO*, Affects Food Intake in Rats. *PLoS One* **5**:e8771. [5]

Turner, R. N., M. Hewstone, and A. Voci. 2007. Reducing Explicit and Implicit Outgroup Prejudice Via Direct and Extended Contact: The Mediating Role of Self-Disclosure and Intergroup Anxiety. *J. Pers. Soc. Psychol.* **93**:369–388. [15]

Twardosz, S., and J. R. Lutzker. 2010. Child Maltreatment and the Developing Brain: A Review of Neuroscience Perspectives. *Aggress. Violent Behav.* **15**:59–68. [12]

Tyrka, A. R., L. H. Price, C. Marsit, O. C. Walters, and L. L. Carpenter. 2012. Childhood Adversity and Epigenetic Modulation of the Leukocyte Glucocorticoid Receptor: Preliminary Findings in Healthy Adults. *PLoS One* **7**:e30148. [7]

Tyzio, R., R. Cossart, I. Khalilov, et al. 2006. Maternal Oxytocin Triggers a Transient Inhibitory Switch in GABA Signaling in the Fetal Brain During Delivery. *Science* **314**:1788–1792. [4]

Tyzio, R., R. Nardou, D. C. Ferrari, et al. 2014. Oxytocin-Mediated GABA Inhibition During Delivery Attenuates Autism Pathogenesis in Rodent Offspring. *Science* **343**:675–679. [4]

UN. 1999. General Assembly: Declaration and Programme of Action on a Culture of Peace. A/Res/53/243. Official Record of the United Nations. New York, September 13, 1999. [1]

UNCRC. 1989. Convention on the Rights of the Child. United Nations Treaty Series 1577 [13]

UNESCO. 2007. Strong Foundations: Early Childhood Care and Education. EFA Global Monitoring Report 2007. Paris: UNESCO. [13]

———. 2010. Reaching the Marginalized. EFA Global Monitoring Report 2010, Education for All. Oxford: Oxford Univ. Press. [1]

———. 2013. Half of All out-of-School Children Live in Conflict-Affected Countries. UNESCO Press Release, July 7, 2013. [14]

Ungar, M., M. Ghazinour, and J. Richter. 2013. What is resilience within the social ecology of human development? *J. Child Psychol. Psychiatry* **54**:348–366. [14]

UNICEF. 2007. Innocenti Report Card 7: Child Poverty in Perspective: An Overview of Child Well-Being in Rich Countries. New York: UNICEF. [1]

———. 2009. United Nations Children's Fund. Machel Study 10-Year Strategic Review: Children and Conflict in a Changing World. New York: UNICEF. [12]

———. 2012. Child Poverty and Inequality: New Perspectives, ed. I. Ortiz, L. M. Daniels, and S. Engilbertsdóttir. New York: UNICEF, Division of Policy and Practice. [1]

U.S. Department of Health and Human Services. 2011. CDC Health Disparities and Inequalities Report—United States. In: Morbidity and Mortality Weekly Report. Atlanta: Center for Disease Control and Prevention. [11]

———. 2014. Patterns in Conflict: Civilians Are Now the Target. http://www.unicef. org/graca/patterns.htm. (accessed June 6, 2014). [18]

Vaish, A., M. Carpenter, and M. Tomasello. 2009. Sympathy through Affective Perspective Taking and Its Relation to Prosocial Behaviors in Toddlers. *Dev. Psychol.* **45**:534–543. [16]

Van den Berg, S. 2010. Current Poverty and Income Distribution in the Context of South African History. A Working Paper of the Department of Economics and the Bureau for Economic Research at the Univ. of Stellenbosch. Stellenbosch: Bureau for Economic Research. [13]

van der Dennen, J. M. G. 1995. The Origin of War. Groningen: Origin Press. [6]

Van der Mark, I. L., M. H. van IJzendoorn, and M. J. Bakermans-Kranenburg. 2002. Development of Empathy in Girls During the Second Year of Life: Associations with Parenting, Attachment and Temperament. *Soc. Dev.* **11**:451–468. [10]

Van der Molen, M. J. W., and M. W. Van der Molen. 2013. Reduced Alpha and Exaggerated Theta Power During the Resting-State EEG in Fragile X Syndrome. *Biol. Psychol.* **92**:216–219. [9]

Vanderwert, R. E., P. J. Marshall, C. A. Nelson, C. H. Zeanah, and N. A. Fox. 2010. Timing of Intervention Affects Brain Electrical Activity in Children Exposed to Severe Psychosocial Neglect. *PLoS ONE* **5**:1–5. [9]

van Ee, E., R. J. Kleber, and T. T. M. Mooren. 2011. War Trauma Lingers On. Associations between Maternal PTSD, Parent Child Interaction and Child Development. *Infant Ment. Health J.* **33**:459–468. [12]

Van Horn, P., and A. F. Lieberman. 2012. Early Exposure to Trauma: Domestic and Community Violence. In: The Cambridge Handbook of Environments in Human Development, ed. L. C. Mayes and M. Lewis, pp. 466–479. New York: Cambridge Univ. Press. [14]

van IJzendoorn, M. H. 1995. Adult Attachment Representations, Parental Responsiveness, and Infant Attachment: A Meta-Analysis on the Predictive Validity of the Adult Attachment Interview. *Psychol. Bull.* **117**:387–403. [11]

———. 1997. Attachment, Emergent Morality, and Aggression: Toward a Developmental Socioemotional Model of Antisocial Behaviour. *Int. J. Behav. Dev.* **21**:703–727. [10]

van IJzendoorn, M. H., and M. J. Bakermans-Kranenburg. 2011. On Embodied and Situational Morality: Neurobiological, Parental and Situational Determinants of Altruism and Donating to Charity. In: Moral Education and Development: A Lifetime Commitment, ed. D. J. de Ruyter and S. Miedema, pp. 13–30. Rotterdam/ Boston: Sense. [10]

———. 2012a. Integrating Temperament and Attachment. The Differential Susceptibility Paradigm. In: Handbook of Temperament, ed. M. Zentner and R. L. Shiner, vol. New York, pp. 403–424. Guilford. [10]

———. 2012b. A Sniff of Trust: Meta-Analysis of the Effects of Intranasal Oxytocin Administration on Face Recognition, Trust to In-Group, and Trust to Out-Group. *Psychoneuroendocrinology* **37**:438–443. [3, 10]

van IJzendoorn, M. H., M. J. Bakermans-Kranenburg, F. Pannebakker, and D. Out. 2010. In Defense of Situational Morality: Genetic, Dispositional and Situational Determinants of Children's Donating to Charity. *J. Moral Educ.* **39**:1–20. [10]

van IJzendoorn, M. H., and A. Sagi-Schwartz. 2008. Cross-Cultural Patterns of Attachment: Universal and Contextual Dimensions. In: Handbook of Attachment: Theory, Research, and Clinical Applications, ed. J. Cassidy and P. Shaver, pp. 880–905. New York: Guilford Press. [2]

van Rompay, T. J. L., D. J. Vonk, and M. L. Fransen. 2009. The Eye of the Camera Effects of Security Cameras on Prosocial Behavior. *Environ. Behav.* **41**:60–74. [10]

van Tuijl, C., P. P. M. Leseman, and J. Rispens. 2001. Efficacy of an Intensive Home-Based Educational Intervention Program for 4- to 6-Year Old Ethnic Minority Children in the Netherlands. *Intl. J. Behav. Dev.* **25**:148–159. [16]

van Zeijl, J., J. Mesman, M. H. van IJzendoorn, et al. 2006. Attachment-Based Intervention for Enhancing Sensitive Discipline in Mothers of 1- to 3-Year-Old Children at Risk for Externalizing Behavior Problems: A Randomized Controlled Trial. *J. Consult. Clin. Psychol.* **74**:994–1005. [11]

Vasquez, V. M. 2004. Negotiating Critical Literacies with Young Children. Mahwah, NJ: Taylor and Francis. [15]

Verkuyten, V., and J. Thijs. 2013. Multicultural Education and Inter-Ethnic Attitudes: An Intergroup Perspective. *Eur. Psychol.* **18**:179–190. [15]

Vestal, A., and N. A. Jones. 2004. Peace Building and Conflict Resolution in Preschool Children. *J. Res. Childhood Educ.* **19**:131–142. [15]

Victora, C. G., P. C. Hallal, C. L. Araújo, et al. 2008. Cohort Profile: The 1993 Pelotas (Brazil) Birth Cohort Study. *Intl. J. Epidemiol* **37**:704–709. [15]

Vlachou, M., E. Andreou, K. Botsoglou, and E. Didaskalou. 2011. Bully/Victim Problems among Preschool Children: A Review of Current Research Evidence. *Educ. Psychol. Rev.* **23**:329–358. [16]

Volbrecht, M. M., K. Lemery-Chalfant, N. Aksan, Zahn-Waxler, C., and H. H. Goldsmith. 2007. Examining the Familial Link between Positive Affect and Empathy Development in the Second Year. *J. Gen. Psychol.* **168**:105–129. [10]

Volkan, V. 2004. Blind Trust. Charlottesville, VA: Pitchstone Publishing. [18]

Vul, E., C. Harris, P. Winkielman, and H. Pashler. 2009. Puzzlingly High Correlations in fMRI Studies of Emotion, Personality and Social Cognition. *Persp. Psychol. Sci.* **4**:274–290. [10]

Vygotsky, L., S. 1978. Mind in Society: The Development of Higher Psychological Processes (translated by M. Cole). Cambridge, MA: Harvard Univ. Press. [17]

Wachs, T., and A. Rahman. 2013. The Nature and Impact of Risk and Protective Influences on Children's Development in Low and Middle Income Countries. In: Handbook of Early Childhood Development Research and Its Impact on Global Policy, ed. P. R. Britto et al., pp. 85–160. New York: Oxford Univ. Press. [13–15]

Wachs, T. D., M. M. Black, and P. L. Engle. 2009. Maternal Depression: A Global Threat to Children's Health, Development, and Behavior and to Human Rights. *Child Dev. Perspect.* **3**:51–59. [15]

Wachs, T. D., and R. Plomin. 1991. Conceptualization and Measurement of Organism-Environment Interaction Synopsis. Washington, D.C.: American Psychological Association. [10]

Wade, N. G., and E. L. Worthington, Jr. 2005. In Search of a Common Core: A Content Analysis of Interventions to Promote Forgiveness. *Psychotherapy* **42**:160. [15]

Wagner, R. V. 2012. Empathy. In: Encyclopedia of Peace Psychology, ed. D. J. Christie, pp. 395–400. New York: Wiley-Blackwell. [15]

Walker, S. P., T. D. Wachs, J. M. Gardner, et al. 2007. Child Development: Risk Factors for Adverse Outcomes in Developing Countries. *Lancet* **369**:145–157. [1, 13, 15]

Walker, S. P., T. D. Wachs, S. Grantham-McGregor, et al. 2011. Inequality in Early Childhood; Risk and Protective Factors for Early Child Development. *Lancet* **378**:1325–1338. [16]

Walsh, F. 2006. Strengthening Family Resilience (2nd edition). New York: Guilford Press. [14]

Walter, W. 2013. Last Ape Standing. New York: Walker and Co. [19]

Wang, A., W. Nie, H. Li, et al. 2014. Epigenetic Upregulation of Corticotrophin-Releasing Hormone Mediates Postnatal Maternal Separation-Induced Memory Deficiency. *PLoS One* **9**:e94394. [7]

Wang, J., M. Imaten, P. Venkatesan, C. Evans, and D. Mendelowitz. 2002. Arginine Vasopressin Enhances GABAergic Inhibition of Cardiac Parasympathetic Neurons in the Nucleus Ambiguus. *Neuroscience* **111**:699–705. [4]

Warneken, F., B. Hare, A. P. Melis, D. Hanus, and M. Tomasello. 2007. Spontaneous Altruism by Chimpanzees and Young Children. *PloS Biol.* **5**:1414–1420. [7]

Warneken, F., K. Lohse, A. P. Melis, and M. Tomasello. 2011. Young Children Share the Spoils after Collaboration. *Psychol. Sci.* **22**:267–273. [7]

Warneken, F., and M. Tomasello. 2006. Altruistic Helping in Human Infants and Young Chimpanzees. *Science* **311(5765)**:1301–1303. [7, 10]

———. 2009a. The Roots of Human Altruism. *Br. J. Psychol.* **100**:455–471. [10]

———. 2009b. Varieties of Altruism in Children and Chimpanzees. *Trends Cogn. Sci.* **13**:397–402. [7]

Weaver, I. C., N. Cervoni, F. A. Champagne, et al. 2004. Epigenetic Programming by Maternal Behavior. *Nat. Neurosci.* **78**:847–854. [3]

Weinfield, N. S., L. A. Sroufe, B. Egeland, and E. A. Carlson. 2008. Individual Differences in Infant-Caregiver Attachment: Conceptual and Empirical Aspects of Security. In: Handbook of Attachment: Theory, Research, and Clinical Applications, ed. J. Cassidy and P. R. Shaver, pp. 78–101. New York: Guilford Press. [2]

Weisman, O., and R. Feldman. 2013. Oxytocin Effects on the Human Brain: Findings, Questions and Future Directions. *Biol. Psychiatry* **74**:158–159. [4]

Weisman, O., O. Zagoory-Sharon, I. Schneiderman, I. Gordon, and R. Feldman. 2013. Plasma Oxytocin Distributions in a Large Cohort of Women and Men and Their Gender-Specific Associations with Anxiety. *Psychoneuroendocrinology* **38**:694–701. [4]

Werner, E. E. 2000. Through the Eyes of Innocents: Children Witness of World War II. Boulder: Westview Press. [14]

West-Eberhard, M. J. 2003. Developmental Plasticity and Evolution. New York: Oxford Univ. Press. [8]

Whiting, B. B., and W. M. Whiting. 1975. Children of Six Cultures: A Psycho-Cultural Analysis. Oxford: Harvard Univ. Press. [7]

WHO. 1999. Report of the Consultation on Child Abuse Prevention, Appendix A. Geneva: World Health Organization. [11]

———. 2005. Integrated Management of Childhood Illness. Geneva: World Health Organization. [13]

———. 2007. Preventing Child Maltreatment in Europe: A Public Health Approach. Violence and Injury Prevention Programme. Copenhagen: World Health Organization. [12]

———. 2009. Violence Prevention: The Evidence. Geneva: World Health Organization. [15]

———. 2013. World Health Statistics 2013. Geneva: World Health Organization. [13]

Wiggins, J. L., and C. S. Monk. 2013. A Translational Neuroscience Framework for the Development of Socioemotional Functioning in Health and Psychopathology. *Dev. Psychopathol.* **25**:1293–1309. [7]

Wilker, S., T. Elbert, and I.-T. Kolassa. 2014. The Downside of Strong Emotional Memories: How Human Memory-Related Genes Influence the Risk for Posttraumatic Stress Disorder—A Selective Review. *Neurobiol. Learn. Mem.* **112C**:75–86. [7]

Wilker, S., S. Kolassa, C. Vogler, et al. 2013. Resilience to the Development of Posttraumatic Stress Disorder Predicted by Common Kibra Alleles. *Biol. Psychiatry* **74**:664–671. [7]

Wilkinson, R., and K. Pickett. 2009. Why Greater Equality Makes Societies Stronger: The Spirit Level. New York: Bloomsbury Press. [1, 15]

———. 2010. The Spirit Level. Why Equality Is Better for Everyone. London: Penguin Books. [10, 13]

Williams, K. D., and B. Jarvis. 2006. Cyberball: A Program for Use in Research on Interpersonal Ostracism and Acceptance. *Behav. Res. Methods* **38**:174–180. [10]

Wilson, D. S., and J. Yoshimura. 1994. On the Coexistence of Specialists and Generalists. *Am. Nat.* **144**:692–707. [8]

Wilson, E. O. 1975. Sociobiology: The New Synthesis. Cambridge: Harvard Univ. Press. [17]

Wilson, F., and M. Ramphele. 1989. Uprooting Poverty. The South African Challenge. Cape Town: David Phillip. [13]

Winter, D. D., and D. C. Leighton. 2001. Structural Violence. In: Peace, Conflict, and Violence: Peace Psychology in the 21st Century, ed. D. J. Christie et al., pp. 99–102. New York: Prentice-Hall. [13]

Wiseman, H., E. Metzl, and J. P. Barber. 2006. Anger, Guilt, and Intergenerational Communication of Trauma in the Interpersonal Narratives of Second Generation Holocaust Survivors. *Am. J. Orthopsychiatry* **76**:176–184. [12]

Wohl, M. J. A., and N. R. Branscombe. 2005. Forgiveness and Collective Guilt Assignment to Historical Perpetrator Groups Depend on Level of Social Category Inclusiveness. *J. Pers. Soc. Psychol.* **88**:288–303. [15]

Woodside, D., J. Santa Barbara, and D. G. Benner. 1999. Psychological Trauma and Social Healing in Croatia. *Med. Confl. Surviv.* **15**:355–367. [12]

Woon, F. L., and D. W. Hedges. 2008. Hippocampal and Amygdala Volumes in Children and Adults with Childhood Maltreatment-Related Posttraumatic Stress Disorder: A Meta-Analysis. *Hippocampus* **18**:729–736. [12]

Wrangham, R., and L. Glowacki. 2012. Intergroup Aggression in Chimpanzees and War in Nomadic Hunter-Gatherers: Evaluating the Chimpanzee Model. *Hum. Nat.* **23**:5–29. [6]

Wright, S. C., A. Aron, T. McLaughlin-Volpe, and S. A. Ropp. 1997. The Extended Contact Effect: Knowledge of Cross-Group Friendships and Prejudice. *J. Pers. Soc. Psychol.* **73**:73–90. [15]

Yagmur, S., J. Mesman, M. Malda, M. J. Bakermans-Kranenburg, and H. Ekmekci. 2014. Video-Feedback Intervention Increases Sensitive Parenting in Ethnic Minority Mothers: A Randomized Control Trial. *Attach. Hum. Dev.* **16**:371–386. [11]

Yehuda, R., and L. M. Bierer. 2009. The Relevance of Epigenetics to PTSD: Implications for the DSM-V. *J. Trauma. Stress* **22**:427–434. [14]

Yehuda, R., S. M. Engel, S. R. Brand, et al. 2005. Transgenerational Effects of Posttraumatic Stress Disorder in Babies of Mothers Exposed to the World Trade Center Attacks During Pregnancy. *J. Clin. Endocrinol. Metab.* **90**:4115–4118. [14]

Yoshikawa, H. 1994. Prevention as Cumulative Protection: Effects of Early Family Support and Education on Chronic Delinquency and Its Risks. *Psychol. Bull.* **115**:28–54. [16]

Yoshikawa, H., J. L. Aber, and W. R. Beardslee. 2012. The Effects of Poverty on the Mental, Emotional, and Behavioral Health of Children and Youth: Implications for Prevention. *Am. Psychol.* **67**:272–284. [7]

Young, M. E., ed. 2002. From Early Child Development to Human Development: Investing in Our Children's Future. In: Proc. of a World Bank Conference on Investing in Our Children's Future. Washington, D.C.: The World Bank. [16]

Young, S. K., N. A. Fox, and C. Zahn-Waxler. 1999. The Relations between Temperament and Empathy in 2-Year Olds. *Dev. Psychol.* **35**:1189–1197. [16]

Yousafzai, A., M. Rasheed, and Z. Bhutta. 2013. Annual Research Review: Improved Nutrition: A Pathway to Resilience. *J. Child Psychol. Psychiatry* **54**:367–377. [15]

Zahn-Waxler, C., M. Radke-Yarrow, E. Wagner, and M. Chapman. 1992. Development of Concern for Others. *Dev. Psychol.* **28**:126–136. [10]

Zartman, I. W. 1993. A Skeptics View. In Culture and Negotiation: The Resolution of Water Disputes, ed. G. Faure and J. Rubin. London: Sage Publications. [17]

Zeanah, C. H., N. A. Fox, and C. A. Nelson. 2012. The Bucharest Early Intervention Project: Case Study in the Ethics of Mental Health Research. *J. Nerv. Ment. Dis.* **200**:243–247. [9]

Zeanah, C. H., M. R. Gunnar, R. B. McCall, J. M. Kreppner, and N. A. Fox. 2011. Children without Permanent Parents: Research, Practice, and Policy. VI: Sensitive Periods. *Monogr. Soc. Res. Child Dev.* **76**:147–162. [9]

Zeanah, C. H., C. A. Nelson, N. A. Fox, et al. 2003. Designing Research to Study the Effects of Institutionalization on Brain and Behavioral Development: The Bucharest Early Intervention Project. *Dev. Psychopathol.* **15**:885–907. [9]

Zeanah, C. H., A. T. Smyke, S. F. M. Koga, E. Carlson, and Bucharest Early Intervention Project Core Group. 2005. Attachment in Institutionalized and Community Children in Romania. *Child Dev.* **76**:1015–1028. [9]

Zevalkink, J. 1997. Attachment in Indonesia: The Mother-Child Relationship in Context. Doctoral Thesis. University of Nijmegen. [2]

Zhang, L., V. S. Hernandez, B. Liu, et al. 2012. Hypothalamic Vasopressin System Regulation by Maternal Separation: Its Impact on Anxiety in Rats. *Neuroscience* **215**:135–148. [4]

Zhang, T. Y., B. Labonté, X. L. Wen, G. Tureck, and M. J. Meaney. 2013. Epigenetic Mechanisms for the Early Environmental Regulation of Hippocampal Glucocorticoid Receptor Gene Expression in Rodents and Humans. *Neuropsychopharmacology* **38**:111–123. [4, 5]

Zhang, T. Y., and M. J. Meaney. 2010. Epigenetics and the Environmental Regulation of the Genome and Its Function. *Annu. Rev. Psychol.* **61**:439–466. [7]

Zigler, E., C. Taussig, and K. Black. 1992. Early Childhood Intervention: A Promising Preventative for Juvenile Delinquency. *Am. Psychol.* **8**:997–1006. [16]

Zimbardo, P. 2007. The Lucifer Effect: How Good People Turn Evil. New York: Random House. [10]

Zoellner, T., S. Rabe, A. Karl, and A. Maercker. 2008. Posttraumatic Growth in Accident Survivors: Openness and Optimism as Predictors of Its Constructive or Illusory Sides. *J. Clin. Psychol.* **64**:245–263. [12]

Subject Index

Abecedarian Project (USA) 13, 308, 310, 311

abusive parenting 107, 131, 138, 139, 204

adaptation 45–49, 68, 114, 139, 142, 148, 253–257, 269, 377–379
  parental 19, 21

addiction 59, 73. *See also* alcohol use, drug abuse

adoption 8, 106, 150. *See also* institutionalized child care

Adult Attachment Interview 198, 207

advocacy xix, 245

affiliation 43, 47, 66, 116, 117, 217

aggression 114, 117, 131–144, 137, 187–193, 231, 261, 309
  impact of gender 61, 189
  impact of social organization on 82, 91, 126
  impact of vasopressin 54, 56, 113
  neurobiology of 44, 45, 331
  predictors 216, 223
  role of group identity 341, 342

Ainsworth, Mary 22, 23

alcohol use 180, 245–247, 282

alloparenting 61, 115, 195, 200

allopregnenalone 70

altruism 26, 137, 165, 174, 217
  in early childhood 121–123, 170
  reciprocal 119, 120
  twin studies on 167

Alzheimer disease 73

amygdala 53, 100, 101, 104, 150–152, 157, 198, 229

Angelman Syndrome 69, 76

animal models 10, 61, 62, 128, 137–143

Anne Çocuk Eğitim Vakfı (AÇEV) 3–5, 15, 28, 63, 127, 312, 319, 342

anterior insula 175

antisocial behavior 162, 163, 177, 180, 201, 242, 252, 261, 266, 270, 278
  cheating 164, 165

Ashland, Oregon xix

attachment 19, 23, 52, 118, 158, 187, 262
  -based interventions 205–208
  secure 274, 295, 339, 342–344, 349–351, 366
  security 22, 23, 166, 169, 196–198, 208
  theory 19, 22, 23, 76, 199, 223

attention 103, 105, 150–153, 169, 197, 225
  deficits in 154, 157, 228

autism spectrum disorders 50, 51, 57, 59, 76, 173

autonomic nervous system 48, 50, 52, 55, 61, 103, 113, 114

Basic Human Needs (BHN) theory 329, 330, 332

Beyond Violence 344

biomarkers 14, 34, 123

bonds 107, 125, 199, 364
  early-life 32–34
  pair 32, 43, 53–57, 137
  social 7, 13, 45, 52, 195

borderline personality disorder 173

Bowlby, John 22, 23, 194, 195, 346

brain development 35, 65–78, 142, 145–147, 150–158
  effect of environment 71–74, 104, 105
  sensitive periods 148, 155, 158
  stress during 100–103
  transgenerational 69–71

Bronfenbrenner, Urie 5, 226, 231, 260, 324, 371

Bucharest Early Intervention Project 8, 145, 148–150, 157–159
  EEG studies 152–157

bullying 35, 190, 265, 266, 301, 309, 328

canalization. *See* neurodevelopmental canalization

cerebellum 151

Chicago Longitudinal Study 13, 308, 310, 311

child abuse 27, 32, 35, 44, 67, 107, 173, 185, 192, 201, 242, 265
    intergenerational 138

child care 20, 262, 270
    cultural differences in 195
    institutionalized 76, 106, 145–160

child health 34, 233, 241–246, 249, 280, 282

child maltreatment 201–205, 213, 215, 229, 246, 261, 262

child mortality 236

child rearing 19, 21, 49, 91, 307
    impact of culture 20, 195, 281
    intrafamily dynamics 318
    surrogate mother 72

children's rights xvi, 90, 233, 238, 240, 242, 324, 368, 371. *See also* Convention on the Rights of the Child

child soldiers 258–263, 268
    rehabilitation 260, 267, 296

Child Support Grant (S. Africa) 238, 243, 246, 247

chromatin 31, 66, 67, 74, 77

chronic stress 53, 114, 156, 187

City of Sanctuary Movement (UK) 381

cognitive behavioral therapy 229

collective narratives. *See* shared narratives

collective violence 214, 215, 228, 229, 275, 285, 332

Combatants for Peace (Palestine-Israel) 344

competition 24, 120, 131–134, 139, 141, 186–192
    intergroup 80, 83

conflict 29, 96, 122, 249, 332, 340–342
    defined 287, 326
    drivers 372
    impact on children 252, 258–260
    preventing 24, 328
    role of identity in 79–82, 266, 292, 299, 341, 342

conflict resolution 4, 27, 30, 126, 254, 263, 287–290, 297, 301, 323, 326

Peaceful Kids Program 335
    role of culture 332
    safe spaces 327, 334
    strategies 91, 140, 142, 195, 320, 333–336
    theories of 329–336

consciousness 52, 114, 153
    "critical" 299, 301

Convention on the Rights of the Child 207, 238, 250, 367, 369, 380

cooperation xvi, 8, 24, 32, 82, 87–89, 122, 137, 186–192, 291, 326, 327, 335, 373. *See also* prosocial behavior

cooperative principle of conversation 198, 199

corporal punishment 187, 202–204

corpus callosum 157

CORT. *See* glucocorticoids (CORT)

corticotropin-releasing factor 53, 54, 100

cortisol 14, 96, 107, 139, 158, 173, 220

Creative Associates International (USA) 331

culture 21, 81, 84, 195, 281, 289, 332, 378

culture of peace xiii–xx, 14, 204, 305, 322, 363, 370, 371, 380, 384
    components of xvii, 90
    defined xvi

culture of war xvii, xix

Cyberball computer game 171–173, 175–177

Declaration and Program of Action on a Culture of Peace xv–xvii, 370, 380

depression 74, 102, 107, 109, 123, 173, 216, 223, 319
    perinatal 52, 277, 279

developmental plasticity 136, 141, 220, 228, 364

diathesis-stress model 169, 207

differential susceptibility 45, 142, 161, 169–171, 188, 207, 208

direct violence 11, 125, 214, 233, 264, 274–276, 285–287
    defined 29, 234
    reducing 96, 126

divorce 21, 25, 221

DNA methylation 66, 67, 69, 72, 99
  differential 9, 73
domestic violence 117, 190, 214, 216,
  221, 222, 224, 227, 230, 289, 290
dominance hierarchies 118, 140, 187,
  189–192, 209, 372
donating behavior 169, 170, 178, 179
  fMRI studies 175
dopamine 62
  -related gene (DRD4) 169, 170
Down Syndrome 154
dreaming 220, 227, 228
drug abuse 44, 117, 245, 247

early childhood development
  defined 28, 29
  impact of structural violence on
    233–250
  relevance to peacebuilding 15, 30–38,
    125, 309, 327, 383
  role of media in 344–347, 369
early childhood interventions 4, 12–14,
  30, 34–38, 126, 127, 188, 198, 238–
  247, 262, 263, 266, 267, 279–281,
  296–299, 305–322
  Abecedarian Project (USA) 13, 308,
    310, 311
  attachment-based 205–209
  Chicago Longitudinal Study (USA) 13,
    308, 310, 311
  Early Head Start (USA) 280, 314, 315,
    320
  Family Foundations (USA) 317, 318
  High/Scope Perry Preschool Project
    (USA) 13, 308, 310, 311
  Huggy Puppy (Israel) 297, 317
  Ilifa Labantwana Essential Package (S.
    Africa) 241–249
  1-2-3 Magic (Canada) 314
  Parental Mediation (Canada) 317–320
  Toddlers without Tears (Australia) 314
Early Childhood Peace Consortium 15,
  383
Early Head Start program (USA) 280,
  314, 315, 320
early learning. *See* education

early-life adversity 9, 57, 99, 102–105,
  107, 116, 127, 145–160, 258–260
  impact on development 45, 50, 72, 173
  preventing 8, 270
Early Years program (N. Ireland) 346,
  369
ecological systems theory 5, 226, 231,
  371
ecology of peace 5, 27–40
education xviii, xix, 9, 226, 238, 261,
  262, 267, 271, 313, 325, 332–336,
  370, 375, 381. *See also* peace
  education
  access to 236
  early learning 36, 242, 243, 246–249,
    277, 280
  school performance 226, 278, 308,
    312, 321
  teacher training programs 194
educational media 345–348, 351,
  355–357
  Beyond Violence 344
  Sesame Workshop 345–351, 369
emotion regulation 44, 49, 104, 105,
  118, 146, 150, 151, 159, 219, 224,
  225, 229, 288
  interventions 296–298
empathy 7, 8, 20, 23, 32, 165–168, 189,
  195, 219, 274, 287–289, 291, 309,
  365
  defined 204
  in newborns 290
  interventions to promote 222, 229, 230
  Leiden longitudinal studies
    (Netherlands) 166, 168
ENCODE project 10, 31, 77
English and Romanian Adoptee study 8,
  148, 152
epigenetic modifications 8–10, 33, 34,
  58, 66, 74, 96, 110, 111
  role of environment 31–33, 97–100
epigenetics 8, 31, 46, 62, 65–78, 142,
  177, 260
epinephrine 100, 101, 105
equity 7, 10–12, 16, 37, 117, 120, 234,
  277, 357, 365

essential package of interventions.
   See Ilifa Labantwana Essential
   Package (S. Africa)

fairness 119, 122, 193, 194, 234, 235,
   274, 291, 327
Family Foundations (USA) 317, 318
family support/interventions 9, 12, 191,
   222–224, 311, 317, 318, 320
   in Afghanistan 289, 290
fathers 35, 117, 204, 222, 227, 277, 307,
   320
   programs for 4, 127, 319, 350, 382
food security 236, 241, 246, 265
forgiveness 123, 220, 230, 231, 288,
   289, 293, 301, 374
foster care 106, 148, 149, 154–157, 190
Fragile X Syndrome 154
frontal cortex 72, 101, 103, 177
future research needs 32, 33, 36, 37,
   59–63, 91, 158, 192, 194, 200,
   204, 208, 270, 271, 300, 301, 336,
   379–382, 384

GABA 62, 70
gene-environment interactions 65–78,
   137, 142, 161, 162, 169–171
Generation R study (Netherlands) 164,
   177
genomic imprinting 10, 66, 68–70, 75,
   142
global citizenship xviii, xx, 6, 7, 14, 79,
   80, 89–91, 339, 348–354, 370, 375,
   384
Global Movement for the Culture of
   Peace xviii, xix
glucocorticoids (CORT) 70, 73,
   100–102, 105, 157
group
   behavior 24, 25, 33, 117, 139, 186
   defined 82
   identity 79–94, 122, 292, 293, 339
   loyalties 82, 84
   neurobiology of 10, 123, 128
guilt 216, 218, 223
   collective 293

harsh parenting 136, 185, 188, 189,
   201–205, 222, 315, 320
Harvard Negotiation Project (USA) 331
helping behavior 121, 162–168, 291,
   301, 302
High/Scope Perry Preschool Project
   (USA) 13, 308, 310, 311
hippocampus 73, 156, 157, 177, 220,
   229
Huggy Puppy (Israel) 297, 317
human development 296, 324
   barriers to 277–284
   role of early experience 137–141
hunter-gatherers 81–83, 195, 237
hypothalamic-pituitary-adrenal (HPA)
   axis 45, 50, 53, 54, 70, 100, 139
   stress response 101, 102, 107
hypothalamic-pituitary-gonadal (HPG)
   axis 139
hypothalamus 51, 53, 65, 74, 101
   fetal 70, 71, 75
   maternal 65, 69–71, 75

identity 298, 372, 375
   group 79–94, 122, 292, 293, 339
   large group 342, 353–357
   manipulation of 341–343
   role in conflict 79–94, 82, 292, 299,
      368
   role in promoting peace 84–87
   social 36, 79–94, 274, 293, 299, 368
Ilifa Labantwana Essential Package (S.
   Africa) 16, 239–243
   components of 244–249
inequality 96, 193, 194, 235–237, 259,
   267, 276
   programs to reduce 240, 241, 282–284,
      289, 296
Infant Health and Development Program
   (USA) 311
in-group bias 80, 82, 122, 292, 293
insecurity 11, 196, 215, 372
   food 237, 242, 277
institutionalized child care 76, 106,
   145–160
   English and Romanian Adoptee (ERA)
      study 8, 148, 152

intelligence, built-in 97, 100, 112–124
interdependence xviii, 7, 20, 85, 87–89, 91, 126, 258, 373
interpersonal violence 214–216, 222, 228, 229, 252, 266, 278, 285
interventions 332, 377, 378. *See also* early childhood interventions
   assessing 302
   community-based 315
   home-based 306, 308, 312, 314
   media-based 351, 352
   principles for 325–327
   windows of opportunity 265, 295
intrafamily dynamics 312–314, 318
   sibling relations 200, 217–222
intranasal oxytocin 55, 119, 162, 171–174, 182
in utero development 7, 65, 67, 69–71, 75
Iroquois Confederacy 85–87

Jamaica Study 13, 308, 312, 313
justpeace 274

kin selection 121
knowledge translation 366, 367, 376, 383. *See also* education

lactation 48–50, 56
language development 10, 29, 76, 147, 277, 278, 315, 364
leadership 89, 191, 192, 268, 343
Leiden Longitudinal Empathy Study (Netherlands) 166, 168
life history strategies 108–110, 112, 124, 125, 131, 136–139
life history theory 135–137, 141, 142
listening skill 197, 218, 222, 327, 335, 375, 382
Longitudinal Israeli Study of Twins 170

malnutrition 74, 242–246
   maternal 68, 278

Mardu (Western Desert society) 85, 86
mass trauma 258–261
maternal behavior 8, 32, 48–51, 102, 277. *See also* attachment
   anxiety 107, 109, 111
   transgenerational 8, 31, 69, 70
maternal-fetal coadaptation 65, 70, 75
maternal health 242, 245–246, 249, 294
   promoting 279
maternal mediation mypothesis 104–112
Mayors for Peace 380
media xvii, xx, 15, 339–360, 375, 376, 382
   -based interventions 15, 298, 349, 351, 352
   Beyond Violence 344
   Early Years (N. Ireland) 346, 369
   Panwapa 15, 349
   radio soap operas 351, 352
   Sesame Workshop 345–351, 369
   Shara'a Simsim/Rehov Sumsum series 346, 348, 350
   social 344, 349, 351, 358, 382
   Tuyour al-Jenne 351
mediation 218, 317, 318, 333–335
   peer 328, 334, 381
memory 219, 227–229
   working 103, 105, 107, 229
mental health 228, 230, 247, 248, 250, 267, 280, 318, 324
   caregiver 277
   children 216, 221, 222, 223
Milgram experiments 178, 181
mindfulness 289, 290
mind-mindedness 196, 197
morality 24, 117, 124, 164, 291, 309, 347, 350. *See also* prosocial behavior
   children's sense of 291, 292, 294
   defined 162
   situational 161–163, 178–180
Mother Child Education Foundation 3–5, 15, 28, 63, 127, 312, 319, 342
   programs 307, 312, 319
multiple intelligences theory 325

nationalism 293

National Youth Service Corps in Nigeria
    378, 379
negotiation skills 126, 127, 140, 190,
    203, 218, 330–334
neocortex 48, 49, 56, 76, 113, 114
  influence of environment 71–74
neurobiology of groups 10, 123, 128
neurobiology of peace 27, 30, 31–38
neurodevelopmental canalization
    98–104, 110
neuroplasticity 46, 47, 51, 99, 260
nomadic foragers 81–84
  Australia Western Desert 85–87
norepinephrine 100, 101, 105
Nurse-Family Partnership Program
    (USA) 35, 262, 307
nutrition 68–71, 187, 193, 241–245,
    249, 255, 277–281, 294–296. See
    also malnutrition

obsessive-compulsive behavior 74, 173
Old World monkeys 138, 139
once-off canalization 98–103, 106, 108,
    110
1-2-3 Magic (Canada) 314–316, 320
orbitofrontal cortex 150, 175
Oregon Social Learning Center 262
out-group prejudice 24, 120, 122, 162,
    164, 186, 292, 293, 372
oxytocin 8, 14, 32–34, 46, 49–58, 60–
    63, 70, 96, 112, 113, 116, 120, 158
  intranasal 55, 119, 162, 171–174, 182
  role in prosocial behavior 171–173
  therapeutic importance of 59

pair bonding 32, 43, 53–57, 137
Panwapa 15, 349
parasympathetic nervous system 55, 61,
    114–116
Parental Mediation (Canada) 317–320
parenting 14, 21, 30, 33, 34, 111,
    137, 165–167, 222–224. See
    also alloparenting
  abusive 107, 131, 138, 139, 204
  harsh 136, 185, 188, 189, 201–205,
    222, 315, 320

intergenerational patterns of 34, 35
role of stress 256
sensitive 171, 185, 189, 196, 197
stress 318, 320
Parkinson disease 67
partnerships xix, 14, 15, 16, 320, 378,
    383
  integrated support system 352–354
Pathways to Peace organization xix
patriotism 293
peace
  biological origins of 44–45
  concept of 299, 321
  defined xiv, xv, 5–7, 27, 29, 43, 45, 95,
    186, 254–258, 363
  measuring 14, 38
peacebuilding 4, 6, 15, 28, 29, 33–38,
    84–87, 110, 125, 213, 214, 230, 253,
    257, 263, 266, 268, 377, 379
  defined 27, 30, 96, 325
  link to early childhood 305–322,
    323–338
  model for 354–358
  National Youth Service Corps in
    Nigeria 378, 379
  role of media 339–360
peace education 323, 324, 375, 380, 381
  curriculum 328, 329, 335, 336
  promoting 327–329
  Resource Center xix
peaceful children 7, 16, 273, 274,
    284–286, 290
  defined 286
peacemaking 6, 27, 28, 36–38, 124–128
  defined 30, 96
Peace Messenger Cities 381
peer mediation 328, 334, 381
peer relations 217–222
peptide systems 43–64
perinatal depression 52, 277, 279
perspective taking 287–289, 291, 298,
    309, 327
Philani Project 281, 282
placenta 48, 60, 65, 69–71, 75, 111, 112
policy 365, 373, 380
  role of knowledge 369–379
posttraumatic cognition 225–227

posttraumatic stress disorder (PTSD) 54,
57–59, 73, 99, 114, 116, 173, 223,
224, 229, 259, 260
poverty 10, 11, 27, 97, 187, 191,
235–237, 249, 262, 285, 372
Prader-Willi Syndrome 69, 76
prairie voles 54, 56, 61, 115
prefrontal cortex 9, 72, 104, 105, 150,
175, 176, 220, 229
prevention of behavior problems
314–317
problem solving 219, 263, 266, 297,
298, 327, 335
joint 333, 377
progesterone 69, 70
PROGRESA (Mexico) 282–284
Project CARE (USA) 311
Project Competence Longitudinal Study
(USA) 256
Project Head Start (USA) 308, 311
promoting peace 263–266, 268, 383
propaganda 339, 341, 355, 356
prosocial behavior 15, 24, 25, 36, 43,
48, 121, 122, 195, 270, 274, 278, 291,
297. *See also* altruism, cooperation
defined 161, 162
development of 161–184
EEG asymmentry in 173–175
evolution of 45
promoting 180–181, 345–348
role of oxytocin 171–173
psychological abuse 214
psychopathology 44, 116, 177, 193, 201
psychosocial deprivation 27, 147, 148,
150–158
psychosocial interventions 213, 223,
229, 230
puberty 65, 73, 74, 131

reciprocity 119–121
reconciliation 203, 230, 299, 333, 335
resilience 12, 16, 23, 35, 45, 118, 200,
214, 251, 255, 256, 269, 289
defining 254–258
-focused interventions 279–281
framework for promoting peace
263–266

mass trauma 258–261
theory 253
Rett Syndrome 72
rhesus monkeys 9, 72, 131, 138–141,
181
Robber's Cave experiment 266, 373
role-playing 297

safety 7, 43, 96, 112, 115, 116, 215, 217,
222, 289, 366, 383
role of oxytocin 52, 63, 113
schizophrenia 51, 57, 59, 72, 74, 173
Search for Common Ground NGO 330,
331
secure attachment 274, 295, 342–344,
366. *See also* attachment
role of media 339, 349–351
security 195, 196, 366
food 236, 241, 246, 265
self-categorization 292
selfish assertiveness 14, 15, 24, 25
self-regulation 103–106, 110, 114, 116,
118, 257, 261, 262, 265, 270, 274,
277, 295, 298, 335, 365
serotonin 62, 71, 139, 229
Sesame Workshop 345–351, 369
Panwapa 15, 349
Shara'a Simsim/Rehov Sumsum series
346, 348, 350
shared helplessness 342
shared narratives 214, 221–223, 228,
231, 284, 289, 348, 351
sibling relations 200, 217–222, 318
Silver-Russell Syndrome 69, 76
situational canalization 179
situational morality 161–163, 178–180
defined 163
social activism in children 274,
299–301, 349
social behavior
biological basis 46–50, 59
social bonds 7, 13, 45, 52, 195
social hierarchy 10, 29, 84, 89, 193, 281
in children 187–191
social identity 36, 79–94, 274, 293, 299
theory 368
social injustice 235, 300, 334, 368

social justice 7, 30, 254, 273, 276, 290, 291, 299, 328, 365, 374
  model for 294–300
social media 344, 349, 351, 358, 382
social norms 39, 119, 321
  children's perceptions of 287–289
social organization 80–89
  hunter-gatherer 81–83, 195, 237
  impact on aggression 82, 91, 126
  in-group loyalty 80, 82
sociocultural context 20, 21
socioeconomic status 8, 20, 97, 104, 105, 165, 177, 187, 189, 277
  inequities in 192–194, 296
stereotyping 36, 122, 126, 330, 341, 343, 346–348, 350, 353, 355, 368, 369, 376
stress. *See also* posttraumatic stress disorder (PTSD)
  chronic 53, 114, 156, 187
  early life 32, 47, 139, 158
  impact on families 256, 259
  inoculation 257
  interventions 297, 317, 318, 320
  model of 169, 207
  neurobiology of 50, 52–54, 70, 112–114, 262
  response 100–108, 228
  toxic 237, 262, 265
structural violence 11, 96, 97, 110, 124–127, 264, 267, 274, 276, 285, 286, 321, 331, 368
  adaptation to 269
  defined 29, 234, 275
  impact on early child development 233–250
  in South Africa 237–240
stumptail macaques 131, 140, 141
subcortex 101, 103, 106
sympathetic nervous system 55, 100, 101, 107, 114, 115, 228

teacher training programs 194
Toddlers without Tears (Australia) 314, 316, 320
toxic stress 237, 262, 265

transgenerational coadaptation 68–71, 75, 111, 112
trauma 35, 116, 223
  impact on development 218–220
  mass 258–261
  neurobiology of 112
  role of memory 219, 227–229
traumatic play 227, 228
trust 8, 32, 47, 91, 118, 125, 171, 195, 229, 274, 293, 294, 327, 334
Turkish Early Enrichment Project (TEEP) 13, 311, 312, 319

uncinate fasciculus 76, 150, 151
underachievement 226, 227
United Nations xiii, xiv, 14, 380
  Convention on the Rights of the Child 238, 246, 250
  Resolution A/RES/53/243 xv–xvii
United Nations Children's Emergency Fund (UNICEF) 3, 236, 258, 261, 344, 381
Upper Xingu peoples 85, 87, 90, 91
us versus them 79–85, 89, 125, 186, 342, 343, 372

vasopressin 8, 32, 46, 49, 53–55, 58, 62, 112, 113
  measuring 60
  sex differences 57, 61
violence 34, 96, 125, 193, 214, 258, 261–263. *See also* direct violence, domestic violence, structural violence, war-related violence
  causes 331, 332, 337
  collective 214, 215, 228, 229, 275, 285, 332
  coping strategies 113, 114
  defined 29, 363
  drivers of 11
  impact on families 222–224, 289
  intergroup 83, 86, 266
  interpersonal 214–216, 222, 252, 266, 278, 285
  memory of 227–229
  political 258–260

role in development 213–232
violence prevention research 261–263

war-related violence xiv, 11, 67, 75, 84,
 213, 216, 221, 258
 biological origins 44–46

impact on development 70, 72
impact on social organization 81–83
interventions for 229, 318
Western Desert peoples 85–87, 90
Williams Syndrome 51, 55
working memory 103, 105, 107, 229